Third Edition

Clinical Assessment and Management of

Childhood Psychiatric Disorders

Third Edition

Clinical Assessment and Management of
Childhood Psychiatric Disorders

Savita Malhotra

MD PhD FAMS FACPsych

Former Professor and Head
Department of Psychiatry
and Dean
Postgraduate Institute of Medical
Education and Research
Chandigarh

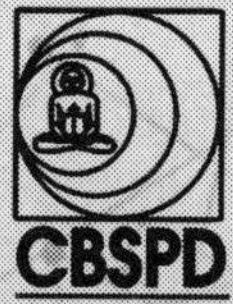

CBSPD

CBS Publishers & Distributors Pvt Ltd

New Delhi • Bengaluru • Chennai • Kochi • Kolkata • Lucknow • Mumbai
Hyderabad • Jharkhand • Nagpur • Patna • Pune • Uttarakhand

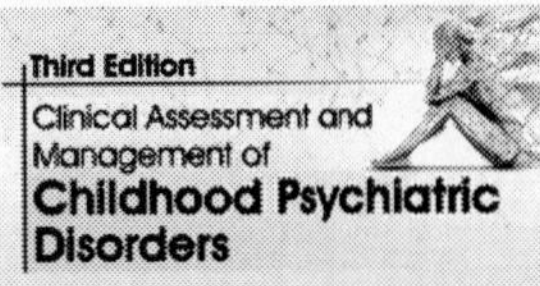

ISBN: 978-93-5466-984-2

Copyright © Author and Publisher

Third Edition: 2025

Second Edition: 2013

   Reprint: 2014, 2024

First Edition: 2002

Published by **Satish Kumar Jain** and produced by **Varun Jain** for

CBS Publishers & Distributors Pvt Ltd

4819/XI Prahlad Street, 24 Ansari Road, Daryaganj, New Delhi 110 002, India
Ph: 011-23266838, 23289259   Website: www.cbspd.com
                                    e-mail: delhi@cbspd.com

Corporate Office: 204 FIE, Industrial Area, Patparganj, Delhi 110 092, India
Ph: 011-49344934   Fax: 011-49344935   e-mail: publishing@cbspd.com; publicity@cbspd.com

Branches

- **Bengaluru:** Seema House 2975, 17th Cross, K.R. Road, Banasankari 2nd Stage, Bengaluru 560 070, Karnataka, India
  Ph: +91-80-26771678/79   Fax: +91-80-26771680   e-mail: bangalore@cbspd.com

- **Chennai:** 18/8B, Subbarayan Street, Shenoy Nagar, Chennai 600 030, Tamil Nadu, India
  Ph: +91-44-42032115, 26681266   e-mail: chennai@cbspd.com

- **Kochi:** 42/1325, 1326, Power House Road, Opposite KSEB, Power House, Ernakulum 682018, Kochi, Kerala, India
  Ph: +91-484-4059061–65   Fax: +91-484-4059065   e-mail: kochi@cbspd.com

- **Kolkata:** 147, Hind Ceramics Compound, 1st Floor, Nilgunj Road, Belghoria, Kolkata 700056, West Bengal, India
  Ph: +91-33-25633055/56   e-mail: kolkata@cbspd.com

- **Lucknow:** Basement, Khushuma Complex, 7 Meerabai Marg (behind Jawahar Bhawan), Lucknow 226001, UP, India
  Ph: +91-522-4000032   e-mail: tiwari.lucknow@cbspd.com

- **Mumbai:** PWD Shed, Gala No. 25/26, Ramchandra Bhatt Marg, Next JJ Hospital, Gate No. 2, Opp. Union Bank of India, Noorbaug, Mumbai 400009, Maharashtra, India
  Ph: +91-22-66661880/89   e-mail: mumbai@cbspd.com

Representatives

• **Hyderabad**	0-9885175004	• **Jharkhand** 0-9811541605	• **Nagpur**	0-8692091830
• **Patna**	0-9334159340	• **Pune** 0-9664372571	• **Uttarakhand** 0-9716462459

Printed at: SRK Graphic, Shahdara, Delhi

Foreword to the Third Edition

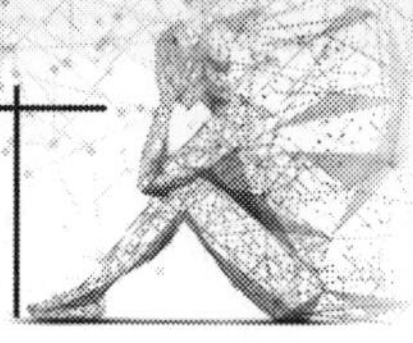

This foreword aims to recognize the contribution which the book makes in facilitating the work of psychiatrists by helping them to deal with mental disorders in children and adolescents in a humane and effective way.

Recent years have been characterized—nearly everywhere in the world—by two trends. The first of these creating much worry to governments is the continuous reduction of natality bringing it below the levels which would guarantee the maintenance of the country's population at a steady or growing level. The second trend is that children are more likely to be born to poor parents who fail to apply measures promoting healthy growth partly because of lacking knowledge and partly because of lacking resources. The second trend is amplified by the lack of perinatal and postnatal care and support which is nearly universally characterizing health care for the poor.

Some governments are taking measures to invert these trends but meanwhile children who have mental health problems only rarely receive the care they need. In part this is due to poverty and parents' limited knowledge about upbringing and education for life and in part also because health workers are failing to provide adequate advice and guidance about helping children which have mental health problems or illnesses. They fail to do so because their knowledge about mental health is poor and their access to information which they need to provide advice is limited. Psychiatrists who have mastered and continue to upgrade knowledge about dealing with mental health problems of children and adolescents can help them by advice and guidance. This book will help psychiatrists to teach others about mental health problems in the young which gives it additional value.

The book which Prof. Malhotra has written many years ago is again more updated. Now, it contains the best of knowledge about child and adolescent mental health which health workers in general and specialists should use in dealing with children suffering from mental health problems. I hope that it will be widely used and that it will contribute to health of children, to the satisfaction of their parents and to the strengthening of their countries' population of tomorrow.

N Sartorius MD PhD FRCPsych

Foreword to the Third Edition

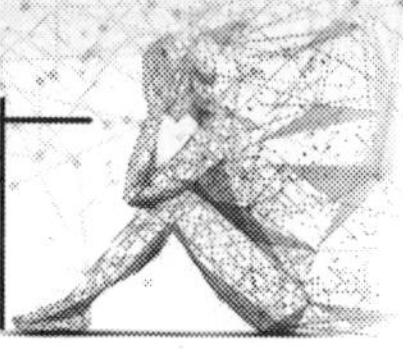

The field of child and adolescent psychiatry has advanced in leaps and bounds since its formal recognition as a subspecialty. Advances in epidemiology and diagnostic classification have enabled a better understanding of the prevalence and onset of psychiatric disorders. Advances in psychopharmacology and psychotherapy have yielded evidence-based treatments that ameliorate symptoms and improve functioning. Advances in genetics and neuroscience continue to illuminate pathways towards prevention and early intervention.

However, the impact of all of these advances is severely limited if front-line practitioners do not have the knowledge or skills to work comfortably with children and adolescents, and/or if there simply are not enough knowledgeable practitioners to meet the needs of the population. This principle is especially true on a global level, where there are significant disparities in the availability of human and material resources available to support youth mental health, as well as in the degree to which children and adolescents are exposed to life-changing stressors and traumas.

Professor Savita Malhotra is an internationally distinguished leader in child and adolescent psychiatry who has devoted her career towards improving child and adolescent mental healthcare in India and everywhere else in the world where there are challenges in ensuring equitable access to care amid formidable resource challenges. Her efforts have focused on ensuring that all psychiatrists, including psychiatrists that primarily serve adults, have the knowledge and skills to contribute to the mental health workforce serving children and their families. Indeed, this may be the single most important approach in providing the nearly 2.5 billion children in the world the best chance for access to mental healthcare and wellness.

This well-written, authoritative, and comprehensive textbook provides general psychiatrists, as well as primary care and other health professionals, the additional knowledge and expertise needed to care for children and adolescents with mental health concerns. It includes concise summaries of the evidence-based literature, readable and relatable guidelines, and locally adapted tools that can practically be implemented in the clinical settings where children and adolescents are most likely to present. In appreciating the truly remarkable focus of this book and the populations that stand to benefit, I join others in the world mental health community in welcoming what may be one of the most seminal contributions, in this era, to children's well-being.

Anthony PS Guerrero MD
Professor
Department of Psychiatry, University of Hawai'i
John A Burns School of Medicine
Chair, Child and Adolescent Psychiatry Section,
World Psychiatric Association

Foreword to the Second Edition

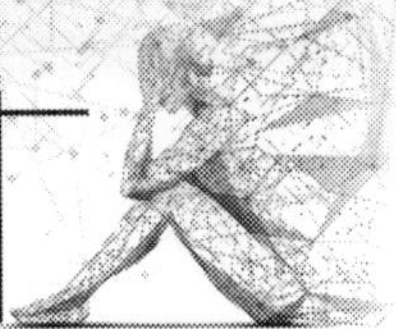

Child psychiatry has evolved over the past 50 years in ways that could not have been anticipated by the pioneers in the field. Rich traditions of clinical care have morphed into a focus on 'evidence-based' care, the focus on psycho-pharmacological, neuroimaging and short-term approaches to care and a host of other 'modern' therapies. Psychotherapeutic approaches, 'talking therapy' is now too often an elective. There is great interest in cultural issues, but too often in an uncritical manner. Even faculties of academic programs find themselves caught between the demands to do research or extensive clinical care and the mandate to teach forcing difficult choices. The integration of what we need to know as child psychiatrists and the comprehensiveness of true child psychiatry is now almost a thing of the past. Prof Malhotra's textbook *Clinical Assessment and Management of Childhood Psychiatric Disorders* is a remarkable accomplishment in this era. It not only acknowledges the need to be modern and incorporate the latest scientific understanding and evidence base but also reminds us of the need to incorporate the valuable aspects of the clinical profession of child psychiatry that makes it so special.

Prof Malhotra's textbook is comprehensive in nature. It could be the single most important reference volume in any student or professional's library. But what makes it special are those sections of the textbook that emphasize the diagnostic process, clinical approach, integration of information, work with the family, and psychological assessment. All of these areas of importance for child psychiatry do not find their way into other treatises in as clear a didactic manner as in this textbook.

This text is extraordinarily useful as a reference. Unlike some texts the reader is given the information about appropriate diagnostic procedures and has at hand the very tests that are discussed. Likewise, the same is true for the diagnostic classifications that are referenced. Thus, both the trainee and more advanced professional need not access additional references which can be a time-consuming or impossible task. There is a section on psychopharmacology that provides principles for care, but does not dwell on esoteric issues or advocacy for a particular psychopharmacological approach. This is refreshing in the modern era.

Prof. Malhotra provides a context for under-standing the diagnostic process. In her development of the chapter that contains information on the diagnostic classifications, she traces the development of the classifications. This is useful for the clinician no matter what level of training to understand the dynamic process and absence of absolute truths associated with our current classifications. Clarity is everywhere in the text. The description of cognitive behavior therapy is the clearest of any textbook and helps the reader to grasp the rationale for use of this intervention.

Perhaps most importantly, the textbook is written from the perspective of a person who knows firsthand about working in low resource environments. While not dwelling on the Indian experience, Prof Malhotra provides very useful information on the collaboration between professionals and nonprofessionals, engagement of families and working in the community. Unlike some other texts, the well-informed guidance comes from firsthand experience.

Prof. Malhotra's textbook *Clinical Assessment and Management of Childhood Psychiatric Disorders* reflects her comprehensive and sensitive understanding of child psychiatry as it should be understood and practised.

Myron L Belfer MD MPA
Professor
Department of Psychiatry
Children's Hospital Boston
Harvard Medical School

Preface to the Third Edition

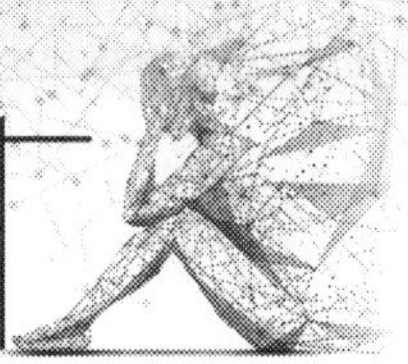

Children can suffer from mental disorders much like adults, rather many psychiatric disorders begin in childhood. Early treatment is the key to promote healthy development and socio-emotional well-being. It has been reported that about 50% of all mental disorders begin before 14 years of age and 75% begin before 25 years of age. Developing brain during fetal, infancy and early childhood phase is the most sensitive to environmental influences and becomes conditioned/patterned accordingly, incorporating the lived experience, and gets built in the process leading to a unique constellation of behavior, emotions and personality. Importance of child mental health has been amply understood by researchers, professionals and societies. In India too in recent years awareness is increasing and the need and demand for professional psychiatric services for children is rising. However, there is great dearth of qualified mental health professionals, i.e. psychiatrists, psychologists, social workers, special educators, speech and language therapists, and occupational therapists in India. Problem is further compounded by the very few training facilities available in the country.

As the theory and practice of child psychiatry is deeply enmeshed in the sociocultural milieu of the child's life, it becomes necessary that approaches and clinical tools for assessments and interventions are ethnosensitive. In my experience of practicing psychiatry and child psychiatry for 50 years, I have felt that the knowledge derived from the work done in the Western countries cannot be directly applied to the Indian population and there is a definite need to adapt such knowledge to make it applicable to the local situation. As a postgraduate teacher of psychiatry, I have often felt that the students find themselves at crossroads due to mismatch between clinical approaches given in the Western textbooks and the practical realities experienced in every day's professional work.

This book has been written to help and guide clinicians such as child psychiatrists, general adult psychiatrists, psychologists and pediatricians to systematically and comprehensively assess and manage psychiatric disorders in children and adolescents. The book is intended to serve as a clinical guide or a manual to provide perspective and assist the clinicians in doing their job effectively. General adult psychiatrists feel a sense of unease or difficulty in approaching children or in psychologically engaging with them in their diagnostic and therapeutic work. The book is written in a simple, descriptive style, providing reasoning for the suggested approach, enabling the reader to understand the frame of reference. As a child psychiatrist deals as much with adults (parents, family, teachers, etc.) all the clinical skills required of a general adult psychiatrist are also required in a child psychiatrist. An introductory chapter on child development outlining various theoretical viewpoints is given to serve as the backdrop within which the clinical assessment, interpretation of signs and symptoms, and planning and execution of interventional approaches can be understood. As the diagnostic process is not merely a labeling exercise, and as the factors contributing towards pathology are equally important for diagnosis, the chapter on family, school, environment and resilience has been given for the reader to know about the most crucial aspects of the child's life that have a bearing on his/her mental health. Chapters on psychiatric assessment and interviewing techniques predominantly provide a skill-oriented flexible system of guidance in conducting a comprehensive examination. Neurodevelopmental assessment is a crucial component of examination, particularly in disorders of neurodevelopment, and a psychiatrist should be well-equipped to carry it out. Psychological assessments in the form of various psychological tests, performed usually by psychologists, provide important supplementary information. However, the psychiatrist needs to know the types of questions that can be answered through psychometry, the types of tests available and their scope and limitations, so as to make most judicious and appropriate use of such tests in clinical practice. Psychological tests can be used for assistance in diagnosis, for assessing the degree of disability or for planning intervention or monitoring effectiveness, etc.

After clinical assessment, the next step of diagnosis and differential diagnosis involves a process of thinking and analyzing the assessment data, interpretation of the signs and symptoms and its summarization into a diagnostic category. A basic knowledge of various diagnostic entities and the rules for diagnosis and classification becomes imperative. The chapter on diagnosis and classification provides a broad framework as well as detailed listing of diagnostic entities and criteria as per International Classification of Diseases (ICD) 10th revision and the Diagnostic and Statistical Manual (DSM) IV revision currently in use that a busy clinician can quickly refer. Introduction has also been made to ICD 11 and DSM 5, with listing of corresponding diagnostic categories keeping the reader updated and well-informed about the latest developments. It is equally important to know about the available Indian scales or tools for assessment even though these are very few and far between. An effort has been made to enlist as many scales as possible and to provide the complete instructions and manual for scoring and administration for those scales that have been developed by me to give an easy and free access to students, researchers and clinicians. These scales have been extensively used in India and remain much in demand. Management has been described in two chapters, one outlining the principles of management and planning process, and the second gives specific treatment methods and guidelines to undertake actual treatment. A separate chapter on psychiatric and behavioral emergencies covering commonly encountered emergent situations in pediatric medicine

or psychiatry and their handling has been included to deal with emergencies even if uncommonly encountered. Issues of adolescence primarily focusing on the special considerations applicable to them have been handled in another chapter.

With growing evidence about the importance of brain development and its psychiatric consequences during fetal stage and infancy stage, a new chapter on 'infant mental health' has been added. This is done to emphasize that the clinician must pay attention to the intrauterine and infancy phase of life in order to understand the earliest neurodevelopmental influences on mental health and illness. Two other major challenges have emerged recently, one is child sexual abuse and the other is substance addiction. Separate chapters have been added to help the clinicians understand and manage these otherwise complex problems. In recent times, there is a great deal of public awareness and outcry about these issues. Drug abuse among children is not only increasing but also occurring at younger age and with newer and synthetic compounds.

Keeping in mind the needs of a practicing clinician rather than that of an intellectual academician, emphasis on practical, realistic and feasibility aspects of treatments is deliberate. Insights gained through my experience of working with children and their families for 50 years in clinical practice has provided the inspiration and quintessence for the book.

Considering the pre-eminence of psychological methods of treatment in child psychiatry, effort has been made to describe various forms of psychological interventions in simple and practical format enabling the clinician to undertake these therapies without much doubt or hesitation. It has been my endeavor to present psychological therapies in the most usable form allowing even the nonmental health clinicians to practice extending the benefits to children and families in need. Unpopularity of psychological interventions with the clinicians on account of these as essentially time consuming or labour intensive, or often difficult or poorly understood interventions, compromising the legitimate interests of child psychiatric patients, is a huge impediment that needs to be addressed and resolved. Throughout the book, effort has been made to include the latest and well-accepted, theories and practices. The term 'child' has been used mostly generically to include infancy and adolescence as well, unless there was a need to specify.

The book was first published in 2002 and the second edition came out in 2013. Now, after 11 years, the book had gone out of print, and it had become necessary to revise and update it. Working on this book has been pleasurable and also challenging. I owe it to my patients and their families who gave me the needed experience and insights and honed in me the clinical art of practicing child psychiatry. I am also indebted to my students for their inquisitiveness and faith, evoking and keeping alive in me a quest for knowledge and excellence.

Savita Malhotra

Contents

Development of the Brain and Mind

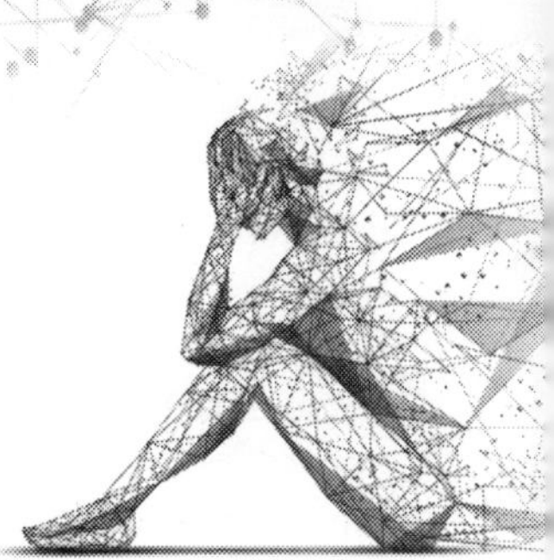

INFLUENCES ON DEVELOPMENT

Development of the mind or psyche through fetal, infancy, childhood, adolescence and adulthood stages, is the most fascinating aspect of human life. Each stage has its own repertoire of neuronal functions and vulnerabilities. Development of the brain incorporates and is driven by two major influences:

1. Evolutionary/Genetic
2. Environmental

Evolutionary past provides a pre-programmed genetic blueprint for organization and structure of nervous system, linking it to phylogeny. Thus, the brain incorporates not only the lived experience but also the evolution. Gene template provides uniform structure of the brain, such as neurons and its connections with major brain regions, unimpacted by the environment. Whereas, environmental influences shape the neural architecture within the context of the environment. There are transcription genes that depend upon environmental triggers for expression. Experience can change the actual structure of the brain. Every experience activates some neural circuits and leaves others alone. Neural circuits used over and over again get strengthened, and those that are not used are dropped resulting in "pruning". Neurons that fire together, wire together.

In a new born, sensory system is more advanced than motor system. There is sequential development of various brain regions and systems. Sensory and motor systems mature first. Association cortex which integrates memory, audio–visual inputs, object recognition mature later. Brain areas involved in complex decision making, impulse control, judgment, mature last. Maturation of brain systems and connectivity continues in adolescence through adulthood. Brain has capacity for neurogenesis throughout life. Neurons generated as a result of experience are not only functional but are associated with better memory and plasticity (Van Praag et al 2002). Brain areas associated with emotions and memory (pre-frontal cortex, amygdala, hippocampus and temporal lobe) are highly plastic, and therefore, amenable to learning even in adulthood.

Contrary to the common belief, the brain of a newborn is the most perceptive, sensitive and adaptable organ that continues to grow and mature into highest levels of complexity involved in the emotional, behavioural and cognitive functioning of an adult, incorporating the experience throughout the various stages of development. Psychological development includes an array of emotions and inner emotional life; myriad behavioural patterns; competencies; skills of interpersonal and social relationships; intellectual and cognitive abilities, in a highly individualistic and unique style. Emotional/social development starts immediately after birth or even before birth. Exposure of the fetus to stress hormones of the mother primes and sensitizes its nervous system leading to patterning of its excitation, inhibition and regulatory functions Thus, the early emotional experiences get embedded in the architecture of their brains. Experience wires the brain through learning and gene expression. Due to repeated exposure and neuronal plasticity, these experiences influence the strength of synaptic connections and embedding of the environment in the neural architecture. This contributes to both "biological evolution" and "cultural evolution". Normal and abnormal development lie on a continuum.

Influences on Development

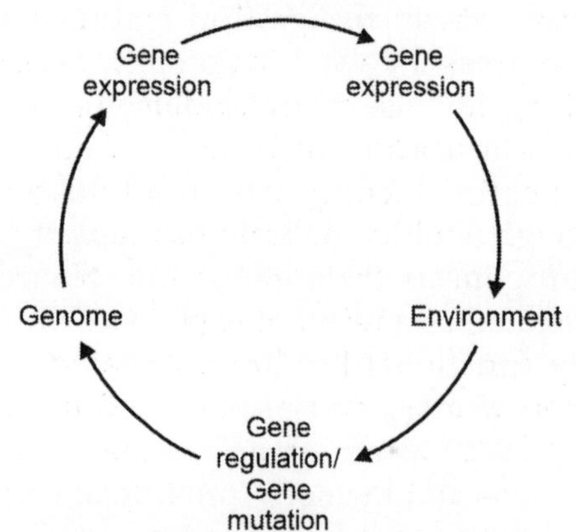

Fig. 1.1: Gene-environment interaction

Genetic Factors

Genetic abnormalities, family history of neurological/neurodevelopmental disorders, parental mental illness, temperamental adversity, low IQ.

Adverse Environmental Factors (Pre and Post Natal)

Diet, toxins, infections, stress, trauma, medications, parenting.

THEORIES OF DEVELOPMENT

Historically, several theories have been proposed to explain the development of mind and personality from early childhood to adulthood. Most of these theories were propounded around the late 19th and early 20th century and have remained in vogue till late 20th century. Each theory, though,

provided only partial explanation, but taken together these have led to considerable accumulated knowledge about the human mind and its emotional, psychosocial, interpersonal and cognitive functions. These developments took place around the beginning and through the course of the last century that led to declaring the 20th century as the century of the child.

Further each of the theories of development have lent themselves to the formulation of therapeutic interventions, corresponding to the theoretical tenets. A brief and quick introduction to the theories of psychological development will always be helpful in understanding the genesis of psychopathology and in planning the therapeutic strategies for the given patient. For the sake of simplification, the explanatory theoretical models, as listed below, can be categorized in accordance with what they can explain best and how these are subjected to treatment formulations.

1. Psychoanalytic theories for intrapsychic functions and inner emotional life.
2. Behavioural theory for social and behavioural learning.
3. Piagetian theory for cognitive development.
4. Attachment theory for emotional attachment and bonding.
5. Temperament theory for stylistic uniqueness of behaviour.

CHILD PSYCHOANALYTIC THEORIES

Sigmund Freud (1859–1936) made a major contribution and founded the psychoanalytic school of thought explaining psychopathology in adults, while focusing on childhood as a crucial phase of life. According to this theory, childhood experiences determined and shaped adult psychopathology and personality. Psychoanalytic theory not only explained the psychological basis of behaviour but also provided a framework for treatment of various disorders. Many others such as Anna Freud and Melanie Klein added a developmental dimension to psychoanalysis making it suitable for assessment and treatment of children and adolescents.

According to psychoanalytic theories, a newborn begins its process of development from the somatic experiences or bodily sensations that it is born with. The infant has the ability to respond to and regulate the influences of internal and external stimuli on its neurological and physiological systems that translate into visceral and emotional experiences. Parental involvement in providing nurturance, fulfilment, relief and safety lays the foundation for development of relationships and emotional reactions in later life. There is a constant interplay between the genetic and biological forces with the experience of the child in the family and social environment, structuring and patterning the child's psyche or mental apparatus. According to Anna Freud, the leading child psychoanalyst, the charting of the mutual influences between the psyche and soma and their representation in mental life provides a framework for understanding both abnormal development and illness (A Freud 1965).

Infant's internal experience involves primacy of certain zones of the body called erogenous zones, i.e. oral, anal, phallic at different stages of development. The infant seeks gratification and relief from mounting tension periodically, till it masters the respective stage to move on to the next stage. Depending on the primacy of the erogenous zone, development progresses along the following phases:

Oral Phase (0–18 months)

During infancy, oral stimulation through feeding, sucking, biting, licking provides utmost pleasure and satisfaction. The child uses this oral experience for feeding and survival as well as for perceiving, regulating and altering his/her inner bodily sensations. Entire effort of the child centers around relief of physical tension and obtaining gratification. As the mother tries to maximize the child's comfort, relieve tension and soothe him/her, there is development of an emotional bond between the mother and the baby and this leads to internalization of the image of the mother. The type of bonding between the mother and the child and the internalized maternal image forms the foundation of subsequent emotional and social relationships in later life.

Any disruption in the relationship between the mother and the child during this phase of life on account of any cause, e.g. separation of mother and child in infancy, mother's physical illness or mental illness particularly depression or schizophrenia, or physical abuse, can generate any form of psychopathology such as failure to thrive, anaclitic depression, stranger anxiety, hypersensitivity to simulation, fear or withdrawal reactions, or developmental lag.

Anal Phase (18–36 months)

At this stage of development, anal sensations are heightened focusing the child's attention to this part of the body. In the acts of defecation and urination, the child experiences bodily sensations, a sense of control on bodily functions; a physical act of doing something. These acts become a source of pleasure and also assume a sense of control that the child can exercise on his body and on the environment. The child sees how what is originally inside "becomes public". This is the age for toilet training where the child has to master control of defecation and urination in accordance with parental rules. Successful mastery over these functions involves internalization of external controls, and conveys a sense of autonomy, a sense of pride and ownership of body in the child. On the other hand, any disruption in parent–child relationship or in toilet training at this stage, can lead to defiance of parental rules, lack of autonomy, obstinacy, aggressiveness and temper tantrums, sense of shame, guilt in the child.

Genital Phase (36–48 months)

During this phase, there is crystallization of gender awareness, preoccupation with anatomical differences in sexes; and attention to sensations arising from penis and testicles in boys and vagina and clitoris in girls. By the age of 3, children are clearly aware of their gender identity and begin to explore theirs' and others' bodies. Children around this age experience pleasure sensation in their genitals and feel the tension arising from genital areas. They can exhibit their genital organs, self-manipulate, or touch or play with each other's genitals. In this phase, children take pride in their genitals, find their bodies pleasurable, a phenomenon termed as "phallic narcissism" (Burgner and Edgecumbe 1975).

Oedipal Phase (4–6 years)

According to the classical psychoanalytic school, children during this phase are concerned with issues of love, sexual or aggressive feelings towards the parents of same or opposite sex, and gender roles. These feelings are a consequence of cognitive, affective, physical and social development at this stage and are resolved by developing mental structures consolidating the realizations that he/she is the child of his/her parents and that the parents have relationship with each other and that the parents have roles and lives of their own which is apart from their role as parents.

Parents are seen as sexual objects. The child clamours for exclusive parental attention and love from the parent of the opposite sex. The child realizes that he can achieve this by being good and compliant, paving the way for development of super ego. Child now understands the virtues of good behaviour and realizes that parents are separate individuals.

Latency Phase (7–10 years)

During this phase, child's concern with erogenous zones of the body, i.e. pre-oedipal phase and the oedipal strivings decrease considerably. Sexual impulses diminish. Intellectual, cognitive, sensory motor and social aspects of development and functioning predominate in the behavioural and emotional expressions. Child begins to acquire several adaptive defense mechanisms such as identification, intellectualization, sublimation and humour to support the diversion and alteration of the original impulses (Bornstein 1951, Freud 1966).

Adolescence (12–20± years)

Adolescence is a period of rapid and profound changes in the biological, psychological and social functioning There is period of pre-adolescence (10–12 years) when sexual curiosity and auto stimulation resurfaces; followed by early adolescence (12–14 years) when biological process of puberty sets in. Along with a growth spurt, there are rapid hormonal and bodily changes, and development of secondary sex characters. This phase is marked by anxiety as the adolescent finds their bodily changes out of control, even unacceptable and external, making them feel embarrassed and secretive about them. In mid-adolescence (14–16 years), sexual function is fully established and there is re-emergence of sexual feelings and fantasies along with awareness that the adolescent is capable of performing sexual functions now. They acquire an aggressive and provocative attitude towards parents and begin to object to any interference by them in their lives. They drift away from parents, moving towards their peer group, both of same sex and of opposite sex with increase in outside home activities. Late adolescence (17–20 years) is marked by development of a stable peer group, involvement in intellectual and academic pursuits, development of athletic or other artistic interests, and extra-curricular activities. By this time, adolescents are able to emotionally disengage from parents to become autonomous; develop their own identity and meaning; try to develop intimacies outside home; and begin to establish heterosexual relationships. Preoedipal and oedipal strivings and fantasies towards parents are surrendered to the heterosexual partner, in which earlier components of attachments to parents such as dependency, exclusiveness, physical intimacy, possessiveness, and jealousy are all subsumed. These relationships move further through a process of maturation and consolidation culminating into development of a sense of self through evolving interests and ideals.

In adolescence, the individual, psychologically re-organizes the representation of the bodily and sexual changes; accepts sexuality and the body with pleasure and pride; develops value system of their own which is separate from that of the parents; learns to regulate drives of love and aggression; and develop intimacies outside family.

In summary, the psychoanalytic theory concerns itself with the child's inner world and intrapsychic functioning, dealing with the child's emotions, thoughts and wishes, frustrations, dreams and fantasies, worries and pleasures.

Psychoanalysis is an exploration into and understanding of child's own private and personal experience of life, his own understanding of persons, issues and the world. Psychoanalytic theory has contributed most to understanding of children suffering from emotional disorders.

LEARNING THEORY OR BEHAVIOURISM

Behaviourism as a movement in psychology was initiated in America by JB Watson (1878–1958) who applied methods of animal research to human behaviour paving the way for use of more objective methods in behavioural analysis as opposed to subjective methods used in psychoanalysis. Behaviourism was based on learning theories propounded by Pavlov's classical conditioning (1927); Thorndike and Skinner's Instrumental or Operant conditioning. According to Watson, learning could shape entire human behaviour and virtually all behaviour could be explained on principles of conditioning (Watson 1919).

According to Pavlov's classical conditioning principles, a stimulus that is neutral or which does not elicit a reflex response, can be made to elicit a reflex response when it is paired with a stimulus that actually elicits the reflex response.

Classical conditioning concerns with stimuli (called unconditioned stimuli) that elicit reflex responses (called unconditioned responses). These unconditioned responses are reflexes, i.e. these are involuntary or automatic and therefore not learnt. However, these reflex behaviours (unconditioned responses) can be learnt as a conditioned response so as to be elicited by neutral stimuli which is termed as conditioned stimulus.

The process by which a new and neutral stimulus gains the power to produce a unconditioned response is called classical conditioning. The concept of conditioning was applied to explain the development of all types of adaptive or maladaptive bahviour. Another type of learning that was described was operant conditioning where the consequences of behaviour were considered more important. Thorndike (1932) formulated Law of Effect which stated that consequences that follow the behaviour help learning. Positive consequences or positive feedback facilitates learning and negative or no consequences produce opposite effect. B.F. Skinner (1953) expanded the concept further. According to him, behaviours are operant, i.e. it influences or operates on the environment; and operant behaviour strengthens (increases) or weakens (decreases) as a function of its effect on the environment.

The process of learning operant behaviour is called operant conditioning. Most behaviour exhibited in everyday life can be considered as operant.

According to learning theories, all behaviours are operationalized into learning paradigms based on classical or operant conditioning principles and these are then subjected to modification techniques collectively called behaviour modifications or behaviour therapies. Here, the focus lies on alteration of behaviour as a means of altering the clinical disturbance. It is assumed that there is plasticity in behaviour, and it is amenable to change under systematic conditions of learning.

Further developments in behaviour therapies emphasized on role of cognition (thoughts and beliefs) in shaping one's own environment and viewed maladaptations as faulty cognitions. Based on these assumptions, a whole new form of therapy called cognitive behaviour therapy was formulated which became the most influential and effective mode of psychotherapy in due course.

Around the same time, experimental research by Ivan P. Pavlov (1849–1936) on classical conditioning formed the basis for learning theory, which was extended to explain the learning of developmental tasks and behaviours. Edward L. Thorndike (1874–1949) explained learning of new behaviours on the basis of consequences that follow which help learning. This learning was described as operant conditioning in which behaviours increased or decreased as a result of consequences that followed them. This led to founding of the behavioural school of psychology as a general theory of child development that explained the processes involved in psychological dysfunction or disorder and stimulated emergence of behaviour therapy as yet another form of psychological method of behavioural change.

PIAGETIAN THEORY

Jean Piaget (1952) propounded the theory of cognitive development which was a stepwise process of evolution of cognitive structures through internal representation of the environment and its organization and integration at successively higher and more complex stages. Piagetian theory explained how children develop the capacity to think logically, how they attribute different meanings to some events at different stages and how they actively contribute to their own experience.

Cognition is a complex concept to describe the "internalized schemas or frames of reference which the child uses in his interaction with the external world" (Daregowski 1977) or in other words it can be construed as the child's mental representations of the world, both physical and social; and of the self. Piaget distinguishes between the "affect which is an energizing force while ... cognition provides the structure for this energy". Cognition has also been understood as information processing system or as the workings of the thought process, or as the higher intellectual processes and structures, or as logical thought.

Jean Piaget (1952) provided a theory of development of intellectual structures which is recognized as one of the most influential theories of cognitive development. According to Piaget, cognitive development involves a continuous process of mentally adapting to and organizing the environment through a process of assimilation and accommodation in the mind of the child. Over time, mental schemas or organized mental structures are created, coordinated and enlarged to involve all aspects and domains of human experience. These schemas are synthesized at each stage of development leading onto the next higher level of organization. Piaget has described four discreet stages of cognitive development:

Sensori Motor Stage
(Birth through 18–24 months)

Child at birth is endowed with sensory motor reflex functioning system devoid of any symbolic or conceptual representations of the world. In their interaction with the environment, these reflexes get patterned, stronger and more and more differentiated through constant process of experience and feedback. For example child roots, sucks and grasps initially the breast, then his own body part, i.e. thumbs (by the second month) followed by other objects in the environment, when simultaneously these reflexes get associated with gaze and touch (by 4–5 months).

Feedback from random movements of limbs, head or eyes give rise to intentional behaviour of repeating the act, thus forming an internal structure for behaviour. Thereafter, the child brings in an element of novelty by slightly altering the behaviour and then looking for feedback. By the second year of life, symbolic function begins to develop when children start playing peek-a-boo and related games. Child develops capacity for symbolic play and use of language.

Pre-operational Stage
(2 through 5–7 years)

This stage is also called intuitive stage or pre-logical state. The child is slowly developing mental images of objects, understands object permanence, learns concept of time and space, acquires enduring memory and symbolic functions which is further facilitated by developing language.

Stage of Concrete Operations
(6–11 years)

At this stage, children learn to deal with concrete objects as they exist or are experienced by the child. Logic begins to develop; thinking is no more intuitive or inconsistent. Concepts are formed as mental operations or structures and these get more and more organized. According to Piaget, mental operation is "any representational act which is a part of an organized network of related acts" (Flavell 1963).

Classification is a form of mental operation where the child constructs cursive relationships according to a property creating vertical hierarchy. Seriation is another example where objects are ordered horizontally in rows according to a particular property. These mental operations get stabilized and get further connected logically.

Stage of Formal Operations
(11 years to Adulthood)

At this stage, children can form hypothesis where reasoning involves hypothetical situations as against empirically derived situations of childhood. Now, the children's thought is not structured by the concept of actual objects or perception. There is development of logical and scientific reasoning. They can distinguish fact from fiction, they can think about their own or other's thinking, taking thoughts as objects.

COGNITIVE DEVELOPMENT IN ADULTHOOD

Several authors believe that cognitive development continues into adulthood even after the fourth stage of Piaget.

DEVELOPMENT OF SOCIAL COGNITION

Cognitive and social development occurs in a parallel and reciprocal manner where cognitive skills mediate social interaction which further provides context for cognitive development. Infants have the ability to recognize emotions in facial expressions and respond accordingly.

Children relate to people as they do to things, moving from external/physical properties of objects to their internal and conceptual attributes. Social cognition incorporates emotional cognition, empathy, and moral reasoning. In social cognition, the child also learns to understand that other people too have thoughts, intentions, and feelings that are separate from their own. This provides the child with what is called "theory of mind" or "mind reading", involving the concept of self and of others and of the relationship between them that has implications for social relationships, empathy and moral judgement. Brain has mirror neuron systems which get similarly activated while watching a certain act or while performing the same act. It means that there is common neural coding for production of an action and perception of same action. This represents the neural basis for imitation, motor learning, learning of gestures, phonetics, actions by observation. Mirror neuron systems are also linked to emotional attachment, recognition of internal emotional states of others thereby serving to develop empathy and theory of mind.

The way children reason about feelings has been analyzed by Nannis (1988) and presented in a sequential manner. Initially feelings are seen as generated by external events or happenings; then these are viewed as being located internally like a body organ with no control over them by the child. At the next stage of development, feelings are understood as diffuse within the person rather than as concrete things in the concrete body. Further, the feelings are conceptualized as being influenced by self. Finally, the most complex conceptualization of feelings evolves and that the "feelings involve regulation and integration of internal processes and external events. Feelings are part of a system with universal laws or principles" (Nannis 1988).

ATTACHMENT THEORY

Attachment is innate, biologically based, enduring emotional bond that unites one person with another. It commonly manifests as seeking proximity and contact with the attachment figure, feeling comforted and secure in presence of attachment figure. Attachment basically serves the purpose of protection and nurturance by the mother or caregiver to the baby providing survival and safety to the young ones. According to Bowlby (1969, 1973), a psychoanalyst and a psychiatrist, mother–infant attachment behaviour is typical to species that evolved to promote infant survival. According to

Bowlby, infants are tuned to respond socially to their social partners, and the attachment process varies according to experience in its intensity and quality on secure–insecure dimension. Secure attachment is derived from the confidence the infant has that his help-seeking signals will evoke adult's response promptly. In case, the quality of care is insensitive, or unpredictable, the infant goes into insecure attachment mode. Many adult personality disorders could be understood as the aftermath of insecure attachment in infancy and early childhood (Bowlby 1973). Attachment theory finds application in clinical and therapeutic situations such as in day-care experience for infant; as a risk-factor for insecure attachment; in determining custody issues in child where the concepts of "best interest of the child" and "psychological parenting" (as against biological parenting) become the determining forces in legal proceedings; and in understanding emotional disorders of infancy and early childhood.

During the middle of the 20th century, animal experiments by Harlow (1958) provided evidence for the psychological phenomenon of attachment which is conceptualized as an enduring emotional bond between two persons manifesting as proximity seeking and contact seeking that serves the purpose of survival, protection and nurturance of the young ones. John Bowlby (1969, 1973) a psychoanalytically oriented psychiatrist brought together ideas from psychoanalysis, developmental psychology and the evolutionary theory, which developed, into an elaborate theory of attachment. Attachment theorists expanded their work and brought into focus, the issues of quality of parent–child relationships. Their understanding of adult personality disorders was described as a long-term consequence of impaired infant–parent attachment. Attachment theory has been an influential and powerful theory of child development that highlighted the importance of early child care.

TEMPERAMENT THEORY

Another significant theory of development came from research on temperament. Temperament is an ancient concept that emphasized the individual differences in behavioural style arising from differences in the constitution and neurobiology.

Temperament refers to unique and innate, psychobiological characteristics in children that underlie a wide array of behavioural and reaction patterns. Temperament is constitutional, present at birth and evident in first few months postnatally, and refers to stylistic aspects (how) of behaviour rather than the content (what) or the motivation (why) of behaviour. Temperament concept serves to tie together a variety of behavioural dispositions commonly used to distinguish one individual from another. Temperament is applicable to children, adults and even to animals (pets, livestock). These are a set of behavioural tendencies that are unique to the individual and are relatively stable across situations and during the course of time.

Temperament acts as a significant force in children in guiding their own development where children are viewed as active participants rather than being passive recipients involved in shaping their environment and experience. Involvement of these biologically endowed temperamental characteristics contributing to children's own development provides a link between the genetic and neuro-physiological characteristics of the child with socially relevant behavioural patterns. Individual differences in behavioural styles evident in neonates and young infants are easily perceived by the primary caregiver.

Pioneering research in this area was done by Alexander Thomas, Stella Chess and others (1968) who undertook an intensive, in depth, observational, longitudinal study of new borns in the New York City called New York Longitudinal Study (NYLS) in 1956. Original cohort comprised of 138 children from 85 families and 97% of the sample was followed up through 30–40 years. They described nine categories of temperament:

1. *Activity level:* The motor component in child's functioning.
2. *Rhythmicity:* Regularity or predictability of biological functions such as sleep-wake cycle, hunger, elimination schedule, etc.
3. *Approach or withdrawal:* The nature of child's initial response to a stimulus (food, toy, person) which could be positive, i.e. approach; or negative, i.e. withdrawal.
4. *Adaptability:* The ease or rapidity with which initial (withdrawal) response is changed in the direction of desired (approach) behaviour.
5. *Threshold of responsiveness:* The intensity level of stimulus required to evoke a discernible response.
6. *Intensity of reaction:* The energy level in response irrespective of its quality or direction.
7. *Quality of mood:* The amount of happy, joyful behaviour, as contrasted to unhappy or crying behaviour.
8. *Distractibility:* The effectiveness of extraneous environmental stimuli in interfering with or altering the direction of the ongoing behaviour.
9. *Attention span and persistence:* Attention span refers to the length of time an activity is pursued by the child. Persistence is the continuation of the activity despite obstacles.

According to Thomas, Chess and Birth (1968), the "degree of fit" between the children's temperament and the environmental expectations and demands determines the degree of stress the child encounters during the course of development. "Goodness of fit" is adaptive and healthy whereas "poorness of fit" can create conditions for maladaptation and problems in the domain of behaviour and emotions.

Several temperamental dimensions have been described by different researchers and some of those with established validity are:

1. *Emotionality:* This may be positive or negative. Negative emotionality (fear, anger, distress) predisposes to maladaptation.
2. *Adaptability* can be high or low and refers to adaptation to novelty. Low adaptability manifesting as shyness, withdrawal and behavioural inhibition and is found to be a risk factor for maladaptation.
3. *Reactivity:* Reactivity relates to Pavlovian concept of the strength of nervous system. It involves the relative strength of stimulus intensity and the response intensity exhibited by individuals in given situations. There are individual differences in how intense a stimulus must be to evoke a reaction; as well as how intense a reaction is to a stimulus of a given intensity.
4. *Activity:* It refers to the frequency and intensity of motor activity in behaviour. To some extent, activity levels are also related to arousal levels where activity helps to regulate the arousal levels or vice versa.
5. *Attention regulation:* This concept refers to the extent to which the child will shift attention from his/her activities or distress in response to external stimuli. To some extent, this concept overlaps with the notion of soothability or distractibility.
6. *Sociability:* Sociability involves appreciation of company of others in the form of socially reciprocal interchange. Sociability is a highly heritable trait.
7. *Difficultness:* This concept was operationalized by Thomas et al (1968) as a sum of five out of nine temperament variables described by them. Difficultness in a child was described as predominant negative mood, withdrawal, low adaptability, high intensity of emotional response and low regularity of biological rhythms.

Temperament concept provides ample understanding of human social development as well as of psychobiology of behaviour and emotions. Developmental psychologists have viewed it as an intervening variable between the genetic constitution and environmental experiences.

Alexander Thomas and Stella Chess (1963, 1977) who carried out empirical studies on temperament and followed-up these children from infancy through adulthood, producing a wealth of developmental data on the vicissitudes and outcomes of the temperament–environment interaction. Temperament theory highlighted the need for attention to the innate biological propensities within the child himself who is not just a passive recipient of the environmental influences but is an active agent in shaping the environmental processes in a dynamic, interactive, reciprocal relationship. Temperament theory helped to explain the developmental course and outcomes in childhood and beyond, and provided a framework for interventions.

DEVELOPMENTAL NEUROBIOLOGY

The central nervous system constitutes the structural as well as functional substrate of the cognition, personality, emotion, consciousness and all other human qualities that constitute human psyche. Life starts at conception and it is clear that both pre- and postnatal influences produce significant effects on the developing brain. Although considered as one organ, brain comprises of several major areas such as cerebrum, thalamus and hypothalamus (diencephalon), midbrain (mesencephalon) and cerebellum; all performing highly specialized functions, interconnected through a higher level organization for a coherent functioning. Further, there are several functional systems of interest to psychiatrists such a limbic system, or basal ganglia. Even though there are separate and specific functional neuronal systems sub-serving consciousness, memory, emotions, perception, cognition, attention, etc., they are also interconnected in a highly complex and interactive manner at a horizontal as well as vertical hierarchical plane.

Brain development starts with neurulation or the establishment of neural plate during the third week of gestation. From 5th to 18th week of gestation, rapid neural precursor cell division is followed by an extensive glial proliferation and subsequent myelination occurring between the 19th week of gestation and 2½ years of age (Dobbing and Sands 1973). The process of myelination of CNS occurs at different rates for different parts of the brain and is also completed at different time periods. Most rapid myelination occurs in first 2 years of life (Dobbling and Sands 1973), primary motor and sensory areas are fully myelinated by the age of 6; and associative areas only in second decade. Myelination of prefrontal cortex occurs the last of all and can go up to 4th decade (Yakolev and Le Cours 1967). Disruption of process of myelination can occur by toxins, nutrition, and other environmental factors. Brain and nervous system are built, neuron-by-neuron, through interaction of genetic programming and environmental influences (Changeux and Danchin 1976). This is a use-dependant development where growth and interconnectivity of neuronal systems is facilitated by continuing use.

Further, the brain is not a static structure; it continues to change and has the potential to change throughout life. Environment plays a crucial role in building the brain where the environmental experience is incorporated in the memory circuits; learning (both implicit and explicit) alters the neuronal functions, establishes newer synaptic connections and modulates behaviour. Emotional memories are located in the amygdala. Eventually, the brain gets specialized into several structural and functional systems such as social brain, emotional brain, and executive brain.

Social brain includes amygdala, anterior cingulate, orbitofrontal areas of the prefrontal cortex and frontal portions of temporal lobe; built between 18 and 24 months of age and is driven by attunement between the right hemisphere of the mother and the right hemisphere of the child (Schore 2000). Early bonding between the mother and the child is primitive, with smell, touch and gaze playing the pivotal role. This early bonding evolves into lifelong patterns of attachment and interactions.

Executive brain incorporates frontal and prefrontal cortices subserving behavioural and emotional executive functions. Parietal lobes organize body image and inner subjective experiences and send projections to frontal lobe. Temporal lobes integrate sensory information with socioemotional aspects and send projections to frontal lobes. Frontal lobes provide the highest level of cognitive and emotional processing (Fuster 1997) and also integrate concepts of time, past and future memories (Fuster, Bonder and Kroger 2000, Ingvar 1985).

Emotional brain is primarily subserved by the limbic system that includes amygdala, hippocampus, cingulate gyrus and septum, connected to anterior thalamic nuclei mammillary bodies and hypothalamus.

Cerebral cortex or the neocortex or the neomammalian brain develops late and much more slowly than most other parts of the brain, and may continue to develop till the third decade of life. On the other hand, the primitive systems of the brain involved in arousal, activation and homeostatic functions, feeding and survival drives are fully functional at birth. The limbic system or the paleo-mammalian brain involved in social and emotional learning, emotional regulation, and memory develops through early childhood experiences. Thus, most of our behavioural patterns and emotional reactions get structured into organized patterns very early in life, much before our ability for conscious awareness, rational thought and reasoning develops. During most of our conscious life, we remain under the influence of emotional brain and not rational brain.

Slow development of human brain allows for incorporation of the environment through prolonged period of education and learning, and for adaptation and change. This fact also underlies the finding that the environment, climate, nutrition, language, culture, parents and parenting factors shape the developing brain in a unique way. Unfavorable environment can lead to formation of maladaptive patterns and psychopathology whereas a favourable and a conducive environment can generate structures that produce healthy, adaptive and resilient patterns of behaviour throughout life.

INDIAN PERSPECTIVE

People in India have reposed much faith in modern medicine and shown concern for physical health and relatively less attention has been paid to psychiatry and mental health. Traditionally, the psyche (mind) and mental health have always been relegated to the domains of philosophy, religion and spiritualism, which are deeply rooted in the lives of people even in the present-day society in India. Therefore, people often do not readily seek medical remedies for psychological problems. Modern psychological theories have been largely derived from the Western thought, such as Hegel's "rationalism", Schopenhauer's philosophy of "will-to-live"; Nietzsche's "Will-to-power" and "assertion of individuality" and William James "pragmatism". The Western psychological theories as applied to modern psychiatry were introduced to the traditional systems of health and healing in India only, recently.

In the Indian Vedanta, the true nature of "self" is construed as the "Atman" (Soul) which is a form of absolute existence that is, immortal, unchanging, eternal, without a beginning or an end, not conditioned by space, time or causation. The physical body that is changing and mortal is the materialization of the results of past "Karma" or the actions. The "Karma" or the actions, which generate our bodies, belong to us and not to others and inevitably result in experiences in the next birth, thus implying continuity in lives and fruits of our actions even after death. Power of action or Karma cannot be destroyed and the same soul continues to materialize in the form of fresh body. Karma determines the character and vice versa. A well-balanced conduct and ordinary nonmoral actions can modify or arrest the fruits of karma (Charaka Samhita). Thus karma theory is not a theory of immutability, just as the phenotypic expressions of genotypes are dependent on the gene–environment interactions, which in itself can modify the genetic code.

This philosophy of life and theory of Karma conditions people to think, perceive and act in certain manner in the face of suffering due to disease or death. Apart from accepting a part of suffering as the necessary penance or expiation, they may ascribe external attributions to its cause and may seek magico-religious remedies for its cure. In many instances, the psychiatric treatment is delayed, at times denied in pursuit of these beliefs. On the other hand, in many situations where psychological distress is an understandable reaction to life's circumstances, problems are contained and resolved within the family or the individual's system of beliefs. It is important to understand these perspectives in order to make a proper judgement about the knowledge people have about mental disorders and the motivations they exhibit in pursuit of psychiatric treatment. One often sees the variations and gradations of these belief systems among people coming from varied sociocultural, geographical and religious backgrounds. Religious and philosophical explanations are more commonly invoked for psychiatric disorders than for physical disorders. The trend is, however, changing with education and urbanization in favour of accepting modern medicine.

Since independence, developments in physical medicine and healthcare in India have made rapid progress. Ironically, till recently, health planning did not include mental health leaving considerable amount of morbidity and incapacitation unattended. Needless to say that mental health is at least as important, if not more, as the physical health.

Psychiatric Disorders of Childhood and Adolescence

Contrary to what many people may believe, mental ill health is not limited only to adults, children are afflicted with it as much (Table 1.1). Population prevalence studies on rates of psychiatric disorders in children in India have shown that, depending upon the method of assessment and the definition and type of psychiatric disorders included, about 6% (Malhotra 2001), 7% (Verghese and Beig 1974); 12% (Srinath, et al) to about 30% (Deivasigamani 1990) of children have a significant disorder at a given time. National Mental Health Survey Data (2015–16) reveals that prevalence of mental disorder among 13–17 years olds was 7.3%; and prevalence was twice as high in urban metros (13.5%) as compared to rural areas (6.9%). Thus, 9.8 million adolescents aged 13–17 years are in active need of mental health treatment (National Mental Health Survey 2015–16). Considering that children and adolescents constitute over 50% of our total population, the burden of morbidity due to psychiatric disorders in children and adolescents in the country is enormous.

It has also been reported that 50% of all mental disorders begin before the age of 14 years, and 75% before 25 years of age. Also, many childhood psychiatric disorders continue into adulthood. There is considerable degree of continuity between the childhood and adult psychiatric disorders. General adult psychiatrists are focusing more and more on earliest phases of life and there is significant blurring and overlap between childhood and adult psychiatric disorders.

Progress in genetics and developmental neuroscience in the last 30 years has revolutionized our understanding of the complex brain functions and its aberrations. There is a significant shift of focus from manifestations to underlying neurobiological mechanisms. Synthesis of all earlier theories of development and developmental neuroscience has led to the emergence of a new field, "developmental psychopathology".

Child psychiatry has been recognized as a medical specialty in its own right only recently. It emerged not from the disciplines of adult psychiatry or paediatrics but from the fields of social work, education and psychology. However, it is necessary to provide it a status of a discipline, independent and separate from adult psychiatry, paralleling a logical distinction between the disciplines of paediatrics and internal medicine. The theory and practice of adult psychiatry is not directly applicable to child psychiatry for various reasons and so are the clinical methods.

It is well-recognized that childhood is the most important period in human life. The transformation of the human infant from a totally dependent state to a fully independent adult takes as long as 25 years, which is the longest time taken by any biological species. The infant not only grows in size but also in the complexity of functions that it attains. The process of development is guided by inherent genetic–biological factors which determine the potential the child is born with, and by environmental experiential factors that determine the realization of the inborn potential. Thus both the nature and the nurture are crucial to optimum development.

Child's mind at birth is not a blank slate. Children are born with unique styles of behaviours, reactions of new environment, patterns of body movements, attention

Table 1.1: When to suspect mental health problems	
Younger children	**Older children**
• Frequent tantrums or irritability much of the time • Often seem fearful, nervous or worried • Frequent crying, easily driven to tears • Complain about frequent stomachaches or headaches, vomiting with no known medical cause • Are in constant motion and cannot sit quietly (except when they are engaged in an activity they enjoy, such as watching videos or playing video games) • Sleep too much or too little, have frequent nightmares, or seem sleepy during the day • Are not interested in playing with other children or have difficulty making friends • Remain self-absorbed, less responsive to environment • Academical difficulties, delayed speech, or poor socio-adaptive skills. • Repeat actions or check things many times (for example, repeatedly checking to make sure a door is locked) out of fear that something bad may happen	Any of the problems mentioned for younger children plus any of the following symptoms: • Have lost interest in things that they used to enjoy • Have low energy • Sleep too much or too little or seem sleepy throughout the day • Have periods of highly elevated energy and activity and require much less sleep than usual • Spend more and more time alone and avoid social activities with friends or family • Diet or exercise excessively or fear gaining weight • Engage in self-harm behaviors (such as cutting or burning their skin) • Smoke, drink, or use drugs • Engage in risky or destructive behavior alone or with friends • Have thoughts of suicide • Say that they think someone is trying to control their mind or that they hear things that other people cannot hear • Using tobacco, alcohol or other substances of abuse.

span and threshold of responsiveness and adaptability, etc. These are referred to as the temperament of the child. Research has shown that infants differ in their temperament style at birth. Their reaction to the environmental and handling patterns are a two-way process, where the mother has to constantly modify her approach of handling of the child depending upon his/her temperament, and the child's behaviour gets moulded by the mother. It requires considerable amount of sensitivity and effort on the part of the mother to recognize the individuality of the child and alter her approach to suit or match it. This is only one example of how the development of children progresses in a complex and inter-active manner.

Another very significant component of the emotional development in children is that of attachment or bonding. Attachment of the young one with the mother is an innate biological characteristic that fulfils the needs of nurturance and security. Any factor that interrupts or interferes in the mother–child bonding process, such as separation, abandonment, abuse, can lead to adverse consequences for the emotional development of the child. The process and pattern of attachment with the mother in childhood also lays the foundations for our social and interpersonal relationships in adulthood. If the infant has secure and adequate attachment with the mother, such a child would be confident, secure, free from anxiety and fear during childhood and would have stable, intimate and fulfilling interpersonal relationships in adulthood. On the other hand, insecure attachment or lack of opportunities for attachment can lead to anxious dependent, demanding, adult social relationships. Such individuals have serious difficulties in getting along with others and remain constantly dissatisfied, unhappy and unstable in their social relationships.

School plays a crucial and a formative role in the development of cognitive, linguistic, social, emotional and moral functions and competencies. However, in the contemporary system of education, schools have to cope with heavy syllabi and curricula, poor teaching facilities, highly competitive examinations, which along with declining social prestige of teaching profession, low priority in national planning, limitations of resources, commercialization of education have seriously marginalized and compromised on their role in guiding and regulating the psychological development of children. School education has become a serious source of stress for children and parents. School phobia, psychosomatic complaints, emotional/behavioural problems, poor sleep, appetite, difficulties in coping and declining scholastic performance are common manifestations of stress in school children.

This situationis in contrast to that where opportunities for education are not available to a large segment of population in rural India. Education may be unavailable, inaccessible, unaffordable and even unattractive. Children are pushed into adult roles and trades such as domestic and industrial labour, prostitution at a very young age depriving them of the opportunities for proper growth and development.

Material, psychological and social deprivation is a serious risk factor contributing to psychiatric disorders in children. Research has shown that deprived children grow up to be more often intellectually deficient, educationally backward, delinquent and drug addicts with inadequacies in personality. They have low level of aspirations, and motivation, low self-concept and poor coping skills. Parental conflict and discord, single parent family, parental alcoholism and antisocial personality, child abuse, living in slums are some of the significant causative factors that contribute to psychiatric disorders in children. Family violence and child abuse, which has been commonly reported from Western countries, is yet to be recognized and acknowledged in India.

Children's mental health has serious implications for the mental health of adults. Many mental disorders of adulthood such as alcoholism, drug addiction, personality disorders, depression, anxiety, social disorders like divorce, violence, abuse, terrorism, crime, etc. are in significant measures, consequences of traumatized and deprived childhood.

Mental health of children is much more intricately rooted in the sociocultural milieu and environment in which they live. Influences of religion, the belief system and the philosophy of life on the mental health of people, though are apparently protective and promotive, but these have not been systematically studied. It is believed that the strong family system that prevails in India has significant positive influence on mental health of children. Child rearing practices that are different in different cultures, guided by the cultural value systems and social norms also play a significant role in development of children.

It is, therefore, imperative that one looks at both the risk and the protective aspect of the given environment in which children live. It is known that a large proportion of children living in adverse circumstances grow up to be healthy adults. There are certain innate or intrinsic factors within the child such as high intelligence, or easy temperament or there may be certain positive and protective influences in the environment that contribute to resilience.

Psychiatric evaluation of children, therefore, must attempt a close and detailed examination of various innate biological, emotional, social and cultural aspects of the case leading to a full understanding of the issues, the causes of morbidity and possible remedies.

BIBLIOGRAPHY

1. Bornstein B (1951). On Latency. Psychoanalytic Study Child, 6: 279.

2. Bornstein B: On Latency. Psychoanal Study Child 6:279; 1951.

3. Bowlby J (1969). Attachment and Loss Vol 1. Attachment. New York. Basic Books.

4. Bowlby J (1973). Attachment and Loss Vol 2. Separation, New York, Basic Books.

5. Burger M, Edgcumbe R: Phallic-narcissistic phase: A Differentiation. Psychoanalytic Study Child 30, 161:1975.

6. Changeux, JP and Danchin, A (1976). Selective stabilization of developing synapses as a mecha-nism for the specification of neuronal network. Nature, 264:705–712.

7. Charaka Samhita. The Charaka Samhita of Agnivesa with Ayurved - Dipika Commentary of Cakra Panidatta. Ed. Gangasahaya Pandeya in 2 vols. Sanskrit and Hindi. Kashi Sanskrit Series, No. 194, Varanasi. Chowkhamba Sanskrit Series Office, 1969.

8. Deivasigamani TR (1990). Psychiatric morbidity in primary school children: An epidemiological study. Indian J. Psychiatry, 32 (3): 235–240.

9. Deregowski JB (1977). Pictures, symbols and frames of reference. In: Butterwroth G (ed): The child's Representation of the World. New York: Plenum Press.

10. Dobbing, J and Sands, J (1973). Quantitative growth and development of human brain. Archives of Disease in Childhood, 48:757–767.

11. Flavell JH (1963). The Developmental Psychology of Jean Piaget, New York, Van Nostrand.

12. Freud A (1966). The writings of Anna Freud Vol 2. The Ego and Mechanisms of Defense. New York International Univ. Press (Originally published 1936).

13. Freud S (1940). An outline of psychoanalysis, New York, WW Norton.

14. Freud S In Strachey J (Ed.) The Standard edition of the Complete Psychological works of Sigmund Freud. Hogarth Press London 1953–66 (Originally published 1914–1920).

15. Fuster JM (1997). The prefrontal cortex. Philadel-phia: Lippincott-Raven Publishers.

16. Fuster, JM Bonder, M and Kroger, JK (2000). Cross-modal and cross-temporal association in neurons of frontal cortex. Nature, 405:347–351.

17. Harlow HF (1958). The nature of Pove. American Psychologist, 13:673–685.

18. Ingvar, DH (1985). Memory for the future: An essay on the temporal organization of conscious awareness. Human Neurobiology, 4:127–136.

19. Jane Costello E (2010). Grand challenges in child and neurodevelopmental psychiatry. Frontiers in Psychiatry. Vol 1, Article 14. www.frontiersin.org

20. Malhotra S, Kohli A, Arun P (2002). Prevalence of psychiatric disorders in school children in India. Indian Journal Medical Research, 116:21–28.

21. Nannis E (1988). Emotional understanding and child psychotherapy. In: Shirk S (ed.) Cognitive Development and Child Psychotherapy. New York, Plenum Press.

22. National Mental Health Survey of India (2015-16). Ministry of health and FW government of India and NIMHANS Bangalore 2016.

23. Pavlov IP (1927). Conditioned Reflexes: An Investigation of the Psychological Activities of the Cerebral Cortex. London, Oxford University Press.

24. Piaget J (1952). The origins of intelligence in children. New York International University. Press.

25. Piaget J (1952). The origins of Intelligence in children. New York International Univ. Press. Skinner BF (1953). Science and Human Behaviour. New York, Free Press.

26. Pavlov IP (1906). The scientific investigation of the psychical faculties or processes in higher animals. Science 24. 613–619.

27. Schore, A.N. (2000). Attachment and regulation of the right brain. Attachment and Human Development, 2(1):23–47.

28. Skiner BF (1938). The Behaviour of Organisms. New York. Appleton - Century - Crofts.

29. Srinath S, Girimaji SC, Gururaj G, et al (2005). Epidemiological study of child and adolescent psychiatric disorders in urban and rural areas of Bangalore, India. Indian Journal of Medical Research, 122:67–79.

30. Thomas A, Chess S (1977). Temperament and Development. New York, Brunner/Mazel.

31. Thomas A, Chess S, Birch HG, Hertzig ME, Korn S (1963). Behavioural Individuality in early childhood. New York, New York University Press.

32. Thomas A, Chess S, Brich HG (1968). Temperament and behaviour disorders in children. New York. New York University Press.

33. Thorndike EL (1932). The fundamentals of Learning. New York, Teachers College, 1932.

34. Thorndike EL (1932). The Fundamentals of Learning. New York. Teachers College.

35. Verghese A, Beig A (1974). Psychiatric disturbances in children: an epidemiological study. Indian Journal. Medical Research 62: 1538–1542.

36. Watson JB (1919). Psychology from the Standpoint of a Behaviourist. Philadelphia, JB Lippincott.

37. Yakolev, P and Le Cours, AR (1964). The myelogenetic cycles of regional maturation of the brain. In A. Minkowski (Ed.) Regional development of the brain in early life (pp. 3–70). Oxford, England: Blackwell.

Risk and Resilience: The Role of Family, School and Environment

FAMILY

Family exercises most powerful and all-encompassing influence on the development of children. "Families render humans … human. It is the family that ultimately embraces the child's maturational promise and through powerful reciprocal, interactive forces, converts tissue and instinct into human development" (Pruett 1991). Family is the primary social group that comprised originally of parents and their biological children. This concept of family as a social institution or unit existed for centuries since the dawn of civilization.

Family is expected to provide nurturance and safety to the growing child; provide a network of social relationships; facilitate attachment and bonding for emotional development; develop patterns of communication; and undertake acculturation through process of imparting social values, norms. All these functions of the family are crucial for the overall psychological development of children which also lays the foundation for development of healthy personality in adulthood.

Parenting and child rearing has been one of the most important functions and occupations of adults till the middle of the present century. However, the concept and the structure of the family has undergone significant change in recent years. The US Census Bureau now has defined families more broadly, as two or more persons residing together, and related by birth, marriage or adoption. Historically, family structures have evolved and changed significantly over the years. There exist several altered family forms such as single parents' family, one biological and one step parent family, foster family, unwed parenthood, same sex parents and so on. Societal acceptance or otherwise will determine what can be considered normal or abnormal. The extent, to which these can be considered as pathological will also depend upon how it influences the fulfilment of psychological and developmental needs of its members including children. Alternative family structures influence the child's broader psychological experience and can be considered far from innocuous. There is clear evidence in literature that children living in these alternative families are at a greater risk of maladaptation and development of disorder. Moreover, it is necessary to consider child's subclinical distress as a part of disruption in family functioning. It is not just the family's structure but also its functioning that contributes to this risk. It is also known that these alternative family forms have greater disruption in their functioning than the traditional families headed by biological parents. In India, the traditional family system still prevails in the form of extended and joint families although there is a change towards greater nuclearization of families in the urban areas.

Other significant change that has taken place is that over the years the family's role in the total development of the child has decreased. With women's emancipation, industrialization, urbanization, increasing demands for working outside home, parents are spending less and less time in parenting functions. Children are looked after in other settings such as crèches, nurseries, day schools, and by other adults like relatives, friends, neighbours, servants, older siblings or even at times, no one. Men are increasingly engaged with child-care responsibilities due to force of circumstances or by choice. It has been seen that there exist difficulties in transitioning from gender specific traditional roles attributed to women and men with regard to child care. For example, it has been seen that women find it hard to discipline children, whereas, men struggle with providing affection and warmth. Single parent of either sex have more troubles in fulfilling the responsibilities traditionally assigned to the opposite sex.

With little time at their disposal, now parents have much less control on the varied environmental influences that impinge the psyche of the child. Children have easy and all pervading access to digital media, television, satellite network, and internet, that has further widened this gap and also added additional risk. Infants and young children are extensively exposed to television and smart mobile phones that hinders development of speech and language and social reciprocity and relationships.

All these influences make a significant impact on the mind of the growing child. Child's innate potentials and propensities unfold or manifest in the psychological environment the child lives in. Interaction between the genetic and biological factors on one hand and the environmental or familial on the other, is a reciprocal, two way interactive process that guides the development towards adaptation or maladaptation depending upon the goodness of fit. Evaluation of these processes is, therefore, crucial to the assessment in children with psychiatric disorders. Detailed analysis of the home environment; family's constitution; patterns of functioning and communication; roles assigned, assumed and performed by its members; needs to be done in order to understand various influences that may be responsible for causation, precipitation or maintenance of maladaptation and psychopathology. Marital conflict or discord; divorce in parents, impaired parent–child relationship; child abuse and neglect, absence of emotional bonds, physical aggression in the context of the family are some examples of dysfunction that contributes to psychopathology.

Adverse circumstances in the lives of children do not always and necessarily lead to disorders. There is evidence in literature that children do have great capacity for resilience and many escape mental disorder (Emery and Kitzman 1995, Werner and Smith 1992, Kolvin et al. 1988). Understanding the sources of vulnerability and resilience requires explorations into various biological, genetic, temperamental, intellectual, socioenvironmental factors. Resilient children, though escape from developing mental disorder, they nevertheless undergo considerable amount of personal distress, social difficulties and subtle deficits in personality (not amounting to disorder), which need detailed study. Any compromise with fulfilment of child's intellectual and creative potential, or development of such personality traits that are detrimental to self or to society, or any deficits in moral or social value systems should also be seen as negative outcomes. Moreover, as mental health professionals, we are not content with the mere absence of disorders; but achieving the highest potential in physical, social, emotional, occupational and spiritual functioning is the ideal goal of holistic health.

SCHOOL

The second major influence on the growing and developing mind of the child comes from another social institution called school.

In many countries, all children attend school. In India, school enrolment rates for children have increased significantly and consistently during the last five decades. In 2013, out of school rate for children of primary school age in India was 2.3% (World Data Atlas India). In 2021, in India over 90% of age 6–17 years in urban areas and 86% of children in rural areas attend school.

Schools contribute to learning and psychosocial development of children. Apart from academic achievement, schools provide an opportunity for building peer relationships, learning discipline, being a part of the social group, learning social skills, and methods of conflict resolution and so on. High intelligence and educational success have positive and protective influences on the mental health of children. Children do best in such schools in which there are good amenities for children, good co-operation and co-ordination between teachers, regular supervision and assignment of tasks, high expectations for achievement, rewarding of good work by children, giving graded responsibility to children, freedom to move about, high rates of praise for good work (rather than reprimand for poor work in the classrooms), more time spent by teachers in teaching rather than keeping order in the class room, flexibility of rules, close co-operation between parents and teachers.

In developing countries, school can serve as a community resource that has considerable potential for exerting beneficial effects on the family life and on the community as a whole. Several mental health programmes can be carried out at the school level. School can provide what is lacking in homes of particularly disadvantaged and deprived children. For example, schools can provide space, provide opportunity and materials for play and recreation, at least one nourishing meal, education to parents on health and education issues, advise parents on the developmental needs of children and proper handling methods and so on. There

have been several enrichment programmes carried out on pre-school children which show that children make significant gains in cognitive development (Zigler 1978); primary prevention of emotional and behavioural disorders can be achieved by interventions such as cognitive problem solving skills (Durlak 1985); reduced aggression can be achieved by teacher and parent training (Hawkins, et al 1991); prevention of school maladjustment is possible through child-oriented-intervention in the form of enhancement of competencies in the child (Durlak 1985). Several such programmes have been reviewed (Price et al. 1989) and methodological difficulties have been high-lighted. However, one most important conclusion is that these programmes have been effective and carry lot of promise for future.

Thus, assessment of child's adjustment and performance in school is an important component of evaluation. It provides a comparison and contrast with the situation at home, an additional at times alternative setting for carrying out intervention, and allows sampling of a broader spectrum and array of behaviours. School also can compensate for what is lacking at home; can complement the efforts of the child and parents in setting, defining and achieving the academic goals; and can provide opportunity to the child to realize potentials and exhibit his/her talents.

ENVIRONMENT

It is clear that the child develops in environment that includes, apart from family and school, the social, cultural, religious, ethnic and ecological systems surrounding him/her. The environment can be construed as forming concentric circles around the inner individual psychological core of the child's mind, comprising of primary care givers, then primary family, secondary extended family, school, neighbourhood, place of residence and so on. Further identity is established based on belongingness to a religion, community, province, nationality and ultimately mankind. All these factors influence the growing mind, creating psychological structures that are internalized to constitute a unique sense of identity and personality constellation. Several factors pertaining to the macro environment of the child, that have been found to be associated with greater prevalence of mental disorders in them, are construed as risk factors (Verhulst 2004). For example, gender is a consistent and robust risk factor across sociocultural, or economic or political differences where boys exhibit more of externalizing disorders such as attention deficit hyperactivity disorder (ADHD), oppositional defiant disorder, conduct disorder, sociopathy and drug abuse; whereas girls manifest more often internalizing disorders like anxiety, depression, somatization. Further, boys show more problems when they are younger (as boys have more neurodevelopmental disorders like ADHD, specific learning disorders (SLD), pervasive developmental disorders (PDD), etc.) and girls show more problems (than boys) in adolescence.

Children from lower socioeconomic status have more mental health problems and lower competencies, attributable to a multitude of associated risk factors such as poverty, poor housing, higher levels of stressful life events, parenting failure, lesser opportunities for education, poor physical health, poor nutrition and so on. Children living in urban slums have very high rates of delinquency, conduct disorders and substance use. Research has shown that living in a disadvantaged neighbourhood increased the risk of developing emotional and behavioural problems. Such risk is mediated through a number of mechanisms, i.e. the absence of social control or norms, poor peer group identification, poor adult role models, presence of a delinquent subculture, high rates of substance use and crime and lack of social cohesion. Further, there are ethnic/cultural differences reported in the rates and patterns of psychiatric disorders in children. Most of these variations are understood to emanate from differences in the social norms and expectations of social behaviour across cultures; parental threshold for perceiving problem behaviour; differences in common ways to understand deviations; culture sensitive methods to deal or cope with behavioural deviations and so on. Sociocultural acceptance and sensitivity threshold for behavioral deviance also varies among families and communities.

Excessive use of screens like computers, tablets, gaming consoles, interactive touch-screens are posing newer challenges and risks to children's mental development. These experiences are captivating, enchanting and powerful. More and more children and adolescents are immersed in this new virtual reality and getting into problems with sleep, focusing attention, becoming aloof, acquiring unhealthy habit patterns, poor diet and so on.

It is, therefore, extremely important to understand the micro and the macrocosm of the child in which he/she is growing and to aim at contextual understanding of the issues and problems. Such understanding will also help in planning intervention suited for each child depending upon his/her circumstances of life. Risk factors pertaining to parents and family, school, peer group and neighbourhood must be targeted for therapeutic as well as preventive intervention.

In a longitudinal study on incidence of childhood psychiatric disorders in India, the incidence was reported to be 18/1000/year, and that children who develop disorder compared to those who did not, were not different any of the parameters such as temperament, parental handling, life stress and IQ at base line (Malhotra et al 2009). In another study on life events in children with psychiatric disorders it was found that these children had more number of adverse life events and more serious events in previous one year as compared to normal children without psychiatric disorders (Malhotra 1993).

RESILIENCE

Resilience refers to maintenance of psychological health and functioning in the face of adversity. It is understood as a person's ability to solve problems and increase resistance to future stress and trauma in the process of overcoming difficulties. Resilience is a skill that is acquired and a strong protective factor.

In contrast to risk factors, there are certain enduring factors that promote resilience and healthy adaptation in the child despite adversity. These are considered as protective factors or factors underlying resilience. These would either mitigate the effect of risk or help the child escape from negative outcomes thus providing a counterbalancing force. There are family factors, individual factors and community factors that contribute to resilience. Family factors that contribute to resilience are:

- Good parenting.
- Low family stress.
- Sound parental mental health.
- Absence of alcoholism, drug abuse, etc.
- Sense of safety.
- Strong moral and religious beliefs
- Strong political ideology

Individual factors as known protective factors are high intelligence; sociable and adaptable temperament; close and positive emotional relationship or bonding with a significant adult in life; favorable genes; good communication skills; good physical health; and cohesive family and social living. Physical illness per se acts as a significant risk for psychiatric illness (Malhotra and Malhotra 1990). There are many community factors that contribute to resilience. These are: positive school environment with high expectations of teachers; safe neighborhood; supportive relationship with a mentor; part of religious or faith community; social support and so on. Both vulnerability and protective factors co-exist in a dynamic balance in every child and should always be evaluated to assess the direction in which one outweighs the other.

BIBLIOGRAPHY

1. Durlak JA (1985). Primary prevention of school maladjustment. Journal of Consulting and Clinical Psychology, 53 (5): 623–630.

2. Emery RE, Kitzman KM (1995). The child in the family: disruption in family functions. In Develop-mental psychopathology vol. 2: Risk, Disorder and Adaptation. Eds. D. Cicchetti and DJ Cohen. Pub. John Wiley and Sons USA; pp 3–31.

3. Hawkins JD, VonCleve E, Catalano JR RF (1991). Reducing early childhood aggression: results of a primary prevention program. Journal of Amer. Acad. Child and Adolescent Psychiatry, 30(2), 208, 208–217.

4. Kolvin I, Miller FJW, Fleeting M, Kolvin PA (1988) Risk/protective factors for offending with particular reference to deprivation. In Studies of Psychosocial Risk. The Power of Longitudinal data. Rutter M Eds. pp 77–95. Cambridge University Press, Cambridge.

5. Malhotra S, Kohli A, Kapoor M, Pradhan B (2009). Incidence of childhood psychiatric disorders in India. Indian J Psychiatry, 51, 101–107.

6. Malhotra S (1993). Study of life stress in children with psychiatric disorders in India. Hong Kong J Psychiatry, 3 28–38.

7. Malhotra S, Malhotra A (1990). Psychological adjustment of physically sick children: relationship with temperament. Indian Pediatrics, 577–584.

8. Price RH, Cowen EL, Lorion RP, McKay JR (1989). The search for effective prevention programs: what we learned along the way. American Journal of Orthopsychiatry, 59 (1): 49–58.

9. Pruett KD (1991). Family development and the roles of mothers and fathers in child rearing. In Child and Adolescent Psychiatry: A Comprehensive Textbook. Ed. Melvin Lewis Pub. Williams and Wilkins Baltimore USA, pp 215–221.

10. UNICEF (1991): Children and Women in India: A situation analysis 1990. Unicef. New Delhi.

11. Verhulst F.C. (2004). Epidemiology as a basis for the Conception and Planning of services. In Facilitating Pathways: Care, treatment and Prevention in Child and Adolescent Mental health by Remschmidt H., Belfer ML, Goodyer I. (Eds). Springer NY (Pub), pp 3–15.

12. Werner EE, Smith RS (1992). Overcoming the odds: High risk children from birth to adulthood. Cornell University Press, Ithaca NY.

13. Zigler EF (1978). America's Head Start program: an agenda for its second decade. Young Children, 33: 4–11.

Approach to Psychiatric Assessment and Interview

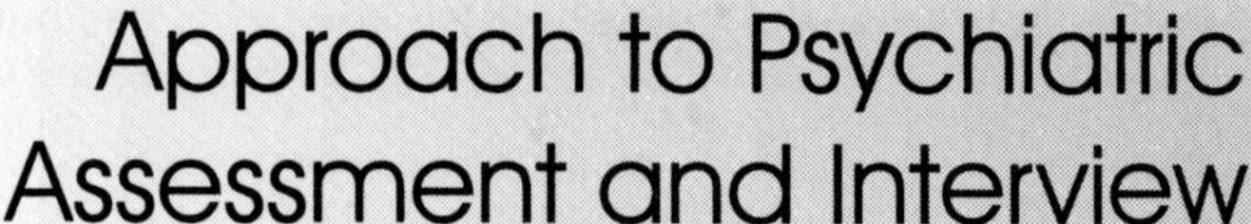

Psychiatric assessment and evaluation are a process of systematic, step by step inquiry, observation, and examination into patient's life history and mental state, through clinical interviewing of the patient and/or family or care givers, to know and understand: (i) the nature of psychiatric disturbance; (ii) how is it affecting the life of the patient and the family; (iii) what factors are possibly contributing to it; and (iv) what can be done to ameliorate it. Clinical interviewing is a highly technical skill learnt through prolonged period of supervised training and experience. Psychiatric assessment and interviewing are the core clinical skills essential for clinical practice of psychiatry. It is a diagnostic tool as well as an investigative tool. It also sets the tone for engaging in therapeutic interaction and procedures.

There can be several approaches to the psychiatric assessment of infants, children and adolescents, varying according to the primary objective or the theoretical conceptualization invoked. For example, there can be psychodynamic interviewing based on psychoanalytic theory; behavioural assessment based on learning theory; or family pathology assessment based on systems theory. The approach may also vary according to the broad areas of assessment as it may be the assessment of the developmental level, neurological functioning, intellectual ability, personality constellation and so on.

Psychiatric assessment also depends upon its main objectives; whether it is to clinically evaluate and treat a child, or to decide on the placement of the child in a particular school or vocation or to evaluate his/her suitability for inclusion in a specific research project. There are variations in the assessment techniques such as interview method, direct observation, structured assessment, psychometric measurement, biological and physical measures and so on. Different techniques are cited for different objectives. For clinical purposes, clinical interview and mental status examination are most appropriate strategy, whereas for research purposes more objective measures such as structured assessment and psychometric assessment are better. Another important determinant of the choice of technique of assessment is the basic qualifications and experience of the assessor. Most methods of psychiatric assessment require specific training and experience before anyone can begin to do it.

Over the years, efforts have been made to make the assessment methods more and more reliable and objective. The element of subjective bias on the part of the assessor should be minimized to its maximum. This has been achieved by making the interviews structured to varying extents, by providing explicit guidelines for interviewing, by providing definitions and descriptions of the phenomenon and signs and symptoms, by laying clear rules and criteria for diagnosis and so on. Some of the structured assessment methods are described in detail in the succeeding chapter. The theoretical basis for the psychiatric interview is described here in detail.

As the present volume seeks to focus on the clinical assessment of children and their families for purposes of diagnosis and treatment, major emphasis is devoted to this aspect.

Psychiatric interview is the basic and fundamental skill in psychiatry that is used primarily as a diagnostic and therapeutic tool. The technique of interview is both art and science and in practice, it is a specialized skill. It comprises of a verbal dialogue in which exploration is done in a systematic manner, into the crucial aspects of the psychiatric problems or illness relating to patient's life. In child and adolescent psychiatry, the patient is generally brought/accompanied by parents who constitute the most important source of information. Parent's presence and involvement is central to not only the diagnosis but also the management of the child or the adolescent. Psychiatric interview aims at eliciting history from parent, the child or other significant adults, and at conducting psychiatric examination.

Reliability is as important as the content of information. It is important to ascertain at the outset, that the informant is able to and is actually providing the correct information. Informant, if capable of giving first-hand information, from his actual observations and interactions, is more likely to be reliable than someone who is reporting a second-hand information. Informants also vary in the degree of accuracy and precision in reporting and may need to be assisted in giving more accurate information, by double checking (looking for consistency) and cross checking with other resources of information. Any information that is inconsistent and does not fit with the chronology or description of events or interactions is more likely to be unreliable. Unreliable and/or incomplete information impedes the diagnostic and therapeutic process.

Psychiatric interview is a systematic and a step-by-step enquiry into child's development, since birth to the present state, covering all relevant areas; in order to understand the nature and the origins of disturbance and to formulate an efficient approach to its amelioration.

Information about child patients is taken on a number of parameters. These are discussed below.

REFERRAL

Most children do not feel the need to consult for themselves. They are commonly referred by someone who could be a friend, a relative, a teacher, or a pediatrician. Some older children and adolescents may feel the need to consult a psychiatrist and may come on their own or with their parents. Source of referral informs about the sensitivity or perception of the referring individual and also of the area of disturbance. When a school or a social agency refers the case, it may be a scholastic or a behavioral issue. Sometimes, the referral is by a pediatrician who suspects that there are significant psychological problems. He is also a source of valuable information through his contact with the family, on the behaviour and upbringing of the child and on the interfamily relationships, as well as on any general health problems.

IDENTIFYING DATA

The biographic information helps orient the psychiatrist to the child, his immediate family and his social milieu. Details are taken about the parents ages, educational status, and occupation. The parent's ages, when the child was born, or the amount of time that elapsed between their marriage and the birth of the child, may be either inconsequential or highly significant for understanding the case. Even seemingly insignificant details may be important here. This information highlights the socio-cultural status of the family, degree of socio-cultural stimulation and values that the child would have been exposed to, that has significant bearing on the social and intellectual development of the child.

INFORMANT(S)

Make note of who the informants are. Depending upon the source of referral, informants can be parents, any other relatives, friends, neighbors, or any social workers or psychologists representing the social welfare agency or police and so on. To obtain a complete and meaningful history of a child, information is taken from the adults who play major roles in his life, usually mother, father and sometimes others like the grandmother. It is important to document the exact relationship of the patient with the informant, and also whether the informant lives with the patient or has first-hand information about the patient's problems and behavior. Informants who can give first-hand and more complete information are more reliable and adequate. It is also necessary to have multiple informants for obtaining information about the life and behaviour of the child in different settings such as home, school, playground, hostel or any institutional setting as applicable.

PRESENTING PROBLEMS AND HISTORY OF PRESENT ILLNESS

This is the most important part of entire history and examination, where one has to know:

What should be the ideal setting for conducting the interview?

What should be the stance or behaviour of the interviewer or how to conduct the interview?

What is the scheme for conducting the clinical interview or what to ask?

Setting

Children do not feel very comfortable in the formal office setting. It is better to have a child friendly office décor and furniture, few toys on the side, and a friendly demeanor of the psychiatrist, that quickly reduces anxiety in the child. There can be small play room kind of setting specially for younger kids or toddlers. There should not be any items or artifacts that are breakable or that can injure the child. It is beneficial to interview parents and child together. Joint interview provides opportunity for father and mother to supplement information, to know about their viewpoints and attitudes, expression of family interactions. For children younger than 6 years most history is taken from parents. Older children and adolescents may not feel comfortable in the presence of their parents and may like to be interviewed alone. Talking to the child or the adolescent first before talking to parents is a good strategy that helps in establishing rapport and gaining confidence of the child. Adolescents are also concerned about the confidentiality of their information which is assured except in conditions where there is possibility of self-harm, suicide, homicide, substance abuse or high risk behaviour.

Stance of the Interviewer

With school-age children, the examiner should introduce himself, explain the purpose of the interview. At the same time the child's understanding of why he has come can be clarified. Every effort should be made to reassure the child who is bound to be somewhat anxious during the first visit. Since children might associate visits to the hospital with injections and other painful procedures, it is often helpful to tell the child that the examiner is "a doctor but not the kind who uses needles". It is best not to sit behind the desk when talking to the child and to avoid taking notes as much as possible. The extent of confidentiality of information offered by the child should be clarified. A general statement that "I will first discuss with you what I will or will not say to your parents," can be used.

Stance of the psychiatrist should be empathic, friendly, engaging, respectful, dynamic, and welcoming. While welcoming the family, one must not forget to acknowledge the presence of the child. In the first few minutes of their entry in the office, do greet the child individually, ask his name, and a couple of general questions about his school, class or home including about who the accompanying informants are. This helps to break the ice and sets the tone for conducting a more detailed interview.

Scheme of History Taking

Interview must start with an enquiry into the presenting problems. It is important that the concerns the parents have about the child should be explored first. In any specific case, some aspect of history may be vitally important and other relatively insignificant depending upon the nature of the problems presented by an individual patient. As in exploring a physical condition, an awareness of the diagnostic possibilities will signal the areas in which detailed data should be obtained. If a child has an educational problem, for example, it may be essential to get full school and developmental histories.

Opening the Interview

Many a times children are not informed by parents that they are taking the child for psychiatry consultation. The child feels confused at why he/she is being asked questions. One must ask the child, whether he knows why he/she is there, or what brings the child to psychiatrists' clinic? If the child says that he does not know why he is brought to psychiatrists' clinic, then ask what can be the possible reasons for psychiatry consultation? Most children are able to then initiate conversation. The opening questions should be simple, non-directive, open ended and broad, leaving scope for a free dialogue. For example, asking "what brings you here?" or "what is the problem for which you are here?" is better than asking. " Does your child have psychiatric symptoms?"

History of Present Illness

It is important to take the history of problems in a chronological order, i.e. which problems appeared earlier and which later. The history of present illness should be roughly divided into three parts.

1. The first part is a verbatim account of the child's problems from the parents. In case of an older child, this can be directly obtained from the patient and supplemented by information from the parents.
2. The second part will consist of enquiries on specific aspects which are relevant to the condition(s) being considered. For example (as stated above) it will be important to explore the birth history of a child with hyperactivity. In a child with possible depression, an inquiry into symptoms such as disturbed biological functions, depressive ideation, etc. may be needed if these have not been reported already.
3. The third part is an assessment of the impact of the illness on the child as well as the parents and the family. Included here will be various areas of the child's functioning, e.g. relationships with parents, other adults, peers, functioning at home and performance at school, etc. After considering each area, a global assessment of functioning (or dysfunction/impairment) is made. The effect of a child's illness on the parents and the family is also important both as a part of the diagnostic process, and in therapy later.

Obtaining the history of present illness starts with information on the presenting complaints first. A spontaneous account of problems is to be obtained. List all presenting complaints in a chronological order with duration of each symptom. Parents arriving at the clinic usually have some preconceived notions about their role in the situation and appear generally discomforted by it. They may be worried, defensive, guilt ridden, angry, annoyed, or, less often appropriately concerned and open minded. Their initial report of the child's symptoms and behaviour will usually suggest further points to be looked into and other questions to be put.

Then ask about the onset of each symptom and the circumstances around the onset, if any. Many a times parents are unable to pinpoint the onset which may mean that the problems are more of developmental in nature. On the other hand, if there is a clear onset, then it shows that the child's development till that stage was fine and that the circumstances around the time of onset may have a significant contribution to problem causation.

After this begins the phase of systematic enquiry. Each complaint is explored further in terms of chronology, associated disturbances, antecedent factors, and consequences. As these problems are presented one after another, they may appear to constitute different facets of the same basic difficulty and a fairly consistent behaviour pattern often emerges from the discussion. For example, the parents may report a series of complaints, such as the teacher says that the child disturbs and annoys his/her classmates; that he/she is constantly picking fights with children; and parents themselves assert that the child cannot be kept from fighting with the siblings. The child may also be described as easily excitable; he/she does whatever comes into his/her head without any regard for the consequences; he/she is accident-prone; he/she destroys household objects or his/her own possessions. All of these particulars create a graphic portrait of a hyperactive, impulsive child whose clash with his/her environment takes varied forms under different circumstances, though all are rooted in the same underlying problem. While listening to the spontaneous account ask the meaning of each complaint that the parents put forth.

Try to elicit entire series of difficulties that the child's behaviour has caused in terms of disruption, distress, or dysfunction in child's or family's functioning. Parents may vary in their assessment of the effect of their child's behaviour on others. Some parents may focus on their own interpretation of child's pathologic conduct, exhibiting either pride that this behaviour indicates high intelligence in the child or much guilt because he/she regards himself/herself as the major cause of the difficulty.

The marked differences in parental attitudes indicate the advisability of pinning down an informant's general statement about a problem with concrete illustrations, even requesting a "blow-by-blow" account of a characteristic episode. Generalities often prove to be more descriptive of a parent's frame of mind than of a child's behaviour. The flat statement that a little girl has no confidence in herself may refer equally well to one who is shy and retiring, to one who gives up easily rather than face an anticipated failure, to a nervous child, or to a child who cannot tolerate criticism. It is helpful to provide alternatives indicating opposing viewpoints to the parent to choose from.

As the pattern of the child's interaction with the environment becomes clearer, the history-taker can make a mental note to pursue certain lines of inquiry. In the case of the hyperactive, impulsive child, for example, a scrutiny of the obstetric and medical history would be in order, to investigate the possibility that this is a child with cerebral dysfunction. The child's temperamental attributes in infancy also need to be looked into. An assessment is made of the intent by frequency and duration of symptoms as also of its effects on the child. For intrapsychic phenomenon, such as sad thoughts, often the child can describe as to its degree of preoccupation, pervasiveness, possibility of self-control. All these indicate severity of illness.

Display of empathy and an understanding attitude in the psychiatrist helps parents to develop confidence in the psychiatrist, which is beneficial for developing a therapeutic alliance. From the parent's initial listing of problems and their explanation of why they are seeking help, the psychiatrist may also obtain valuable insight into their readiness to accept real responsibilities for an appropriate resolution of the behavioural difficulty. Immersing oneself in guilt more often leads to avoidance of responsibility than to its assumption, since one may well expend all one's energy in discharging the intense guilt feelings. The opposite attitude that of blaming the neighbours, playmates and teachers for the child's problems is certainly not a better approach to an examination of a patient's own role in creating or maintaining a destructive situation.

In the investigation of each problem presented, it is important to ascertain its duration, the circumstances, which seem to have initiated or contributed to its development, whether or not it is recurrent, and the relative intensity of the present manifestations.

Comprehensive history taking involves assessment of:
- Predisposing factors
- Precipitating factors
- Perpetuating factor
- Protective factors

Finally, a list of all treatments up to the present consultation should be enquired into, also taking into account which of them succeeded (and to what extent) and which failed. Reports on any previously conducted psychiatric examinations or psychological tests should be obtained wherever possible. Parents who have "shopped around" before may be reluctant to come forth with previous reports fearing that the present therapist may be influenced by a "bad opinion". Nevertheless, it is important to obtain details of previous examinations or investigations in order to assess the exact significance of the latest reading. The opinions of earlier investigators do not have to be accepted uncritically, but a careful study of their findings will tell a great deal about the cause of the child's behaviour. It is also a good idea to ask at this point why the child was brought to the clinic at that particular juncture. There are usually several different reasons for this, some of which are applicable to the child, e.g. worsening of his/her problems; and some to the parents, e.g. an impending separation and some to others such as the family (e.g. a major life change) or the school (e.g. teacher's suggestion). This information is important as it provides a better understanding of the problem.

PAST HISTORY

This should include both physical illnesses and psychiatric problems that the child has suffered from in the past.

To begin with, one should inquire routinely about operations and childhood illnesses and delineate a year-by-year pattern of health or illness. Whenever possible, the therapist should obtain confirming reports of physical illnesses. Past history of any psychiatric problems should also be asked for at this point if they have not been gone into already.

BIRTH AND EARLY DEVELOPMENT

The parents' ages and the length of the marriage at the time of the child's birth may contribute to an understanding of the atmosphere into which he was born. A striking difference in the ages of the parents or the information that both were no longer youthful when the child was born may highlight the existence of special circumstances such as low fertility, miscarriages, negative attitude towards having children or any practical difficulties in child care, which may prove to be crucial data for further investigation.

The number of times the mother was pregnant before the patient was conceived, and the history of miscarriages, stillbirths or living children with congenital anomalies may point to possibilities of subclinical organic factors in the child and also the expectations centred on the child.

The history of the mother's pregnancy, labour and delivery, as well as data on the child's weight at birth and events of the neonatal period, may reveal the presence of early organic difficulties. Entries about the infant's care should note who took care of him. Details of the feeding history should include whether he/she was breastfed or bottlefed, the age at which weaning began and the time required for its completion, and comment on the introduction of new foods and the development of self-feeding. Whether a baby was breastfed or bottle fed may or may not be significant. Bottle-feeding represents an aspect of the urban middle class pattern of infant care today.

The child's individual style of indicating hunger, satiation and food preferences, and the mother's response to his behaviour are all aspects of the feeding history that may be instructive. The interview should also note the child's reaction to special or newer diets that may have been instituted from time to time.

Recommended techniques and schedules for weaning a baby vary from one generation to the next and from one culture to another. It is important to learn which person or combination of persons was responsible for the baby's day-to-day care. If the mother was employed outside the home or had another outside responsibility, one should investigate how this affected her relationship with the baby and his daily schedule.

The next series of questions comprise an evolution of developmental history. This encompasses vital steps in maturation, i.e. the ages at which the child became capable of sitting, standing, walking, and saying his first word, and also the salient facts about his toilet training. The information in this category often gives valuable clues to diagnosis. Normally, there are variations in the ages at which different children achieve various milestones.

A significant lag in motor maturation may point either to specific neurological difficulties, which may not have been previously recognized, or to mental retardation. The combination of such a lag with normal or precocious development in language would suggest that the cause is something other than mental retardation. On the other hand, extreme variability in the pattern of language development and a delay in speech itself do not necessarily imply that there specific delay in development and general intellectual development is not sluggish. Even children of normal or superior intelligence may not utter their first word until they are two and a half years old. Characteristically, in that case, a speedy pick-up of language function follows so that, within a short period of time, it is impossible to distinguish such children from those who started to speak earlier. Whereas if the whole speech pattern is uniformly delayed, there is no babbling during infancy, no exploration of sounds during the first eighteen months, the first word spoken after the age of three, and thereafter a very gradual develop-ment in the use of language, one would suspect that the delay has been caused either by general retardation or specific maturational lag in the area of language.

SOCIAL AND PERSONAL HISTORY

Included here are habits, neurotic traits, behaviour problems, play and sexual history. Relevant parts would already have been covered earlier. Any additional information can be documented here.

EDUCATIONAL HISTORY

The information obtained about the child's schooling usually conveys an impression of his adjustment to other children and to the learning process. A child presumed to have been normal in every respect may give the first indication of behaviour problems when he enters an organized group. The parents may have become so used to adapting themselves to him/her that they failed to realize that he/she would experience some difficulty in adjusting to social situations, to sharing objects or attention with other children, and to fighting for his/her rights. A child whose personal reactions seemed alert to his/her parents may be revealed as mentally retarded when he/she begins to function for the first time in formal learning situations. Data of this sort can contribute significantly to an understanding of the presenting problems. Assessment of the child's performance at school is also important for several other reasons. The school is an area where it is possible to come to know about how the child accomplishes several tasks required of him/her independent of the family. It is thus an extremely important part of his/her development. Some problems may be more common or more evident at school than at home and vice versa. Academic performance, social skills, relationships with peers and teachers are all important parts of the child's global functioning. One would expect any kind of illness or disturbance to affect these aspects as well.

TEMPERAMENT IN INFANCY

Following the taking of a basic clinical history, systematic inquiry can be made into the child's temperamental characteristics during infancy. Most parents are unable to judge the intent of the general questions about temperament of the child and end up in saying that the child was fine.

It is therefore necessary to ask description of behaviours from which judgements of temperament may be made for each of the temperamental attributes one by one. Given below are the suggested questions appropriate to each of the temperamental category.

Activity Level

"How much did your baby move around? Did he/she move around a lot, was he/she very quiet, or moderately so? If you put him/her to bed for a nap and it took him/her ten or fifteen minutes to fall asleep, would you have to go in to rearrange the covers, or would he/she be lying so quietly that you knew they would not be disarranged? If you were changing his/her diaper and discovered that you had left the powder just out of reach, could you safely dash over to get it and come right back without worrying that he would flip over the surface and fall? Did you have trouble changing his/her diaper, pulling his/her shirt over his/her head or putting on any other of his/her clothing because he/she wriggled about?"

Rhythmicity

"How did you arrange the baby's feedings? Could you tell by the time he/she was six weeks (two months, three months) old about when during the day he/she would be hungry, sleepy or wake up? Could you count on this happening about the same time every day or did the baby vary from day-to-day? If there was any variation, how marked was it? About when during the day did he/she have his/her bowel movements (time and number) and was this routine variable or predictable?"

Parents can generally recall such events. They will say, "he/she was regular as clockwork", or," I could never figure out when to start a long job because one day he/she would have a long nap and the next day he/she wouldn't sleep more than fifteen minutes", or, "I never could figure his bowel movements because his/her time changed every day."

Adaptability

"How did the child respond to changed circumstances? When he/she was shifted from one room to another, did he/she take to the change immediately? If not, could you count on his getting used to it quickly or did it take a long time?" (Parents should be asked to define what they mean by "quickly" and what they mean by "a long time" in terms of days or weeks)". If his/her first reaction to a new person was a negative one, how long did it take the child to become familiar with the person? If he/she did not like a new food the first time it was offered, could you count on his/her getting to like it and most other new foods sooner or later? If so, how long would it take if the new food was offered to him/her daily or several times a week?"

Approach Withdrawal

"How did the baby behave with new events, such as when he/she was given his/her first tub bath, offered new foods or taken care of by an unfamiliar person? Did he/she fuss, did he/she do nothing, or did he/she seem to like it? Were there any changes during his/her infancy that the mother remembers, such as a shift to a new bed, or a visit to a new place? Describe the child's initial behaviour at these times."

Threshold Level

"How would you estimate the baby's sensitivity to noises, heat and cold, things he saw and tasted, and textures of clothing? Did he/she seem very aware of these things or was he/she unresponsive? Did you have to tiptoe about when the baby was sleeping lest he be awakened? If he/she heard a faint noise while awake, would he/she tend to notice the sound by looking towards it? Did bright lights or bright sunshine make him/her blink or cry? Did the baby's behaviour seem to show that he/she noticed the difference when a familiar person wore glasses or a new hair style for the first time in his/her presence? If he/she did not like a new food and if something familiar that he/she liked very much was put with it on the spoon, would the baby still notice the taste of the new one and reject it?"

Intensity of Reaction

"How did you know when the baby was hungry? Did he/she squeak, did he roar, or were his/her sounds, somewhere in between? How could you tell that he/she did not like something? Did he/she just quietly turn his/her head away or did he/she start crying loudly?"

"If you held his/her hand to cut his/her fingernails and he/she did not like it, did he/she fuss a little or a lot? If he/she liked something, did he/she usually smile and coo or did he/she laugh loudly? In general, would you say he/she let his/her pleasure or dis-pleasure be known loudly or softly?"

Quality of Mood

"How could you tell when the baby liked something or disliked something?" (After a description of the infant's behaviour in these respects is obtained, the parents should be asked if he/she was more often contended or more often discontented and on what basis they made this judgement.)

Distractibility

"If the child was sucking on the bottle or breast would he/she stop when he heard a sound or if another person came by or would he continue sucking? If he/she was hungry and fussing or crying while the bottle was being warmed, could you divert him/her easily and stop his/her crying by holding him/her or giving him/her a toy? If he/she was playing, gazing at his/her fingers or using a rattle would other sights and sounds get his/her attention very quickly or very slowly".

Persistence and Attention Span

"Would you say that the baby usually stuck with something he/she was doing for a long time or only momentarily? For example, describe the longest time he/she remained engrossed in an activity all by himself. How old was he/she and what was he/she doing? If he/she reached for something, say a toy in the bathtub, and couldn't get it easily, would he/she keep after it or give up very quickly?"

TEMPERAMENT AT LATER STAGES OF DEVELOPMENT

After completing the inventory of the child's temperamental characteristics in infancy, the next step is to identify those attributes, which appear extreme in their manifestations and those which seem clearly related to the child's current pattern of deviant behaviour. This is followed by an inquiry into the expression of these temperamental attributes at succeeding age-stage periods of development. Thus, if the history in the period of infancy suggests a pattern of marked distractibility, it is desirable to gather data on behaviour related to distractibility at succeeding age periods, and in varied life situations, such as play, school or homework. Similarly, if the presenting complaints indicate that the child currently finds it difficult to undertake new activities or to join new groups, and if the early temperamental history suggests a characteristic pattern of initial withdrawal coupled with slow adaptation, it is important to obtain descriptions of his/her initial responses to situations and demands at various points in his developmental course.

The final step in assessing the child's temperament is the evaluation of his/her current temperamental characteristics. The information obtained for current functioning is usually more valid than that obtained for past patterns of behaviour, since the problem of forgetting and retrospective distortion are minimized. The inquiry into present behaviour, while attempting to cover all temperamental categories, should concentrate on those which appear most pertinent to the presenting symptoms.

Activity levels may be estimated from a child's behaviour preferences. Would he/she rather sit quietly for a long time engrossed in some task or does he/she prefer to seek out opportunities for active physical play? How does he/she fare in routines that require sitting still for extended periods of time? For example, can he/she sit through an entire meal without seeking an opportunity to move about? Must a long automobile ride be broken up by frequent stops because of his/her restlessness?

Adaptability can be identified through a consideration of the way the child reacts to changes in environment. Does he/she adjust easily and fit quickly into changed family patterns? Does he/she have difficulty adapting to the routines of a new classroom or a new teacher? Is he/she willing to go along with other children's preferences or does he/she always insist on pursuing only his/her own interests?

Approach-withdrawal or the youngster's pattern of response to new events and people can be explored in many ways. Questions can be directed at the nature of his/her reaction to new clothing, new neighbourhood children, a new school, and new teachers. What is his attitude when a family excursion is being planned? Will he readily try new foods or activities?

Threshold level is more difficult to explore in an older child than in a young one. However, it is sometimes possible to obtain information on unusual features of threshold, such as hypersensitivity to noise, visual stimuli and rough clothing, or remarkable unresponsiveness to such stimuli.

The intensity of reactions can be ascertained by finding out how the child displays disappointment or pleasure. If something pleasant happens, does he/she tend to be mildly enthusiastic, average in his/her expression of joy, or ecstatic? When he/she is unhappy, does he/she fuss quietly or bellow with rage or distress?

Quality of mood can usually be estimated by parental descriptions of their offspring's overall expression of mood. Is he/she predominantly happy and contended or is he/she a frequent complainer and more often unhappy than not?

Distractibility, even when not a presenting problem, will declare itself in the parents' descriptions of ordinary routines. Does the child start off to do something and then often get sidetracked by something his/her brother is doing, by his/her coin collection or by a number of circumstances that catch his/her eye or his/her ear? Or once he/she is engaged in an activity, is he/she impervious to what is going on around him/her?

Data on persistence and attention span are usually easier to obtain for the older child than for the infant. The degree of persistence in the face of difficulty can be ascertained with regard to games puzzles, athletic activities and schoolwork. Similarly, after the initial difficulty in mastering these activities has been overcome, the length of the child's attention span for and concentration on these same kinds of activities can be ascertained.

The delineation of the child's temperamental characteristics at different age-periods may indicate that changes have occurred over time. There are normal variations of temperament and the fate of any temperamental attribute is dependent upon a host of influences.

The process of socialization may blur the individual behavioural style evident in new situations and experiences. In other words, certain patterns of response, once they are adapted to a cultural norm, may serve to minimize individual variations. For example, the first attempt at toilet-training will cause one child to scream and struggle violently, another to fuss mildly while he/she sits on the seat for only a few minutes, and a third child to smile and play while sitting on the seat for many minutes. A year later, when all three children are fully trained, their behaviour on the toilet seat may show comparatively slight differences.

Similar blurring of initial differences may occur with a variety of other experiences, such as entry into nursery school, the beginning of formal learning, changes in the family group, new living quarters. Therefore, when the behavioural history suggests an apparent change in a child's temperament over time, the data should be scrutinised to determine whether the change remains in evidence or disappears when the responses to new situations at the different age periods are compared.

In many instances, querying teachers or other adults familiar with the child's behaviour can obtain additional data on temperamental organization. For such inquiry, the history-taking protocol for the parents can be utilized if it is appropriately modified to permit a focus on the areas of the child's functioning with which the adult is acquainted.

FAMILY HISTORY

Essential here is a family tree (using standard notations) with age, sex and very brief personality descriptions of each member. Family history of mental illness or any significant physical illness needs to be mentioned.

Data on the patient's sibs will help to clarify his/her own position in the family hierarchy and will alert the history-taker to the existence of any special stresses or strains produced by that position. Unusual facts about each sib, and about any other children who may be permanent members of the household, should also be secured.

Two other broad areas to be covered are those of "family functioning" and "parent–child interactions". Family functioning will include an enquiry into how the family copes with various tasks, patterns of communications, etc. Any discord, lack of communication between members as well as problems the family faces as a whole, e.g. poverty or discrimination should be highlighted if present.

Interactions between various members are also important. Areas to be focused on are negative interactions such as lack of warmth, hostility towards or scapegoating of the child, sibling rivalry, etc. The possibility of abuse, physical or sexual, should always be kept in mind. Exploring these areas will need considerable tact and patience.

PARENTAL FUNCTIONING

At this point in the interview, the examiner may have become aware of patterns that were not evident earlier. More precise inquiry into the nature of the behaviour disorder may now become possible. Enquire into areas such as amount of time spent in care of the child; degree of over protection or indulgence; degree to which demands of the child are fulfilled; degree and methods of discipline employed; degree of autonomy allowed or fostered; any behaviour indicating infantilizing or babying; consistency *vs* inconsistency in disciplining across time or across care-givers. Pathological parenting or care giving patterns are an important source of maladaptation and psychopathology in children. Correction of pathological parenting patterns is a major method of treatment.

SOCIAL AND ENVIRONMENTAL CONDITIONS

It is useful to obtain an idea of the current living conditions of the child's family. This would include physical aspects such as type of housing, degree of overcrowding, etc. and socio-economic data such as the financial status of the family, and also the constellation of family at the given time. These factors have significant bearing on the child's state of health. If any aspect of the living conditions found to be stressful for the child, this should be mentioned.

SPECIAL ENVIRONMENTAL CIRCUMSTANCES

Life events contribute to development and exacerbations of psychiatric illness and this is true for children as well. Thus, it is important to enquire into significant events or life changes that might have occurred in the recent past such as change in living arrangement, change in school or city, any major illnesses, bereavements, separation, divorce, family conflict, failure, disappointment, broken relationship etc. The relation between the event and the child's illness should be explored. An attempt is to be made to assess what impact a particular event has had on the child.

PHYSICAL EXAMINATION

One should look for evidence of any physical disorder as indicated in history or as may be evident in observation of the child such as any neurological signs, abnormal gait, abnormal movements, or any dysmorphic features or any neurocutaneous stigmata. Recording of weight, height and head circumference helps to plot the growth status. Any evidence of physical injury, neglect, deficiency, trauma or abuse should also be noted.

MENTAL STATUS EXAMINATION

Age and developmental level of the child will determine both the technique as well as inferences made from the mental state examination. Every opportunity, thus, should be taken to observe the child's behaviour. This should be noted down systematically and objectively. Observation of infant or preschool children is best done in the playroom situation in the presence of parents. Parent–child interactions should also be noted.

As in any mental state examination certain types of questions are more likely to elicit information from the child. These include:

- Open-ended questions (How did that make you feel?)
- Facilitatory questions (You must have been upset, could you tell me a bit more about that?)
- Clarifications (Have I got this right?)

Mental state examination starts with observation of the child from the point of entry in the clinic. Make note of the following:

General Appearance and Behaviour

Stature, physical deformities or stigmata and nutritional state should be noted. Dress gives an idea of the care the child receives or has much he cares for himself. Tics, stereotypies, mannerisms, abnormal movements if any should be described.

Relationship Capacity

Children will usually relate to the examiner cautiously at first. They might be shy or anxious. Adolescents might be rejecting. With a gradual buildup of trust, more often than not, a working relationship is established. This might take one or several sessions. Some children, who are deprived or abused are indiscriminately friendly and shallow from the beginning. Does the child know the purpose of interview?

Separation Anxiety

The ease with which the child separates from his/her parents has some diagnostic value. Difficult separation may be due to pathologic ties between the parents and the child or the child' anxiety in response to new situations and new people. Separating the child from the parents is thus often tried at some point during the interview. It is important to explain to the child that you would like to chat with him alone and his/her parents will be waiting just outside the room. If separation is too problematic, it should not be insisted upon and can be tried on a subsequent visit. The age of the child is a major factor in deciding whether or not to try out this procedure.

Motility/Psychomotor Activity

Can the child sit still? Does he/she move from one thing to another? Is this to the extent that it is disruptive? Is it associated with a short attention span, low frustration tolerance and labile emotions? All these could be indicative of a hyperkinetic disorder. Over activity can also be a normal variant or a manifestation of other disorders such as anxiety or psychosis.

Affect

Shyness or anxiety is normal reactions during the initial phases. As a child feels more reassured and learns he/she can trust the examiner these usually subside. Any evidence of fear, anxiety, sadness, distress, or undue happiness, irritability. Any verbal or physical aggression? Some abnormal affects might be evident from the onset, e.g. sadness, inappropriate smiling. It is useful to determine whether the child is displaying the whole range of affects or is there a restriction in the type of emotions displayed. Thus, it would be necessary to observe his affective display during various parts of the examination and in relation to different questions, objects, situations, etc.

Speech/Language

Assess general level of speech proficiency, fluency, vocabulary, articulation and communication. Does the child talk in complete sentences, or what is the developmental level of speech acquisition? Assessment of speech should also include reading and writing (whenever appropriate). If any developmental problems are suspected a more detailed evaluation including CNS examination, hearing tests, IQ, etc. should be done.

Thought Content

Several areas need to be covered, attitudes towards family, peers and teachers are enquired about. The examiner might ask the child who in the family he gets along with best/worst. Pleasant and unpleasant aspects of the relationship with sibs and parents can be asked. What kind of things makes the family members (especially parents) angry? How is this anger expressed? What makes them happy and how is this expressed?

Peer relationships give an idea of the capacity to relate to others, identifications, social awareness and level of independence. The child can be asked if he has one/few/ many best friends. How often do they meet? What do they do together? Look for any obsessions (thoughts, impulses, doubts, images) or compulsions. If indicated in the history, look for delusions, hallucinations or thought disorder as in adults. Children often lack clarity in content, are inconsistent in reporting, and often present these as fantasy.

Attention span, persistence, concentration, impulsivity: Assess attention, concentration and persistence, degree of frustration tolerance and oppositionality.

Fantasy

Much of the spontaneous content of the interview may be the child's fantasies. None of these fantasy productions is particularly characteristic of any specific condition but gives general impressions about the child's contact with reality, his/her intelligence, predominant feelings, self-concept, etc. To elicit fantasies several techniques can be used. Any topic that the child introduces can be pursued. He/she could be asked about his/her favourite animal (sport/videogame) and what he likes about it. A standard technique is the "three wishes test". The child is asked what he/she would wish for if a fairy granted him three wishes. Sometimes, the wishes reveal a direct problem situation, e.g. "I would wish that my parents stop fighting". Or the child might give a 'popular' response, "I wish to be rich". This can indicate that the child is in tune with the aspirations of his/her peer group. An alternative to the "three wishes test" is to ask the child what he/she would do if he/she had three bags of money to spend. The ability to distinguish fantasy from reality needs to be assessed as well. Some degree of blurring, especially in younger children, would be normal. Gross distortions are however indicative of psychosis in a child with average intelligence. If such distortions are present an enquiry into psychotic symptoms such as delusions and hallucinations should be made.

Assessment of self-esteem and problem solving capacity are other important areas to be covered in this part of the examination.

Intellectual Capacity

A fair estimate of intelligence can be made based on the overall assessment of developmental history, educational history, level of speech and language functioning, and current level of functioning in comparison to the chronological age.

As in adults, general knowledge, calculating ability, comprehension is used in estimating the level of intelligence. A referral to the psychologist should be made if IQ tests are indicated.

Judgment and Insight

Depending on the age the child, it may be possible to assess judgement and insight. Child may be able to say what he/she thinks is wrong but most of the time they see their problem as emanating from the environment. They invariably exhibit external attribution as they lack the cognitive and emotional maturity for internal attribution.

OBSERVATION OF PLAY

Playing is the principal activity of childhood and has much more personal significance than a mere relief from other activities. It may be the only form of expression in a younger child. Form and content of play, affective reactions during and accompanying fantasies are all important parameters which help in gaining a better understanding of the child's problems and conflicts. It can also be a useful indicator of the child's attention span, distractibility, frustration tolerance, etc. Ideally toys and other materials should be available in every examining room. When this is not possible, a special room and a therapist are often designated. To understand the child better, an attempt should be made to join the play therapist in observation of the child, whenever this is possible.

Conclusion

Always ask the child at the end of the interview if he has any questions or anything else to tell you. Inform him about what is going to happen next, e.g. IQ testing. Parents should be similarly asked and told about the next set of procedures.

Interview Technique

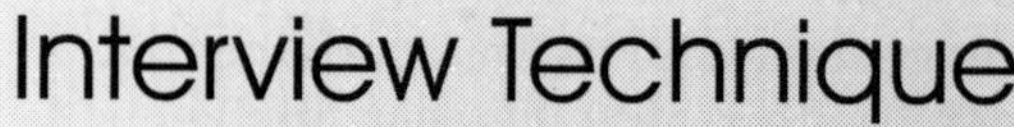

The child, in addition to being smaller in dimensions, differs from adult qualitatively both in its physical and psychological characteristics. From psychological point of view, the child has relatively 'fluid' psyche where his/her emotionality, thinking and reaction patterns are not fixed or deep rooted. It is more pliable and susceptible to outside influences. It is also important to be continuously aware of the developmental dimensions involving biological maturational processes which in its interaction with the environmental factors, in a step wise manner, determine the course of development. Children behave differently at different ages, so it is important to know the range of normal behaviours at different ages.

When a particular behaviour is age inappropriate we can ascribe it a pathological significance. A particular behaviour may be normal for one age and abnormal for another, e.g. fear of animals occur normally in early childhood (about 5–6 years of age) and its persistence in later childhood indicates pathology. Manifestations of the same disorder vary as the child goes along the developmental ladder. A clear example is that of hyperkinetic syndrome. During infancy and preschool years a child with hyperkinesis is unusually active, hyperalert, very difficult to soothe and may be irregular and unpredictable in his/her biological needs of hunger, sleep and elimination. As he/she grows during childhood, he/she is impulsive, impervious to disciplining,

and has poor understanding of danger. Later on, in late childhood or adolescence, it manifests as poor academic performance and antisocial behaviour. It highlights that development exerts pathoplastic influence on psychiatric symptomatology.

The emotional conflicts in children are more superficial in contrast to adults. With minimal probing or even without it, the problems are seen on the surface with such clarity sometimes that one may be led to think it is a deliberate behaviour. But it is partly due to the poor ability to formulate and verbally express emotions in children and a tendency to take refuge in bodily language in the form of somatic symptoms. For example, a child with school phobia may present with vomiting or pain abdomen, which on probing is generally found to occur in the mornings, which is the school time.

For the assessment of the psychiatric problems in a child, there are certain differences worth noting as compared to the routine adult work-up.

1. The child is generally brought for the psychiatric consultation by parents and it is the others (parents, teachers, or relatives) who feel the need for the same rather than the child himself. Very often he/she is not even told or may have been given a misleading reason for consultation with psychiatrist. The child obviously is confused and at times embarrassed when confronted with the psychiatrist and may not co-operate fully for examination.

2. There is a greater need to depend on the indirect methods for assessment. In children, the verbal medium of expression is limited because of their biological immaturity. Therefore, the interview with parents and the other significant adults like teacher, caretaker is taken into account more often.

3. Observations in the natural environment or in the play setting are useful, at times integral components of assessment.

As is obvious, for psychiatric assessment, the main investigative tool is "talking". In addition to knowing about 'what to talk', it is as important to learn 'how to talk'. Psychiatric interview consists essentially of two aspects:

1. The obtaining of information about events, happenings and behaviour, i.e. the factual data.

2. The observation of feelings, thinking, attitudes and motivations concerning these events and the individuals participating in them.

INTERVIEW SETTING

Psychiatric interview should be conducted in quiet secluded rooms, adequately lighted and lightly furnished. Too much of noise, hustle-bustle of people or equipment around, or a busy telephone inside the room are not conducive for a good interview. The patient and the relatives should be assured of adequate privacy and confidentiality. Effort should be made for an uninterrupted conversation which facilitates for psychological exploration.

BEHAVIOUR OF THE CLINICIAN

How the clinician behaves during the interview is very important and generally sets the tone for the subsequent development of the therapeutic relationship based on which the patient is either going to accept or reject the advice, specially the psychological intervention. Do not appear in a hurry. Make the patient and the relatives comfortable by offering the chair. Initial introduction as to who the patient is and who are the others accompanying the patient should be done. Keep only the key informants (parent or the parent surrogate, and the others who have been with the child during his/her illness) for interview and ask others politely to wait outside.

The clinician should be non-judgemental, empathic, interested and warm in his approach. Avoid emotional let outs or exclamations. Keen observation right from the beginning like the manner of coming in and the behaviour of the patient during interview, provides considerable insights into the emotional undercurrents and motivations of the patient.

OBJECTIVES OF THE PSYCHIATRIC INTERVIEW

Generally after history taking, we tend to stop at arriving of a diagnosis. Aim of the interview is not just diagnostic. As summarized below the psychiatric assessment must address the following issues:

1. What is wrong? For example, to arrive at a diagnosis and differential diagnosis.

2. What possibly has caused it? (Indicating the etiological factors.)

3. What can be done about it?

One should be able to set a tone for psychological intervention (if needed), after a skilful interview. These questions should act as the guiding elements for the subsequent interview.

BEGINNING OF INTERVIEW

First of all enquire about the identification data, i.e. name, age, educational level attained and the residential address of the patient and the parent or the relative accompanying the patient. It makes the patient and the relative more comfortable and provides a reference point regarding the patient's sociocultural background.

Make a note of the source that made the psychiatry referral. In addition to serving as an important resource for taking information, it will also indicate the specific area of maladjustment. If the referral is made by the teacher, the problems are likely to be in the academic field or in behaviour, if it is a paediatrician the problem is likely to be certain somatic symptoms with absent or insufficient organic basis.

HISTORY OF PRESENT ILLNESS

Start with the presenting complaints: What has brought the patient to the hospital? Enquire from the patient and the relatives separately. Attention should be paid to the actual words used to describe the complaints, (record verbatim as far as possible), because that will reflect the area of utmost concern as well as his/her attitude and understanding of the problem to some extent. Parents often make general statements like "his/her mind does not work"; "his/her mind is not developed", "he/she shows abnormal behaviour", etc. Each of these complaints might mean many different things, e.g. "his/her mind does not work" may be true of mental sub normality or of an impulsive child who is highly distractible or even a quiet, shy and inhibited child or it may just be an apprehension of over expectant parents about a normal average child. Generalities indicate the parent's frame of mind more often than the actual problems the child has. Therefore, it is very important to find exactly what the parent means by the stated complaints, taking the illustrative examples. Ascertain with regard to each symptoms, specifically, as far as possible, the duration, severity, frequency, relationship with the situational factors which initiated or contributed to its development and how is it dealt with by parents? Generally, based on the details of the complaints, one is able to understand the likely nature of the disturbance and also it will give hints towards the specific areas in which further exploration is necessary. For example, in a child presenting with scholastic backwardness, details of the developmental and educational history would be in order. Similarly, in a child

presenting with shyness, withdrawal and anxiety it will be worthwhile to explore into the temperamental attributes of the child and the patterns of parental handling.

If the symptoms are present since birth then start the history from conception through early and later development.

History of present illness, in the end, should address the assessment of the level of functional disabilities of the child and the degree of impairment in him/her. How far have the child's interpersonal relationships with parents, sibs, peers; scholastic and leisure time activities; self-care and other activities, etc. been affected by the symptoms or the problems he has come with? The amount of functional disability or the impairment in the area has implications not only for the assessment of current severity of illness, but also for future development. The future growth and development of the child can be arrested, retarded, or even deviated on account of continued or persistent impairment in any functions. Any problem that can potentially jeopardise child's growth and development is a matter of serious concern. Assessment of the severity of present illness, therefore, must take into account the severity, intensity, persistence and pervasiveness of symptoms; the degree of distress or disability caused by these; as well as the degree of functional disability and impairment.

PHYSICAL HEALTH

After the history of present illness, exploration into the physical health of the child should be done. Enquire routinely about any childhood illnesses, operations, accidents or any other illness the child has had. Descriptions of physical illnesses and of how they were dealt with would reveal the attitudes of overprotection/underprotection vs the proper handling by parents. For example, during the period of physical sickness the children often become irritable, demanding, clinging and the parents become more indulgent and permissive. A child who is emotionally insecure earlier might find this situation satisfying and continue to exhibit demanding behaviour and temper-tantrums even after the physical illness is over, in order to get the attention of the parents. Similarly, if the parents get very anxious about the child's illness; thus, after recovery might impose certain unwarranted restrictions on his activity to create feelings of inadequacy and in extreme cases it interferes in the subsequent psychological development.

It is worthwhile to contact the paediatrician or the general practitioner who looked after the child during the physical illnesses and considerable amount of relevant information can be obtained which may not have been told to the parents.

SIGNIFICANCE OF THE SYMPTOMS

All the symptoms reported by the parents are not pathological per se. In children, many of the problems are developmental in nature and hence self-limiting. For example, around the age of 1½ to 3 years, when the child is rapidly acquiring speech, mastering motor skills, becoming increasingly autonomous, he may want to do everything himself and refuse what parents ask him to do. At this stage they may become negativistic and stubborn causing worry to the parents who want the child to be compliant and amiable. Whether the complaints are a function of normal developmental process or emotional pathology is judged in reference to the following:

1. Is the behaviour appropriate to the chronological age of the child?
2. Is the behaviour appropriate to the mental age of the child?
3. Is it impairing his further development?
4. Is the behaviour appropriate to the sociocultural background?
5. Is the behaviour distressing or disturbing to the child and/or the family.

Behaviour not in keeping with the age (chronological and mental), sociocultural milieu is pathological. Behaviour that hampers the further development or causes significant distress or disruption to the normal routine functioning also is abnormal.

DEVELOPMENTAL HISTORY

It includes the history of birth and infancy; milestones of development; habits of sleep, eating, personal care; presence of neurotic traits; play and educational history.

To begin with it is important to understand the circumstances and the atmosphere into which the child was born. Was it a wanted pregnancy or unwanted, was the child born when the parents were not yet ready emotionally or otherwise to accept him or was he born after a long and anxious waiting being childless after many years of marriage. It will highlight the existence of special anxieties in parents, which may be crucial data for further exploration.

The history of mother's pregnancy and labour, child's weight at birth and the events of neonatal period may reveal the presence of early organic difficulties. Details of the feeding history should include whether he was breastfed or bottlefed, the age at which weaning began, and comment on the development of self-feeding, introduction of new foods, etc.

Schedules of feeding and weaning vary with sociocultural background and also from one generation to the next. Therefore, one must not assume an automatic correlation between certain factual data and its pathogenic significance.

It is important to know who all were responsible for the baby's day-to-day care. In Indian joint families system, it may be the grandparents or other aunts and uncles, in addition to the mother. However, if the mother is employed, one should further investigate into the effectiveness with which she was able to combine her work schedule and childcare. Did she have any specific difficulties or were there other family members to support her? This will have implications for child's development. There is no evidence to believe that a "working mother means a rejecting mother".

A detailed study of the development of motor skills, language and other social, adaptive functions' comprises the next series of questions. A global lag in the development of all functions will indicate mental retardation whereas a significant lag in motor maturation with normal development of language and other skills will indicate some specific neurological difficulties. There is a great variability in normal children as far as the acquisition of the various milestones is concerned. Sometimes children of normal or superior intelligence may not utter their first word until they are two and a half years old. A speedy pick up of language follows in such a case, so that within a short time, it is impossible to distinguish such children from those who started to speak earlier. Whereas, if, the whole speech pattern is delayed uniformly, e.g. no babbling during infancy, no exploration of sounds during the first eighteen months and a very gradual development in the use of language, one would suspect that the delay has been caused either by general retardation or a specific maturational lag in the area of language.

Enquiry into the various habit patterns of sleeping, eating, personal care and the presence/absence of neurotic traits during early childhood generally reflects on the child's adjustment through the various phases of development.

Among the, preschool years the child is moving gradually from a state of dependence to autonomy, i.e. he/she is learning to eat himself, acquire the skills of dressing up, explore actively into the environment, and the parents are teaching him the right ways of behaving. The conflict between the child and the parents at this stage is likely to produce the disorders like being fussy about food, sleep problems, temper-tantrums, and enuresis, nail biting, etc. At this stage, going to the school further expands the social circle as the child starts gradually preferring group play than solitary play. Child's inability to play in a group or develop peer relationships indicates a serious disturbance of socialization as would be seen in psychosis or severe conduct disorders. Whether the play is organized, meaningful and age appropriate will point towards the child's intellectual level.

In the educational history enquire into when the child was first sent to school, his/her initial reaction to going to school, subsequent educational performance, the level obtained, any failures, or problems of adjustment with other schoolmates or teachers, any disciplinary problems. If there is poor school performance along with a generalized delay in development it will be in keeping with a diagnosis of mental retardation whereas in the absence of generalized delay it will signify the presence of specific learning disabilities.

School report forms another source of information regarding the child's behaviour and conduct. Any disparity between the parent's report and the teacher's report will show that the problem is more specific limited only to home or school.

TEMPERAMENT OF THE CHILD

It has been observed uniformly by all those professionals involved in the care of the children (paediatricians, psychologists, psychiatrists, parents, and teachers) that the children are different physiologically and psychologically right from the early infancy. Accordingly they need different sort of handling in an individual case. Research on the temperament of children has shown that these differences become apparent and can be identified in the behavioural style of the child, e.g. the amount and the tempo of motor activity, reaction to new situations, people or objects, intensity and quality of emotional reaction, adaptability, attention span and persistence, and threshold of responsiveness. Details of the temperament variables and their definitions are given in the preceding chapter as well as in the chapter on temperament measurement.

After completing the inventory of the child's temperamental characteristics in infancy, assess the temperament now and compare what changes have occurred. There are normal variations of temperament and the fate of any temperamental attribute is dependant upon a host of influences. The process of socialization may blur the individual behavioural style. The relevance of the temperamental assessment lies in finding out the "goodness of fit" between the child's temperamental attributes and the parental handling which will determine whether the emotional development is normal or deviant, e.g. a child who is of withdrawing nature temperamentally and the parents expect and pressurise him to mix up and socialise soon, the child will develop emotional problems. Here, the parents will have to learn that the child will take his/her own time and pushing him hard will only damage him/her psychologically.

FAMILY HISTORY

Traditionally, information pertaining to the parents and siblings, their ages, sex, personality characteristics, education and occupation is taken. Specifically, enquiry is to be made into the family history of mental illness, patterns of parental functioning, special environmental conditions and circumstances if any. The crux of the matter lies in understanding as to what kind of parents and family are we dealing with. If there is considerable age difference between parents then they are likely to have their own problems which would reflect in the child rearing. Similarly, personality constellations of each of them will also have a direct bearing on their behaviour and attitude towards children. In most cases parental attitude and behaviour are as much a part of the child's problem as the child's own feelings and thoughts.

Guidelines along which to explore the patterns of parental functioning are whether the disciplining is strict or liberal; permissive or rigid; consistency of parental behaviour *vs* inconsistency; protectiveness *vs* non-protectiveness; approval *vs* disapproval of the child and their expectations for him. Details regarding each of these areas would generally bring forth the faults in child rearing practices and attitudes indicating the origin of the problem and areas for intervention.

Similarly, the assessment of the child's social environment is made by enquiring into the type of dwelling degree of overcrowding, affluence of the family and the financial stresses. Question should also be asked whether there had been any special environmental stresses, temporally related like birth of a sibling, death, illness of the mother or any of the significant family members, accidents, divorce, hospitalisation, etc. in the family. If present, these factors might act as precipitants. Lastly, any family history of mental illness, mental retardation, epilepsy suicide, etc. is taken as relevant because their presence indicates genetic or constitutional predisposition.

In the end, the parents should be asked as to their understanding and insight into the problem because that will reveal their expectation regarding the treatment. If the parents believe that the problem is mainly physical, they would be reluctant for psychological intervention unless we have discussed with them in detail about the possible psychogenicity. On the other hand if the parents believe that the fault lies with the child himself or his/her school environment the knowledge of their contribution to the problem may come to them as a shock. Synthesizing the historical data we can formulate as to:

1. What sort of a child are we dealing with? (Genetic, temperamental and developmental data.)

2. What sort of parents and family are we dealing with? (Attitudes, relationships and child rearing practices.)

3. What sort of sociocultural environment are we dealing with? (Socioeconomic status, cultural background, etc.)

Usually, a complicated interplay between all these three sets of factors best explains the condition of the child.

EXAMINATION OF THE CHILD

Physical Examination

Generally, a paediatrician or a family doctor should be responsible for the general medical care of the patient. However, psychiatrist should be able to interpret and integrate the general medical data with the other historical data. If the children are referred from non-medical sources like school or parents themselves, a detailed medical assessment and examination is mandatory. The clinician should have a good knowledge of normal child development.

It is easier to detect any gross physical disorder if present. However, even the minor deviations such as mild visual or auditory disturbances, poor motor co-ordination, are often as significant as the gross lesions, in producing psychological decompensation. The assessment of the minimal disturbance of CNS function may be done by observing the child in his/her activities more than on carrying out a routine neurological examination. Any history suggestive of brain damage should generally be pursued by a detailed neurological examination.

Psychological Examination

In addition to the mental state examination by interview, other aids in psychological examination are play observation and psycho-logical testing.

Mental State Examination

Before coming to the mental state examination, the examiner has had sufficient briefing about the child's problems. In the first place the clinician should provide an emotional setting within which the child can express himself. Exhibit sympathy and acceptance, use reassurance and suggestion. Observe and listen carefully. Manner of the interview depends upon child's age and his/her prior emotional set. Overcoming his initial inhibitions, generally the child will be able to express freely. It is also necessary to attempt interview of the child without parents. Certain children may be more free to talk in the absence of parents who may have been very domineering and strict, whereas some other child may feel too insecure and anxious without them and therefore has to be interviewed along with parents. In case of older children some degree of confidentiality is to be ensured, the child should be made to feel that he/she can trust the examiner and only certain information, which is likely to help him/her, will be discussed with his/her parents. Absolute confidentiality is unrealistic with young children. Mental State Examination is carried out and reported under the following headings:

General Appearance

Start with the life-like description of the child's size, its relationship to age, dress, physical handicaps if any, etc.

Relationship Capacity

Describe the reaction of the child to the interview situation and his/her relationship to the examiner. Generally, it is possible to establish some rapport with the child. In case, the child does not show any emotional response towards the examiner, it will indicate a severe psychopathology even amounting to psychotic illness.

Also note his response to the separation from parents. Responses of anxiety, fear and crying will indicate presence of dependence, insecurity.

Spontaneous Motility and Speech

The amount and quality of motor activity spontaneously exhibited by the child will immediately provide evidence for hyper-kinesis. The complexity of verbal speech and vocabulary reflects on the intellectual status of the child when there is evidence for global retardation whereas inappropriate or ineffective use of language might point towards a pervasive developmental disorder or psychotic illness.

Affective Behaviour

Note any evidence of anxiety, fear, depression, and shyness during the interview situation.

Attitude Towards Family, School and Playmates

An attempt must be made to enquire into how the child feels towards his/her various family members, school, studies, teachers and others. Take a note of the obvious liking or dislike for any of these.

Stated Interest and Content of Thought

Include the child's evaluation of the problems specifically referred to in the history; for example if the child is referred for scholastic backwardness, he/she should be asked what he/she thinks about it. Also explore into other disturbances of thinking like obsessions, delusions, etc.

Attention Span and Distractibility

It is the best evaluated by assigning the child some simple task like drawing, writing, etc. Evidence is also taken from his/her general activity, behaviour and ability to engage in conversation. Deficits of attention are generally apparent.

Intellectual Capacity

Clinical assessment of intelligence takes into account the developmental history and language development; and current intellectual functioning is assessed by asking certain questions of general information, calculations; judging the comprehension of commands of varying complexity.

Most of the behavioural symptoms are judged with respect to the intellectual level of the child.

Motivation

Look into the child's knowledge of the reasons for his/her attendance, desire for help and his/her sense of own capacity for change.

Mental state examination, thus, encompasses assessment of various sensory-motor, behavioural, intellectual, affective and cognitive functions.

Play Observation

Play acts as a medium of expression in children. In those children where interview is not very successful, like for example, a very young child, very shy and inhibited child, anxious or uncooperative child, observation in play setting will reveal the disturbances in various areas of functioning. The child should be left with toys in a room along with as observer. Spontaneous choice of toys; whether organized or unorganised; age appropriate or not, apparent emotional interaction; general activity level; attention span and concentration, relationship capacity, can all be observed during play. Children often indulge in role-playing with toys, assigning the roles of mother, father and sibs to various toys. The imaginary interaction between these reflects on their actual home situation. Therefore, for the assessment of all the children play observation has a complimentary role.

Children enact their stresses and concerns through play, they express their emotions and display their intellectual abilities, skills, and creativity during play sessions. Although, in large measures, play observation is non-directive but the therapist can make an attempt to engage the child in diverse activities in order to observe different mental functions and behaviours. The parent may be allowed to be with the child to start with but later on the child should be observed alone. Play observation supplements mental state examination and in many cases it is the proper setting for the examination of the child.

PSYCHOLOGICAL TESTING

Psychological tests provide objective and clinically relevant information about the psychological attributes. Although the administration and scoring of tests are technical skills but their interpretation and integration into clinical practice is more than merely a technical job. Testing is an investigative method that assists the wider process of assessment and treatment.

There are readily available sets of tests useful for common clinical problems. These include a range of intelligence tests appropriate for children of different ages; diagnostic tests used to identify broad clinical syndromes such as "brain damage", schizophrenia and the like. The choice of the tests depends upon the age of the child as well as the nature of the problem.

All the psychological tests ultimately involve the observation of behaviour, which is quantified and compared with some criterion, or what are called "norms". The commonest examples are the intelligence tests where an individual child's performance is compared with that of a group of similar children and IQ derived from such tests is simply a number, which expresses how successful the child is relative to comparable children on the same sets of tasks.

Individual tests measure various aspects of functioning or abilities and generally a group of tests is chosen. For example, some tests of intelligence require spoken answers (verbal skills), whereas others tap performance abilities. Most commonly used intelligence tests are Sequin form Broad, Gessel's drawing test, Vineland's Social Maturity Scale, Malin's Intelligence test for Indian Children, Wechsler's Intelligence test for Children. Details of psychological assessment are discussed in a separate chapter.

DIAGNOSTIC FORMULATION

The data from the clinical history, examination and investigation, is synthesized into a diagnostic whole and a suggestive differential diagnosis. Various positive and negative findings are accorded significance and interwoven into a diagnostic mesh. Care is taken to reflect on the psychosocial factors, which could be responsible for initiating or perpetuating the illness. Diagnostic formulation involves an abstract and reflective analysis of the findings and not merely a summary. It should further lead to the directions to be followed and areas to be explored; in other words, suggest a management plan.

Example: An 8-year-old child, born into a middle class, urban family, much pampered being the youngest of the sibs, presents with symptoms of school refusal, obstinacy and temper tantrums since 5 years of age. Mother is a strict disciplinarian and has high expectations from him/her whereas father is lenient and both parents often get into arguments about his/her bad behaviour and hold each other responsible for it. The child has had normal developmental milestones and there is no evidence to suggest organic brain involvement. According to the teacher's report the child is well-behaved in school, average in studies but appears a little tense and aloof. Intellectual assessment reveals an IQ of 108. On examination, the child appeared nervous, afraid of parents, insecure and looked at parents for approval before speaking or undertaking any task.

Diagnosis: Anxiety disorder: School phobia, separation anxiety.

Differential Diagnosis

Once we know that we are dealing with abnormal behaviour, the symptoms are considered to be the non-specific indicators of pathology and the efforts are to be made to understand the etiological contributors. Another caution that needs to be observed is that every behavioural symptom can occur as a direct result of an organic disease. Therefore, adequate attention should be paid to the organic aspects of the illness and a careful medical history in many cases will be sufficient to rule it out. On the other hand if there is an internal inconsistency in the history and physical findings, there is an apparent "secondary gain" to the child; temporal relationship of the symptoms with some precipitating event; apparently disturbed family relationships, one should suspect emotional disorder. Again, all these indices are relative not absolute, these are suggestive not definitive. Emotional disorders and organic illness are not mutually exclusive. These can coexist as well. In children, the emotional disorders are rooted in the family relationships involving the parents and the child or the parents with each other.

Understanding of the psychopathology in the child, would automatically suggest the plan of management. A semi-structured sample proforma for taking history and doing mental state examination is given at Appendix 1.

Neurodevelopmental Assessment

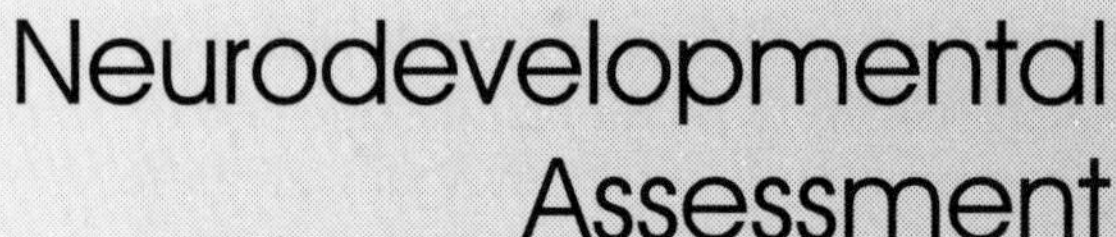

Abnormalities of brain function affect child's development in one or several areas. These difficulties become apparent very early or later during the course of development. Sensory deficits, most common of which are vision and hearing loss, leads to restriction or absence of sensory input to the brain leading to impairment of integration of several information and severe developmental difficulties. Structured and functional integrity of brain is the necessary biological condition for normal developments. Any abnormal pattern of development seen in the child will point towards the possibility of brain insult or dysfunction, which could be diffuse involving the entire brain or focal involving certain specific areas of the brain.

Impairments of development can also vary in grades or severity. More severe developmental disorders are identified early whereas less severe impairments of development often have associated problems like academic under-achievement, behavioural difficulties, cognitive deficits, social adjustment difficulties.

Assessment of neurodevelopmental status is an integral part of the psychiatric assessment of the infants and children. Neurodevelopmental assessment comprises:

1. History taking;
2. Physical examination and neuro-developmental assessment; and
3. Neuropsychological assessment.

HISTORY

General aspects of history taking apply here. Current concerns the parents have generally point towards the possibility of developmental delay. Most infants and children brought to pediatricians for routine health check, immunization, growth monitoring are examined for presence of any developmental delays. At what ages did the child acquire various milestones such as motor, social and language skills? These are evaluated in comparison to normal expected patterns of development. There may be delay in acquisition of one or more milestones or there may be evidence of loss of acquired milestones which is called as regression. Depending upon pattern of acquisition of milestone or of regression, various disorders of development can be diagnosed. Effort should be made to date the onset of regression as it has diagnostic significance.

It is important to assess the current level of functioning of the child in several areas like play, speech and language comprehension as well as expression, social and adaptive skills, gross and fine motor skills and the social behaviour. It is important to inquire into all the areas of development as there may be patchy or discrepant pattern of development where only some skills are delayed and others are normal. History of general health and illnesses is also important and should be inquired. Certain developmental disorders are associated with neurological conditions such as epilepsy, or cerebral palsy.

Family history is extremely important in this regard as several neurodegenerative disorders, which have hereditary or familial pattern, can be diagnosed early.

Social history is taken to understand the family's reactions to and coping with the presence of a handicapped child. Family's knowledge about the nature of the disorder and expectations from treatment need to be understood and accordingly modified making it more realistic and acceptable.

DEVELOPMENTAL EXAMINATIONS

Routine history and unstructured and informal observations of the child during routine well baby check often provides a rough estimate of child's level of development. Here, the clinician relies on the parental report and informal brief clinical observations. Information is obtained on child' hearing, vision, behaviors, temperament and activities. This method of informal screening is quick, practical and is generally useful for screening low-risk populations in busy clinics. However, systematic developmental screening is recommended for greater reliability of assessment. There are several structured tests or developmental screening instruments, which can be used. Detailed screening should be done for children who exhibit higher than expected risk of developmental problems due to certain biological or psychological risk factors.

Biological risk factors are: Low birth weight (<1500 g); birth asphyxia, Apgar score of 0–3 at 5 minutes; seizures, congenital abnormalities; sensory deficits such as blindness, deafness; meningitis or other chronic infections, maternal illness during prenatal period, etc. Child abuse and neglect is another major psychobiological risk factor that can hamper development.

PHYSICAL EXAMINATION

Physical examination should be done to assess:

1. Height, weight and growth rate
2. Motor problems, such as those of tone, reflexes and power
3. Hand preference
4. Head circumference
5. Vision and optic fundi
6. Hearing
7. Congenital malformations or body dysmorphic features
8. Behaviour, activity level, attention span

Findings of physical examinations generally supplement information obtained on developmental screening tests and provide clues to possible sources of pathology.

DEVELOPMENTAL SCREENING INSTRUMENTS FOR PRESCHOOL CHILDREN

Most extensively and widely used test is the Denver Developmental Screening Test (DDST) and the Revised Denver Developmental Screening Test (Frankenburg WK Thornton SM 1989) applicable to preschool children (0–6 years). Denver II (Frankenburg et al. 1990) has also been released. This test identified children with motor or cognitive deficits from any cause. A wide range of developmental tasks that can be performed by young infants and children at specific ages are looked at and evaluated for the index child's ability to pass or fail. Failure to perform developmental tasks at an age at which most other children can do it, i.e. performance below a norm indicates possibility of developmental delay and requires further in depth evaluation. These are standardized tests with well-defined guidelines for assessment and scoring; norms are provided, and are available with the publishers. DDST basically assesses the current status rather than predicting poor performance later on.

Arnold Gessel (1950) established norms for gross motor, fine motor, adaptive, language, personal–social functioning of children during their first five years of life (Tables 5.1 and 5.2).

Table 5.1: Development during the first year of life	
Neonatal period (First 4 week)	• Lies in flexed posture; turns head from side to side; head sags on lifting from body suspension • May fixate face or light in line of vision: movement of eyes on turning of the body "doll's-eye" • Grasp reflex active • Visual preference for human face
At 4 week	• Holds chin up; turns head; lifts head momentarily, head lags on pull to sitting position. Watches person; follows moving object. Begins to smile
At 8 week	• Raises head slightly farther • Follows moving objects • Smiles on social contact; listens to voice and coos
At 12 week	• Lifts head and chest, arms extended; head above place of body on ventral suspension • Reaches toward and misses objects; waves at toy • Early head control back rounded • Makes defensive movements or selective withdrawal reactions • Sustained social contact; listens to music: says "aah, ngah".
At 16 week	• Lifts head and chest, head in approximately vertical axis; legs extended • Reaches and grasps objects and brings them to mouth • No head lag on pull to sitting position; head steady, enjoys sitting with full truncal support • When held erect, pushes with feet • Laughs out loud; may show displeasure if social contact is broken; excited at sight of food
At 28 week	• Rolls over, crawls • Lifts head; rolls over; squirming movements • Sits briefly, with support of pelvis • May support most of weight while standing, bounces actively • Reaches out for and grasps large object; transfers objects from hand to hand • Polysyllabic vowel sounds formed • Prefers mother; babbles; enjoys mirror; responds to changes in emotional content of social contact
At 40 week	• Sits up alone without support • Pulls to standing position, walks holding on to furniture • Crawls • Grasps objects with thumb and forefinger; pokes at things with forefinger • Repetitive consonant: sounds (mama, dada) • Responds to sound of name; plays peek-a-boo or pat-a-cake; waves bye-bye.
At 52 week (1 year)	• Walks with one hand held (48 wk); rises independently, takes several steps • Picks up pellet with unassisted pincer movement of forefinger and thumb; releases object to other person on request or gesture • A few words besides mama, dada • Plays simple ball game; makes postural adjustment to dressing These have formed the basis for several other scales or modifications for screening of preschool children for developmental delays, (Knobloch and Pasamanick 1974), and revised developmental screening inventory (Knobloch, Stevens and Malone 1980).

Table 5.2: Development from 1 to 5 years of age	
15 months	• Walks alone; crawls up stairs • Makes tower of 3 cubes; makes a line with crayon • Follows simple commands; may name a familiar object (ball) • Indicates some needs by pointing; hugs parents
18 months	• Runs stiffly; sits on small chair; walks up stairs with one hand held; explores • Makes a tower of 4 cubes • Speaks about 10 words; names pictures; identifies parts of body • Feeds self; seeks help when in trouble; may complain when wet or soiled; kisses parent with pucker. • Handles spoon, helps to undress; listens to stories with pictures
30 months	• Goes up stairs alternating feet • Tower of 9 cubes • Refers to self by pronoun "I"; knows full name • Pretends in play • Rides tricycle; stands momentarily on one foot • Tower of 10 cubes; imitates construction of "bridge" of 3 cubes; copies a circle; imitates a cross • Knows age and sex; counts 3 objects correctly; repeats a sentence of 6 syllables • Plays simple games (in "parallel" with other children); helps in dressing (unbuttons clothing and puts on shoes); washes hands
48 months	• Hops on one foot; throws ball overhand, uses scissors to cut out pictures, climbs well • Copies cross and square; draws a man with 2 to 4 parts besides head • Counts, tells a story • Plays with several children with beginning of social interaction and role-playing; goes to toilet alone • Skips • Draws triangle from copy; names heavier of 2 weights • Names 4 colours; repeats sentence of 10 syllables; counts up to 10 • Dresses and undresses; asks meanings of words; role-playing.

Table 5.2 provides the developmental norms on Gesell and revised by Knobloch.

These have formed the basis for several other scales or modifications for screening of preschool children for developmental delays, (Knobloch and Pasamanick 1974); and Revised Developmental Screening Inventory (Knobloch, Stevens and Malone 1980). The following table provides the developmental norms based on Gessel and revised by Knobloch.

DEVELOPMENTAL ASSESSMENT OF SCHOOL AGE AND OLDER CHILDREN

As the child grows, developmental functions become more complex and fall in the broad domains of motor skills (gross motor, fine motor, and hand writing); language and communication (receptive, expressive, usage); visuospatial and perceptual skills; sequential concepts; problem-solving reasoning and moral development and social skills. The following Table 5.3 gives levels of developmental attainment at different ages. Developmental difficulties may manifest in several general areas of functioning particularly:

1. Academic performance
2. Social interactions and peer relationships
3. Family interactions
4. Extracurricular interests
5. Self-esteem.

Table 5.3: Agewise developmental attainment				
Category	**5–6 years old**	**7–9 years old**	**10–12 years old**	**13+ years old**
Gross motor skills	Hops on one foot; can walk on heels or toes	Secure balance during stressed gaits; begins to learn complex motor tasks' sports	Involvement with sports increases; good eye-hand coordination; more strength	Much increased strength, endurance, coordination
Fine motor skills	Pencil grasp becomes sure; capital letter formations automatic; colors neatly with crayons	Prints capital and lower case letters neatly; improved pencil control; uses tools awkwardly	Cursive writing becomes automatic; works well with tools and implements; can do complex crafts, mechanical, or art projects	Writes or types with ease; can work with small parts and tools, build difficult models; increased refinement of crafts, artwork
Sequential concepts	Remembers four digits or objects in sequence; knows past and future future tenses; knows alphabet, days of week in order; counts to >20	Remembers five digits or objects in sequence; uses before and after correctly; counts backward 20–1; knows days of week backward; tells time to the minute on analogue clock	Remembers six digits or objects in sequence; knows months of year; can alphabetize automatically to use telephone book, dictionary, card catalogue	Remembers six to seven digits or objects in sequence performs multi-step tasks or problems; writes organized essay with appropriate introduction, development, and conclusion.
Receptive language skills	Understands "where", "when", "why" questions	Understand passive verb forms ('the car was hit by the train")	Understands multiple meanings of words; knows meaning of figurative language (simile, metaphor, parody, analogy)	Understands linguistic explanations of abstract concepts; appreciates "deep structure" humor ("Call me a cab", "Okay", "you're a cab")
Expressive language skills	Sentences average six words in length, uses noun plurals and possessives, narrative has cause–effect sequence	Uses temporal prepositions ("before, "after"), uses past and future tenses; narrative has proper sequence, development and resolution	Changes style of language to fit several contexts (formal versus informal) and listeners (peers versus principal or parent)	Complex sentence structure: Uses idiomatic language; can speak and write about abstract concepts
Visuospatial and perceptual skills	Matches identical shapes or figures; copies Discriminates left versus right consistently	No reversals of a, b and d persist; copies Sight word vocabulary increases	Attempts three-dimensional shapes in artwork; copies complex figure Begins to understand maps, geography; good sight word vocabulary	Understands architectural plans, complex spatial relationships; artwork matures; uses and creates maps, schematic drawings of circuits, concepts, relationships.

Contd.

Table 5.3: Agewise developmental attainment				
Category	**5–6 years old**	**7–9 years old**	**10–12 years old**	**13+ years old**
Problem solving, reasoning, moral development	Compares lengths, sizes; simple, concrete problem solving; turns to adults for answers	Compares volumes, begins to reason, attempts simple conceptual problems; limited capacity for empathy; right and wrong defined in terms of punishment; interest in rules of complex games	Abstract reasoning skills developing; begins to attempt varied problem solving strategies; can solve two-step abstract problems; can empathize (imagine what others feel); understands rules of complex games and can anticipate action (chess, sports)	Flexible, abstract reasoning skills fully developed: understands and discusses concepts (liberty, justice, freedom) and ideals (utopias); right and wrong defined in terms of impact on individuals and society
Social skills	Cooperative group play, simple games; limited verbal interaction	Plays in same-sex pairs or groups; uses social conventions ("please", "thank you"), identifies him or her-self on telephone (automatically)	Group activities focus on areas of competence or common social interest; usually plays in pairs or groups of same sex	Interactions involve intense exploration of feelings with friends; social activities more adultlike (sports, shopping, going to events); peer approval important; early interest in sexual relation-ships emerges.

Busch (1992), Developmental assessment of children of school age and adolescents, pp 624–632.

Academic Performance

This is one of the most frequent and significant problem reported by children with developmental delays. It may manifest as:

- Poor academic grades
- Slowness and inability to complete work in the class and at home
- Dislike for school and school refusal
- Poor reading, writing, mathematics
- Inattentiveness, impulsiveness, carelessness
- Poor memory, poor concentration
- Untidy, messiness in work
- Disinterest in studies

Neurodevelopmental functions involved in academic skills are listed below and should be tested in detail. These are:

- *Attention:* Inattention, impulsivity, distractibility and restlessness are common neurodevelopmental dysfunctions.
- *Memory:* There may be problems with registration, short-term memory, consolidation of long-term memory or active working memory.
- *Language:* Language difficulties such as problems of fluency, vocabulary, discrimination of sounds, syntax and active listening are very common.
- *Neuromotor function:* Poor motor coordination, poor drawing and handwriting may occur as a result of neuromotor dysfunction.
- *Visual–spatial ordering:* Children with visuo–spatial deficiencies may have

difficulties with recognition of letters, configuration of words, problems in discriminating between right and left or motor clumsiness.

- *Temporal sequential ordering:* Children with difficulties in temporosequential ordering may have problems in following multistep commands, organize material or narrative, sequencing of steps in order. Such children also have difficulties in adhering to time schedules.

- *Higher order cognition:* This function consists of high level of thinking skills including concept formation, problem solving, critical thinking, brainstorming, creativity and metacognition. All these are highly complex and abstract abilities, which are involved more and more in intellectual and academic tasks with growing age.

- *Social cognition:* Several social skills such as ability to form new relationships, sensitivity to social needs and cues, maintaining effective social interaction, resolution of social conflict without aggression, social reciprocity, effective use of language and communication, sharing and negotiation comprise what is termed as social cognition.

All these academic skills directly affect a child's language, reading, writing, spelling and arithmetic abilities. These dysfunctions can occur in varying degrees of severity and combinations and are generally grouped under the broad category of specific developmental disorders of scholastic skills (involving reading, spelling, arithmetic and mixed disorders) and disorders of speech and language (speech articulation disorder, expressive and receptive language disorder, acquired aphasia and other mixed disorders). There is delay or impairment in acquisition of these skills due to abnormalities in biological maturation and cognitive processing rather than due to other disorders (such as mental retardation, visual or hearing impairment, gross neurological disorder) or due to lack of opportunity for learning and education (as in children with no formal education or those with poor teaching facilities).

Specific reading disorder manifests as slowness in reading; omission, substitution, distortion of words or parts of words; inaccurate phrasing; reversal of words, inability to draw inference from the material read. There may be specific spelling disorders. In disorder of arithmetic skills, the child is unable to understand the concept underlying arithmetical operations; fails to understand mathematical symbols for numerical symbols; finds it difficult to align members, place decimal points; may be unable to learn tables satisfactorily.

Disorders of speech and language are very common and may manifest as misarticulation of speech, omission, substitution or distortion of words in speech. They may fail to respond to familiar names or follow simple verbal instruction, or fail to understand the tone of voice and gestures.

Apart from impairments of academic skills, there may be specific developmental disorder of motor function characterized by motor clumsiness, delay in development of motor milestones; awkward gait; slowness in running, hopping or climbing stairs; inability to tie shoe laces, fasten or unfasten buttons, tendency to drop things, unable to throw and catch bells; poor drawing and poor hand writing, etc. On examination, such children are likely to exhibit 'soft' neurological signs.

Non-academic impact of neuro-developmental dysfunction occurs in wide ranging behavioral/emotional domains. They may have maladjusted behaviour, aggressive or disruptiveness in class, poor peer relationships, problems of discipline, difficulties in accepting rules and behavioural limits, and highly provocative behaviour. Some children exhibit excessive anxiety, social phobia, high performance anxiety, depression, low self-esteem, low motivation, disinterest and even suicidality.

There are several standardized instruments for neuropsychological/neurodevelopmental assessment which can be used by pediatricians, i.e. pediatric early elementary examination (PEEX); pediatric examination of educational readiness at middle childhood (PEERAMAID); pediatric evaluation of educational readiness (PEER); pediatric extended examination at three (PEET). There are also tests by psychiatrists, psychologists such as goodenough harris drawing test, peabody picture vocabulary tests (PPVT); Wechsler intelligence scales for children-revised (WISC-R); stanford binet test and other standard tests of IQ assessment. Psychological tests to assess the neuro-cognitive and neurodevelopmental tests are described in the succeeding chapter in this book (chapter 6).

Evaluation is generally multidisciplinary. Data obtained from several sources of information and examination is collated to obtain a profile of child's level of development in comparison with the standard norm expected for that age. Depending upon the predominant area of dysfunctions a diagnosis is put forward. Simultaneously, hypotheses about the etiology of dysfunction are considered to complete the diagnosis as well as to prepare a management plan. Attention is paid to child's assets or area of strength as much as to areas of dysfunction.

Management does involve strengthening of the area of strength as also to use these in remediation. Parents are given feedback and understanding of the child's strengths and weaknesses in a descriptive manner. The child also should be given the information about his problems. Often the child perceives his/her problems as more severe than what it actually is. Child should be made to accept and understand his role and contribution in the total treatment. Treatment requires active participation of the child, the parents, teacher, pediatricians and specialists where child is as much responsible for resolving his/her problems as others. Details of management and specific interventions for

neurodevelopmental disorders is given in the chapter on Management in this book.

Specific disorders of learning and neurodevelopment, pervasive developmental disorders, mental retardation and ADHD are the most common neurodevelopmental disorders of childhood seen in psychiatric clinics. These can occur in the background of a known neurological condition like tuberous sclerosis, cerebral palsy, fragile X syndrome, neurodegenerative disorders, epilepsy and so on. Full neurological assessment is mandatory in all such cases.

BIBLIOGRAPHY

1. Blackman JA. Developmental screening of infants, toddlers and preschoolers. In Levine MB, Cary WB, Crocker AC (eds). Developmental and Behavioural Paediatrics. IInd Edition WB Savnders Company. Philadelphia 1992.

2. Busch B. Developmental assessment of children of school age and adolescents. In Levine MD, Cary WB, Crocker AC (eds). Developmental–behavioural Paediatrics IInd Edition. WB Saunders Company, Philadelphia 1992; 612–24.

3. Crystal D. 1986. Listen to your child. Penguin Books, Middlesex Gesell A 1950. The first five years of life. Methuen, London. Harris, D.B., 1963. Children's drawings as measures of intellectual maturity. Harcourt, Brace and World, New York.

4. Day RE. Psychomotor and intellectual development. In Cambell AGM, Mc Intosh N (eds) Forfar and Arneil's Textbook of Pediatrics. Fourth Edition, Churchill Livingstone, Longman Group UK ltd. 1992; 447–468.

5. Frankenburg WK, Dodds J, Archer P; et al: Denver II. Denver, Denver Developmental Materials, 1990.

6. Frankenburg WK, Jhornton SM: A child development program for a busy office practice. Contemp Pediatr February: 90, 1989.

7. Knobloch H, Pasamanick B (eds): Gesell and Amatruda's Developmental Diagnosis, 3rd ed. Hagerstown, MD, Harper and Row, 1974.

8. Knobloch H, Stevens F, Malone AF: Manual of Developmental Diagnosis, Hagerstown, MD, Harper and Row, 1980.

9. Levine M. Neurodevelopmental dysfunction in school aged child. In Nelson WE, Behrman RE, Kliegmun RM, Arvim AM (eds). Nelson Textbook of Pediatrics. 15th Edition. WB Savanders Company 1996;100–108.

10. Levine MD, et al. The Pediatric Assessment System for Learning Disorder (Questionnaires and Neurodevelopmental Examinations). Cam-bridge, MA, Educators Publishing Service, 1982.

11. Levine MD. The pediatric early elementary Examination (PEEx); The Pediatric Examination of Educational Readiness (PEER AMID). Cambridge, MA, Educators Publishing Service, 1985.

12. Levine MD. Attention and memory: Progression and variation during the elementary school years. Pedaitr Ann 1989; 18:366.

Psychological Assessment of Children

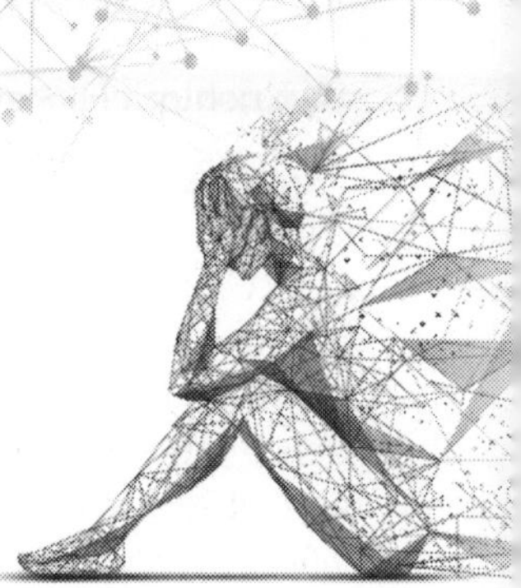

Psychological assessment refers to the observation of a sample of child behaviour or evaluation of its capacities in a wide variety of domains. This is obtained through standardized techniques which are analyzed, scored and interpreted according to well-accepted rules, finally leading to quantitative and/or qualitative description of some aspect of behaviour or mental function. In other words, psychological assessment covers both qualitative and quantitative aspects of measurement. In children and adolescents, the most important areas for assessment include intellectual ability, adaptive behaviour, visuomotor coordination, and personality and intrapsychic conflicts.

Psychological assessment is invariably an important and significant component of a comprehensive psychiatric evaluation. There are several clinical questions that are addressed to the clinical psychologist who is a part of the multidisciplinary team treating children and adolescents for a better understanding of their problems and for making appropriate treatment decisions.

Psychological testing is generally directed at the specific question that is posed to the psychologist. In the absence of such a question, it would be difficult to decide on the course of action to be adopted for a given case. The questions referred to the psychologist could be wide ranging and include: Assessment of the child's developmental level, and/or its intellectual ability; assistance in diagnosis and differential diagnosis in cases with evidence of anxiety, depression or psychosis, and understanding of psychological conflicts, particularly in situations where a child is not articulate enough in the interview setting; decision on the type and technique of psychotherapy suitable for a child; and to predict the course and outcome of therapy. As already mentioned, psychological testing can be most helpful when a clear and specific question is referred to the psychologist. Access to the clinical history of a case is essential for the psychologist in order to interpret the test findings. Many a times, after going over the clinical history of a case, the psychologist can help formulate the question for referral.

Psychometry, which is also a method of measuring mental capacities and processes is a more narrowly defined term that deals primarily with issues of technical and methodological outputs of measurement, such as reliability, validity and standardizations whereas psychological testing or assessment is a broader term that deals with clinical questions.

Assessment tests can be variously classified according to the type of functions involved and the purpose for which they are required, as also the age, education, ability levels and other sociodemographic and clinical characteristics of the sample and the population served. For convenience, these tests have been classified here according to the type of functions involved.

COGNITIVE FUNCTIONS

Cognitive functions broadly include several abilities such as intelligence, attention and concentration, memory, abstraction, judgment and perceptuomotor functions. There are separate methods for measuring each of these functions. Children differ in their abilities to learn, form concepts and benefit from past experiences, and in their capacity to adjust to novel situations. These cognitive functions are markedly affected in certain psychiatric disorders of children like learning disabilities, hyperactivity, brain damage, mental retardation, etc.

A. Tests of Intelligence

Intelligence is a global term that denotes the relative capacity of the child to think rationally, act purposefully and deal effectively with the environment (Wechsler, 1981). It grows with age up to a certain level (say 14–16 years) after which it remains more or less constant and then declines in old age. This age-related growth and decline of intelligence varies in its rate for different abilities—as also in children—it is faster for the very bright but slower for dull children. It also declines in brain damage due to certain disease conditions and accidents and does not develop fully in cases where there is cultural deprivation or lack of a stimulating environment. Intelligence is assessed and described in terms of the IQ, which is a ratio between the mental (or developmental age) and chronological age of the child. This ratio (mental age over chronological age) is multiplied by 100 to remove the fraction. There are two kinds of IQs:

a. Classical IQ (in which mental age is used and the MA/CA ratio is multiplied by 100), and

b. Deviant IQ where the means and standard deviations for each group are calculated and transformed into IQ scores with a mean of 100 and standard deviation of 15 to 16). Both the methods give some stability to the assessed IQ scores, which

sometimes vary among tests due to variations in the type of abilities assessed.

Given below are some of the commonly used intelligence tests in India. All these tests are properly standardized, published and extensively used. Details about administration, scoring and interpretation of these tests can be obtained from the test manuals which are available with the respective publishers.

a. Intelligence Tests for Infants

- Developmental screening test (Bharath Raj 1983)
- Gessel's developmental schedule (Gessell 1949; Indian adaptation by Muralidharan 1969)
- Denver developmental screening test (Frankenburg, et al. 1992; Indian adaptation by Puri et al. 1994–95)
- Gessel's drawing tests (Bakwin and Bakwin 1960; Verma et al. 1972)
- Nancy–Bayley scales (Bayley 1969; Indian adaptation by Phatak 1969)
- Vineland Social Maturity Scale (Doll 1965; Indian adaptation by Malin 1972)
- Vineland Adaptive Behaviour Scales (Sparrow et al. 1984)

b. Intelligence Tests for Children

- Bhatia's Battery of Performance Tests of intelligence (Bhatia 1955; Murthy 1966)
- Coloured Progressive Matrices (Ravens, 1965)
- Seguin Form Board Test (Indian norms by Verma et al. 1980)
- Draw-a-man scale (Indian adaptation by Phatak 1984)
- Malin's Intelligence Scale for Indian Children (Indian adaptation of WISC by Malin 1969)
- Porteus Maze Test (Porteus 1962)
- Standford-Binet Test (Indian adaptation of Kulshreshtha 1971)
- Wechesler's Intelligence Scale for Children—Revised (Wechsler 1974)
- Kaufman Assessment Battery for Children (K-ABC) (Kaufman and Kaufman 1983)

Sources

- First mental measurement handbook of India (Long and Mehta 1966)
- Handbook for psychological and social instruments (Pareek and Rao 1974; Pestonjee 1988, 1998)
- Tests in print, published periodically by the NCERT and the ICSSR, Delhi
- Firms dealing with psychological tests (see Annexure)
- National test library, NCERT, Delhi

In testing very young children, particularly below 2 years of age, the clinician would have to depend upon developmental milestones and on developmental age (DA comparable to mental age) and developmental quotient (DQ comparable to IQ). Some tests give us just one DQ, while others give two or more.

The salient features of some of the tests mentioned above are as follows:

Developmental Screening Test (DST)

Based on the developmental milestone-especially that of language and speech development – Dr J. Bharat Raj developed this scale in 1983 at the All India Institute of Speech and Hearing, Mysore. Though this is an age scale, starting from birth to 15+ years, it seems more valid for children below 10 years of age. Better tests are available for higher age groups. It gives Mental (Developmental) Age and a single IQ (DQ) score, which can be read directly from a dice provided with the manual (IQ calculator). Items vary from 3 to 7 for each age: 3, 6, 9, 12, 15 months and thereafter at 2 to 13 and 15+ years.

Gessel's Developmental Schedule (GDS)

This developmental schedule, based on the monumental work by Arnold Gessell, has been ably adapted to Indian conditions by Muralidharan in Delhi. It provides 5 scores or DQs, viz. motor, language, adaptive, personal–social DQs and finally an overall DQ. This is also an age scale and developmental milestones are grouped into these four areas for each of the selected ages, i.e. 4, 16, 28 and 40 weeks, 12, 15, 18, 21, 24, 30, 36, 42, 48, 54, 60 and 72 months. This schedule is based on the four developmental areas: motor (gross and fine motor coordination), adaptive (perceptual, orientation, manual and verbal adjustments), language (all means of communications) and personal–social (reactions to others).

Denver Development Screening Test (DDST)

This developmental screening test measures development of children between 3 and 36 months of age, in the following four areas: gross-motor, fine-motor, language and personal–social. It has been well adapted in simple Hindi for use with Indian children. It can give a DQ (Puri et al. 1995) which is found to be normally distributed and significantly correlated with the Vineland Social Maturity (VSMS), thereby demonstrating the validity extending the utility of this screening instrument.

The DDST provides a profile of milestones achieved rather than just the DQ and has been adapted in India by Puri et al. (1995) in Chandigarh.

Gessel's Drawing Test (GDT)

Gessel's studies on drawings of children by copying/imitation suggested that these geometrical shapes and forms can be used as rough, simple, and reasonably accurate measures of maturation and intelligence in children, e.g. an average child of 11 months could imitate vertical strokes, at age 2 could copy vertical and circular strokes, at age 3 could copy a circle, at age 4 a cross, etc. These geometrical shapes are available till the age of 12 (Bakwin and Bakwin 1960; Verma et al. 1972). It showed highly significant correlations with the VSMS and the Seguin Form Board Tests.

Nancy-Bayley Scales

The Nancy-Bayley Infant Scales for motor and mental development are point scales. The motor scale has 67 points and the mental scale has 163 points. The items in the two scales are distributed unevenly. The month-wise norms are for infants up to 15 days, 16 days to 1 month, 2 to 30 months (with age placement of the items 50 percent is pass percentage). It has been found that Indian babies tended to perform about 50 percent of the motor items and about 35 percent of the mental items earlier than the American babies in Dr. Bayley's sample. There are separate DQs for motor and mental development but if a single DQ is required, it can be obtained by getting a mean of DQs for motor and mental development.

Vineland Social Maturity Scale (VSMS)

This scale consists of 89 items, arranged in age scales from birth to age 12 at yearly intervals and then from ages 12 to 15. The number of items vary widely (between 3 and 17) across the ages, being highest during ages 0 to 1 and 1 to 2 (1 each) followed by ages 2 to 3 (10 items) and lowest at ages 9 to 10 and 11 to 12 if we ignore the 5 items in the age group 12 to 15. The items mostly cover social milestones, hence the obtained age is called social age (SA) and the quotient as social quotient (SQ) to differentiate it from MA and IQ. The scale was adapted in Nagpur, India by Malin (1972) and gives a developmental profile in different areas like self-help in general; self-help at eating; self-help at dressing, self-direction, communication, locomotion, occupation, and socialization. Information on specific deficiencies in the scale is also available (Doll 1965).

Vineland Adaptive Behaviour Scales (VABS)

This is a revision of the Vineland Social Maturity Scale. It is a semi-structured inter-view assessing psychological functioning in the four domains of communication, daily living skills, socialization, and motor skills applicable to children and adolescents from 0 to 19 years of age. Separate norms are available for normal, mentally retarded,

visually handicapped and emotionally disturbed children. The test is available in three forms: The survey form, expanded form, and the classroom edition. The survey form is generally sufficient for most of the clinical work. So far, it has not been adapted in India.

Bhatia's Battery of Performance Tests of Intelligence (BBPT)

This test is mainly meant for children between the ages of 11 and 16 and consists of 5 subtests: Block design, pass along, pattern drawing, digit span (letter span for illiterates) and picture construction. The first two subtests are borrowed from Alexanders battery of performance tests (Koh's block design and Alexander's pass-along test). Immediate memory for digits, pattern drawing and picture constructions are devised by the author. Separate norms are available for literate and illiterate children. Age-wise norms (at 6 monthly intervals) are provided. For calculating IQs, all the 5 subtests have to be used and norms are given separately for literates and illiterate population. For calculating PQs, only 4 subtests (excluding digit span) are used. Raw scores are first converted into weighted scores, which when added can be read from the accompanying tables but are only available for the literate groups. A shorter version of the scale is available where only the first two subtests (Block Design and Pass-along) are used. Raw scores are multiplied by 2.5 for IQ conversions and weighted scores are doubled to convert them into PQ scores (Murthy, 1966).

Coloured Progressive Matrices (CPM)

This test measures the clarity of perception and thinking in children and consists of the general factor ('g') of intelligence and is "culturally fair". It can be used with people who, for any reason, cannot understand or speak the English language, with people suffering from physical disabilities, aphasias, cerebral palsy or deafness. The

CPM has 36 items which are arranged in 3 sets, of A, AB and B. Each set progresses from the easiest to most difficult tasks: For completion, comparison and reasoning by analogy. It is a non-verbal, non-performance test of intelligence, and has no time limit. It can be self-administered and also be group administered. Norms are provided for children of 5½ to 11 years of age. The scores can be converted into comparable scores of the larger 5 set version-standard progressive matrices (60-item adult scale) that has IQ equivalents (Burke, 1972).

Standard Progressive Matrices (SPM)

This can be administered on children in the age range of 12 to 15 years to assess intellectual functions. It measures educative ability which is the ability to forge new insights to perceive and identify relationships. It consists of 60 problems divided into five sets (A, B, C, D, E) where each build on the argument of the previous one and become progressively difficult. Number of correct responses in all five sets constitutes the core for SPM (Raven, Raven and Court 2000).

Seguin Form Board Test (SFB Test)

This performance test of practical ability consists of 10 blocks of geometrical shapes, which have to be inserted into their respective slots in the board, with the preferred hand. The test has a time limit. Norms start with children who are 3½ years of age and as the child grows older, time taken for completing the test decreases, i.e. from 45 seconds, the shortest time for three trials by a 3½ years old to about 10 seconds by normal adults. From the conversion table one can calculate the mental age of the child, which then can be converted into classical IQ. It is an age scale and a reliable and valid test for children up to 11 years of age, although norms are also given for higher age group.

Draw-a-Man Scale (DAM Scale)

Goodenough's Draw-a-Man technique has been adapted well in India by Phatak (1984) in Baroda providing age-wise norms for children between the ages of 2½ and 16. It is an age scale with no time limit. The instructions are easy to follow and scoring is based on points for different body parts, their correct proportions, motor coordination, dress, action, etc. Although its variations like draw-a-cow, draw-a-cycle or draw-an-elephant test, etc. are also available, and described in the literature, the Draw-a-Man test is the most popular and frequently used in India (Verma 1996).

Malin's Intelligence Scale for Indian Children (MISIC)

This is an Indian adaptation of Wechsler's Intelligence Scale for Indian children by late Dr. A.J. Malin from Nagpur. It has 11 scales: 6 verbal and 5 performance scales (information, comprehension, arithmetic, similarities, vocabulary and digit span for verbal and picture completion, block design, object assembly, codes and mazes for performance scales). Norms are provided for children of 6 to 15 years of age. Each of the 11 subtests can be directly converted into what Malin describes as Test Quotients, whereas the IQ is a mean of these. This is unlike the original test where each raw score is first converted into a weighted score which is then combined to give the verbal, performance and total (mean of VQ and PQ) IQ scores.

Porteus Maze Test (PMT)

Porteus has, in his work of over 50 years, reported on the use of his mazes as a reliable and valid test of intelligence aged from 3-year-olds to adults. The mazes are designed for ages 3 to 12 at yearly intervals and then for 14-year-olds and adults. Full credit is given to the subject for success at the first attempt and half credit for later successive attempts. This is also an age scale with no time limit.

Stanford-Binet Test (S-B Test)

There are a number of revisions of the Binet-Simon Test, its third revision has been translated into Hindi by Kulshreshtha (1971) and is the most frequently used test in the Hindi speaking belt of North India. This age scale starts with 2-year olds and goes up to adults with a mixture of items at each age level. An overall IQ is calculated that is based on the mental age (basal age is where all items included under it are passed, terminal age is where all items are failed, and credits are given for some items that are passed between these two extremes). In the latest edition of the test age adjustment has been provided.

Wechsler Intelligence Scale for Children–Revised (WISC-R)

This is a comprehensive test of intelligence applicable to children from 6 to 16 years of age, that gives separate scores for verbal and performance IQ tests, as well as full scale IQ. There are 12 subtests, each of which measures a specific skill or ability. Verbal tests are information, similarities, arithmetic, comprehension and digit recall. Performance tests are picture completion, picture arrangement, block design, object assembly and coding. This is the most widely used and extensively researched test. Intelligence defined as the broad ability to understand and cope with the world forms the basis for this test.

Kaufman's Assessment Battery for Children

This is a relatively new test that measures cognitive abilities in children aged 2½ and 12½ years. The two broad domains of achievement and mental processing are measured through the Achievement Scale and Mental Processing Scale. These have 10 subtests, which provide a profile of abilities. The Mental Processing Scale is equivalent to the WISC-R's full scale IQ and the Achievement Scales tests measure acquired knowledge in a child. If a child scores high in the mental processing scale, it would indicate a high intellectual capacity, which if coupled with lower score in the Achievement Scale will point towards the possibility of a specific learning disability.

Most of the developmental schedules that we have just examined are age, scales and can be easily converted into development quotients.

The following brief IQ tests can be conducted by any general practitioner/paediatrician/psychologist for a quick assessment of a child's intelligence.

a. Ask the child to show/point his body parts one by one (DA = 2½ years).
b. Ask the child to pick/identify common objects placed before him (key, coin, pencil, spoon, match box, scissors, etc.) (DA = 3 years).
c. Ask the child to pick-up things according to their use (DA = 4 years).
d. Place pencils or other objects of primary colours (red, green, yellow, blue, black and white) before the child and ask him to point the colours by name (all 6 correct answers would mean a DA = 6 years; 5 correct answers = 5 years and 4 correct answers = 4 years).
e. Put a blank sheet of paper before the child and give him a pencil. Draw a circle slowly on the paper and ask the child to copy it (successful = DA = 3 years). Draw

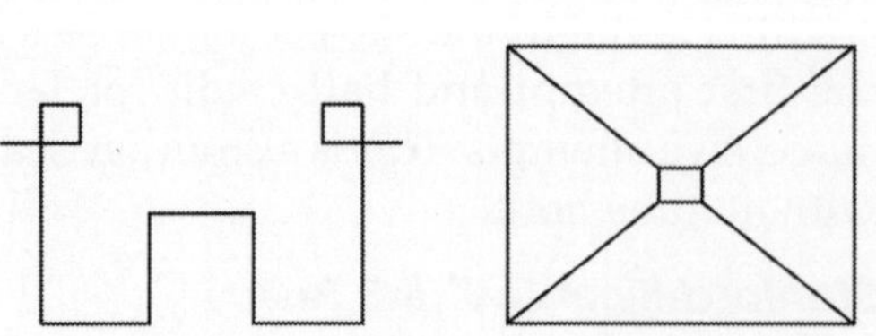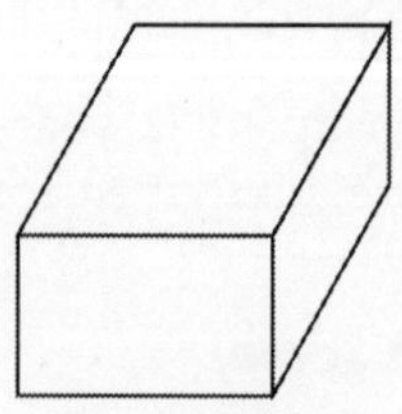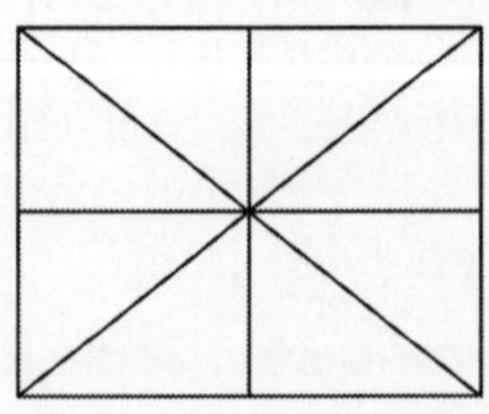

Fig. 6.1: DA = 8 years and above

and ask the child to copy a cross (DA = 4 years), square (DA = 5 years), triangle (DA= 6 years) and a diamond (DA= 7 years). If the child can draw the following figures shown below, his DA would be 8 years and above.

If the mental or developmental age of a child is more than 8 years, there is little sense in continuing with this test, as better, more reliable and valid tests are available, which may be time consuming but are worthwhile due to greater accuracy and precision in their results.

A brief list of IQ tests commonly used and available in India is given Table 6.1 below:

Table 6.1: Commonly used IQ tests in India		
Test name	**Age**	**type**
Seguin Form Board	3–16 years	Performance test
Binet-Kamath Test of Intelligence	3 years to adulthood	Age scale; Predominantly verbal
Stanford-Binet Intelligence Scale	3 years- adulthood	Age scale; Predominantly verbal
Malin's Intelligence Scale for Indian Children	6–16 years	Has verbal and performance tests
Developmental Screening Test	0–15	Developmental tasks
Vineland Social Maturity Scale	0–15	Social Quotient
Progressive matrices a. Standard b. Coloured	11 years to adults 5 to 11 years	Non-verbal and non-speed
Gessel's Drawing Test	18 months to 8 years	Performance test
Bhatias's Battery of performance Test of intelligence	11 years and above	Performance test
Wechsler intelligence scale for children- fourth edition (India)	6–16 years 11 months	Contains both verbal and performance scales

Most of these tests are commercially available from firms dealing with psychological tests like the Manasayan, Psycho-centre, Rupa Psychological Centre, National Psychological Corporation, Agra Psychological Research Cell, etc. (A list of these firms is given in Annexure.) In a classified list of tests, the National Council of Educational Research and Training (NCERT), Delhi, has included both Indian and foreign tests along with critical evaluations. The NCERT has also established a National Test Library, which is open for consultation and includes a large number of tests, e.g. the Draw-a-Cow Test, Draw-a-Bicycle Test, Knox Cube Imitation Test, and many other (group) verbal intelligence tests.

B. Evaluation of Cognitive Functions

Another important area of psychological assessment in children involves evaluation of cognitive functions.

The measurement of cognitive functions usually serves the following five functions:

1. For assessing cognitive deficits which help in psychiatric diagnosis and in assessing the type and degree of organic damage.

2. For making rehabilitative plans, identifying areas of damaged and intact cognitive functions.

3. For providing cognitive retraining and other correctional procedures, e.g. in hyperactive, brain damaged children and children with learning disabilities.

4. For evaluation and comparisons of various therapies.

5. For assessing improvements over time and the rate of improvement with and/ or without treatment.

Cognitive functions include cortical/ lobar functions, attention and concentration, memory, judgement and abstraction, and intelligence. Several test batteries are available to assess these functions. Specific tests to assess neuropsychological functions are described below:

1. A full-length neuropsychological battery for children was developed by Bhoomika R Kar et al. 2004 at NIMHANS Bangalore with the aim:

    i. To aid in the detection of brain dysfunction for the purpose of differential diagnosis.

    ii. To provide a precise specification of the behavioural effects of known brain injury.

    iii. To help in identification of specific underlying dimensions of dysfunction in particular handicaps.

    iv. To use assessment data for formulating effective strategies and

    v. To assess the child's prognosis and risk for certain developmental outcomes.

2. NIMHANS Neuropsychological Battery for children has been developed giving due consideration to the developmental perspective of brain functions. This battery is standardized in the age range of 5 to 15 years (age range varies for different subtests).

3. Lobe functions: Reliability and validity of the Battery: All the tests showed significant test-retest reliability co-efficient suggestive of temporal stability in scores. The test-retest reliability coefficients of the various tests ranged from 0.53 to 0.92 that reveals a fairly good test-retest reliability of the battery. The battery was found sensitive in terms of localization and lateralization of brain dysfunction.

Different neuropsychological functions assessed and the tests used to assess them are given in Table 6.2. The localization of the brain functions to the major lobar region is also depicted in the Table 6.2.

Table 6.2 Neuropsychological functions and related tests for assessment

Lobes	Functions		Tests
Frontal lobe	Motor functions		
	Motor speed		Finger tapping test (Reitan 1970)
	Motor coordination		Hand tapping (Luria 1966)
	Attention		
	Sustained attention		Colour cancellation test (Kapur 1974)
	Focused attention		Colour, trails test, trail A and B (D'Elia, Sat, Uchiyama and White 1996)
	Clinical rating	Arousability	Clinical observation
		Distractibility	
		Fatiguability	
	Expressive speech	Repetitive speech	Repeating sounds, repeating words
		Nominative speech	Categorical naming, object naming
		Narrative speech	Sentence construction (Luria 1973)
	Executive functions	Verbal fluency	Phonemic Fluency (Lezak 1995)
		Design fluency	Design fluency (Jones-Gotman and Milner 1977)
		Verbal working memory	N-back test-verbal (Smith and Jonides 1995)

Contd.

Table 6.2 Neuropsychological functions and related tests for assessment			
Lobes	**Functions**		**Tests**
		Visuospatial working memory	N-back test-visual (Smith and Jonides 1995)
		Planning	Porteus Maze test (Porteus 1965)
		Self-shifting	Wisconsin Card Sorting Test (Heaton, Chelune, Talley, Kay and Curtis 1993)
		Motivation	Clinical observation
		Behaviour change	Clinical rating
			Parental interview
Parietal lobe		Visuo-perceptual ability	Motor-free visual perception test (Collarusso and Hammill 1972)
		Visuo-conceptual ability	Picture completion (Malin 1969)
		Visuo-constructive ability	Block Design (Malin 1969)
		Visual recognition	Recognition: Pictured objects (Lezak 1995)
		Apraxia	Symbolic and sequential acts (Lazek 1995)
	Somatosensory perception	Tactile finger localization	Finger Localization (Boll 1974)
		Tactile form perception	Tactile form perception (Lezak 1995)
		Reading	Reading a passage
			Reading comprehension
		Writing	Writing to dictation, copying
		Calculation	Age appropriate sums
Temporal lobe		Verbal comprehension	Token test (De Renzi and Vignolo 1562
		Verbal learning and memory	Rey's Auditory Verbal Learning Test (Maj et al 1993)
		Visual learning and memory	Memory for designs (Jones–Gotman and Milner 1986)

C. Attention and Concentration

Tests to measure levels of attention and concentration in a child include a variety of tasks.

a. The Digit Span Test

This is the most frequently used test for assessing attention and concentration in children. It assess their ability to repeat the maximum number of digits of a set of numbers after its single presentation plus the maximum number of digits repeated backward after its single presentation. As the age of the individual tested advances, the total number of digits forward and backward increases. Digits may be substituted by alphabets for rural children, with no formal education.

b. Eysenck's Digit Test of Concentration

It consists of repeating in the same order the last four digits of the eight series of varying number of digits presented—one score is given for each correct response in its proper place. The maximum score is 32.

c. *Colour Cancellation Test*

From a standard page of numerous dots of varying colours, the child is asked to cancel two specific colours. The score is calculated by the maximum number of correctly cancelled colours minus the incorrect ones. Colour Cancellation Test has been adapted in India (Kapur 1974). The test measures attention, concentration and impulsivity. The test consists of a sheet with 150 coloured dots—red, blue, yellow, black and grey equidistant from each other, each occurring randomly 30 times. The child is asked to cross all the dots in black colour with pencil as far as he can (simple colour cancellation); or cancel all yellow and red dots within the time limit of one minute (complex colour cancellation task). Variations of this test can include picture cancellation, letter cancellation, number cancellation or symbol cancellation.

d. *Symbol Substitution Test*

In this test, each digit is assigned a different symbol. After a practice session with a limited set of numbers, the child is asked to substitute symbols with numbers in a fixed time period, say 60 seconds. The scoring is done in the same manner as in the colour cancellation test.

e. *Simple Additions or Subtractions*

In a limited period of time, a maximum number of sums, simple additions or, subtractions a child can do would be its concentration score.

f. *Knox-Cube Limitation Test*

It consists of five cubes; four are placed in a straight line and one is used either by the examiner or, the subject. The examiner touches the four cubes in a certain order, which the subject is asked to repeat. Each of the correct series constitutes one score. The maximum score is 12 (Catell 1946).

All these are structured by relatively unstandardized tests and norms are only available for the first few. Some of them are also used as intelligence tests. These are mentioned in some of the books on psychological tests but not in much detail (Catell 1946). They are used as subjective measures, depending upon one's experience.

D. Tests of Physical and Mental Alertness or Retardation

Children differ in their psychological and motor activities. Some are quick, alert and fast while others are hesitant and slow, particularly those with emotional or behavioural problems showing psychomotor retardation. In addition to the observation of behaviour, which is rated during psychiatric interviews or while testing is done, there are some structured tests, which are used but rated by one's own subjective experience. Some of these tests are as follows:

a. *Minnesota Rate of Block Reversal Test*

It consists of a board with some blocks which are red in colour on one side and blue on the other. The required task is to reverse all the coloured blocks in the shortest possible time. It usually takes about a minute and is a very simple and easy test.

b. *Pencil Tapping Test*

The scoring in this test is based on the number of pencil taps by a child on a standard sheet of paper, within the standard time of 30 seconds. The subject is asked to tap as quickly as possible.

c. *Reaction Time*

Simple reaction time should be noted while administering any test. Alternatively, an apparatus is available to measure simple, discriminant reaction time. Though gross retardation is visible to the naked eye, is milder form and the degree of retardation can only be measured with the help of these psychological tests. (Since the test is used as comparison across time and within group, norms are not required and are not available.) Usually, comparisons across time (before and after) and group comparisons (chi-square or t-tests) do not require norms, hence agewise norms are not available.

E. Memory

In children, memory is tested as part of intelligence, tests for some memory functions like the immediate memory span (digit span test), memory for words, sentences, stories, etc. form part of intelligence tests like the Standord Binet Test, Malin's Intelligence Scale for Indian children and Bhatia's Battery for Performance Test of intelligence. The norms for these subtests are sometimes used to assess memory functions in children, e.g. memory for recent events, remote events, mental control, memory for new associations, recognizing sentences and words, etc. These are also used with adolescents. However, there is need for development of specific tests for memory in children. Assessment of various processes involved in memory functions such as attention, concentration, registration, retention, recall of various types of information involving varied inputs like auditory, visual, perceptuomotor, etc. will help considerably in understanding the deficits occurring in information processing and specific learning disabilities. Variations in ability to memorize different types of information will help in neuropsychological assessment.

There are few published tests to specifically and comprehensively measure memory functions in children.

1. PGI Memory Scale for Children

This is a simple clinical test in Hindi comprising of 10 subtests, *viz.* remote memory, recent memory, mental balance, attention and concentration, delayed recall, immediate recall, retention for similar pairs, retention for dissimilar pairs, visual retention and recognition of common objects. The authors have reported test-retest reliability after one month as 0.82 (Kohli et al. 1998). The scale is applicable to children aged 7 to 12.

2. Memory Test for Children (Barna Das IP, Kapur M, Uma H, Sinha UK, (2006)

This is a battery of 12 subtests assessing memory of children in the 7–11 age group. 12 subtests are:

1. Personal information;
2. Mental control;
3. Sentence repetition;
4. Logical memory;
5. Word recall-meaningful;
6. Digit span;
    a. Digit forward;
    b. Digit backward;
7. Word recall—nonmeaningful;
8. Delayed response learning;
9. Picture recall;
10. Benton visual retention test (BVRT);
11. Paired associate learning;
12. *Catell's retentivity test:* Test retest reliability varies between 0.51 and 0.97 for different subtests and validity ranges between 0.27 and 0.78. Complete test battery is given in the source book, under reference.

F. Tests for Perceptuomotor Functions

Children with brain damage often show disturbances of perceptuomotor functions for which the Bender-Gestalt Test is frequently used. The test provides nine cards with geometrical designs. The child is asked to copy these designs from the cards. Norms are available for children from several sources (Bender 1938; Bhargava and Sandhu 1987; Koppitz 1964; Dwivedi 1987). The tests are also used to find out if a child is ready for school and to assess learning disturbances (Koppitz 1964). Another test that is commonly used for assessment of the perceptuomotor functions is the Benton Visual Retention Test (Benton 1974). The test consists of 10 cards with geometrical designs which are shown to children aged 8 or above for 10 seconds, after which they are asked to draw the design from memory. Scoring is done on the basis of number of errors committed.

G. Tests for Abstraction, Judgement, Thought Disorder and other Related Concepts

The capacity for abstract thinking and judgement is reported to be impaired in certain groups of psychiatric disorders in children. These disorders lead to concrete thinking in some children which may be attributed to a faulty filtering mechanism in the brain, and in others it may be a case of over generalization. Many of these tests which focus on interpretation of proverbs, as also identification of similarities and absurdities in pictures and statements have already been mentioned like the Standford-Binet Test, MISIC, and the WISC-R. Since intelligence is often associated with the capacity for abstract thinking, some of these tests which focus on it form a subpart of many intelligence tests.

PERSONALITY

Personality is broadly and operationally defined as all those distinctive characteristics that help in predicting what a given person would do, in a given mood and situation. For the sake of convenience, we have presently defined personality in a limited sense to only include non-cognitive functions, as cognitive functions and their measurements in children have already been described earlier in this chapter. The instruments for personality testing can be broadly grouped into:

a. Personality questionnaires/inventories/rating scales and interview schedules and

b. Projective techniques.

(a) Personality Questionnaires

Some of the personality questionnaires that have been developed for children in India are as follows. A brief description is provided of some of these questionnaires.

- Temperament Measurement Schedule (Malhotra and Malhotra 1988)
- Thakur's Death Anxiety Scale (Thakur and Thakur 1984)
- Learned Helplessness Scale (Dhar et al. 1987)
- Sarason's General Anxiety Scale for Children—GASC (Nijhawan 1971)
- Sarason's Test Anxiety Scale for Children—TASC (Nijhawan 1971)
- Preadolescent Adjustment Inventory (PAS) (Pareek et al. 1976)
- Self-esteem Inventory
- Children's Personality Questionnaire
- Developmental Psychopathology Checklist (Kapur et al. 1995)
- Reporting Questionnaire for Children (Giel et al. 1981).

Since it is not possible to provide descriptions of all available personality questionnaires, only a few are described here. A comprehensive listing with details may require another book rather than a chapter.

Temperament Measurement Schedule (TMS)

Following "Thomas and Chess" (1977) New York Longitudinal Study, Malhotra and Malhotra (1988) developed a 45-item scale for Indian children. The scale is available both in Hindi and in English and is for children of 4 to 14 years of age. Scoring is done for factors such as rythmicity, approach withdrawal, attention span, activity, adaptability, mood, intensity, distractibility and persistence with 5 items each being rated on a 5-point scale. Through factor analysis the questionnaire isolates the five factors of sociability, emotionality, energy, attentivity and rhythmicity. Details have been given in the subsequent chapter on structured assessment and some Indian scales.

Thakur's Death Anxiety Scale (TDAS)

It is a simple questionnaire in Hindi to measure anxiety about death (Thakur and

Thakur 1984). The scale is reported to have high reliability and validity in measuring this form of anxiety in Indian children.

Learned Helplessness Scale (LHS)

This is a 15-item simple scale for measuring a feeling of helplessness. The scale consists of three alternatives right, wrong and uncertain. It is available both in English and in Hindi. It has high reliability and validity (Dhar et al. 1987; Verma et al. 1988). It is based on the fact that there are people who are unable to face new problems not because of their lack of capacity to deal with such problems but because of an acquired sense of helplessness from their earlier experiences. Hence, the scale is called learned helplessness scale.

Sarason's General Anxiety scale for Children (GASC) and Test Anxiety Scale for Children (TASC)

These two scales of Sarason have been translated and adapted in Hindi and Punjabi languages by Nijhawan at the Punjab University, Chandigarh. These scales are simple, easy to score and have been usefully employed in a number of studies as reliable and valid measures of anxiety in children. One is a general test of anxiety while the other measures anxiety in a specific situation, *viz.* Anxiety Before Undertaking any Achievement or Scholastic Performance Test (Nijhawan 1971).

Developmental Psychopathology Checklist (DPCL)

This checklist consists of 124 items in 6 major areas, *viz.* developmental history, developmental problems, psychopathology, psychosocial stressors, temperamental profiles and social support including the assets in a child. The application of cluster analysis on this checklist in the course of a study yielded seven distinct clusters such as conduct disorders, hyperkinesis, autism, emotional disorders, learning disabilities, hysterical syndrome and childhood psychosis (Kapur et al. 1995).

Reporting Questionnaire for Children (RQC)

This questionnaire consists of ten items and is a simple, quick and easy to administer screening scale dealing with speech/language problems and disorders such as fits, headaches, running away from home, stealing, nervousness, backwardness, social withdrawal, soiling, etc. It has a satisfactory record of reliability and validity as a quick screening instrument for children (Giel et al. 1981).

Children's Personality Questionnaire (CPQ)

The CPQ (Porter and Cattell 1972) is one of the few tests that are available for assessment of personality in children aged 8 to 12. This is an extension of Cattell's work on 16 PF and provides information on personality factors such as extraversion, anxiety, etc.

Minnesota Multiphasic Personality Inventory (MMPI)

The MMPI (Hathway and Mckinley 1943) is a personality test for adults and adolescents aged 16 or above. It consists of following subscales, i.e.

1. Hypochondriasis
2. Depression
3. Hysteria
4. Psychopathic deviate
5. Masculinity—famininity
6. Paranoia
7. Psychasthenia
8. Schizophrenia
9. Hypomania
10. Social introversion.

It can be used as a screening test for a variety of psychiatric disorders.

Millon Adolescent Personality Inventory (MAPI)

The MAPI (Million et al. 1982) is applicable to adolescents aged 13 to 18 and is an improvement over MMPI. It generates scores on variable such as personality style (introversive, sociable, inhibited, sensitive, etc.); expressed concerns (self-concept, body comfort, peer security, academic confidence, etc.) and behavioural correlates (impulse control, social conformity, etc.).

The long list of these tests does suggest that considerable amount of work has been done in this area. Some of these instruments are also used for screening purposes, for group comparisons and for evaluation of various therapeutic techniques like reduction in anxiety, depression, or increase in school adjustment following behaviour modification. However, very little work seems to have been done in the area of personality disorders in children.

There are also inadequately standardized screening tools, semi-structured interview schedules, rating scales, based on the observations of play therapists, school teachers, parents and relatives, which form an integral part in the assessment of a child's behaviour and sometimes they do come up with useful and meaningful information. At times, such information is merely descriptive, nevertheless, these sources need to be examined in a systematic fashion. In certain situations some information, however, crude may be better than not having any information. At least, it can provide useful insights for developing more reliable and valid techniques in the future.

Adjustment Inventories

A large number of adjustment inventories for school children have been devised following Bell's adjustment inventory and some of them are translated into Indian languages (Kapur 1995; Malhotra et al. 1992; Verma 1992, 1996; Pareek and Rao, 1974; Pestonjee 1988; 1998). One such inventory by Pareek et al. (1976) has 40 items and claims to be a reliable measure in assessing adjustment levels of Indian students towards home, school, peers and general matters. (For details on other inventories, which are too numerous to be described

here, see latest lists of firms dealing with psychological tests given in Annexure at the end of this chapter.)

The problem with many such measurement tools is that they are only available in the English language or, have been translated in local languages other than the national language Hindi, which limits their use. Moreover, a large number of these tools remain unpublished and exist in the form of research project reports (unpublished manuscripts which are available from only authors on request) or presented at regional conferences. The following are some examples of the unpublished questionnaires.

Self-esteem Inventory (1981)

- Ittelsan centre family interaction scales (Behrens et al. 1969)
- SRA junior inventory (remmers and Baurnfeind 1951); Pleasure Scale (Kazdin 1989)
- Achenbach checklist (Achenbach and Edelbrock 1983)
- Children's behaviour questionnaire (Rutter 1967)
- Children personality questionnaire (CAQ) by Porter and Cattell (1972)

In general, there has been a dearth of instruments to measure personality in children and adolescents. In addition, at the theoretical and conceptual level it is argued that personality cannot be reliably assessed in children who are still developing and changing as individuals. Further, any personality constellation does not stabilize till the age of 16 to 18. However, it is necessary and useful to assess general traits and tendencies even in children so that their behaviour and psychopathology can be more clearly understood. Moreover, certain tests are available for personality assessment in adolescence.

(b) Projective Techniques

Projective techniques are indirect measures of assessing a child's personality and psychopathology. They are essentially based on the Freudian psychoanalytical theory and also on the "gestalt approach" (as opposed to the psychometric approach) where personality of an individual is viewed as a dynamic whole rather than a sum of different parts. These are more descriptive (qualitative measurement) as opposed to the quantitative and precise measurement as in the typical statistical approach. In this qualitative approach, personality seems to merge with psychopathology as is evident in Freud's discussions in his essays on "Psychopathology of Everyday Life" and defense mechanisms explaining the sources of human behaviour—normal as well as abnormal. This technique has certain advantages over the more limited and subjective distortions (lies, malingering, response biases, motivational distortions) found in the questionnaires and rating scales. But it would be incorrect to describe projective techniques as faultless, their excessive dependence on subjective intuitions and insights is a limitation. The use of projective techniques in clinical settings is a controversial issue as strongly different views are held on the subject. There are some clinical psychologists who do not approve the use of these techniques without intensive and prolonged training under professional supervision with a large number of subjects. On the other hand, there are psychologists who have no interest in these techniques—would be happy to throw them away as invalid and useless tools. Truth, however, lies somewhere in between these two warring positions. The projective techniques in competent hands do provide useful information but obviously they do not provide answers for everything and cannot be blamed for all the alleged pitfalls or limitations of the psychometric approach to human behaviour. Judiciously used, they can play a useful role in the personality assessment of children particularly as they tend to play out their problems whereas adults talk about their problems. Projective techniques, when used for children, are introduced in the form of a game (come, let us play a game). This make-believe play often helps children to express their innermost motives, desires, wishes, fears as well as goals and attitudes, however, temporary they might be.

In projective techniques, the situation is usually vague, relatively unstructured and open to a variety of interpretations by children. There are some tests, which are more unstructured than others, for instance, the Rorschach Test is more unstructured than the story making test, *viz.* the Children Apperception Test. While the Rorschach uses a series of ink blot designs and can be described as an interpretation (vague stimulus) test, the Children Apperception Test can be classified as a completion test. The Draw-a-Person test (Draw-a-Person followed by Draw-a-Person of the opposite sex) is a production test in which test material that is required is just a paper and a pencil. The following are some of the commonly used projective tests in India.

List of Projective Tests for Use with Children:*

- Rorschach ink blot test (Indian norms for children are available, Bagh 1955).
- Children apperception test (Indian adaptation by Uma Chaudhury 1960).
- Draw-a-person test (Karen Machover's DAP Test, 1949).
- *Rosenzweig picture:* Frustration study (Indian adaptation of child form by Pareek 1958).
- Make-a-picture story test (MAPS).
- *Make-a-wish test:* Three wishes test (children asked to prioritize their three most important wishes along with assurance that they would be fulfilled immediately).
- A projective question test. (If in the next birth you were to be an animal, what animal would you like to be and why?)
- House-tree-person test
- Sentence completion test
- Play observation, etc.

Brief descriptions of some of these tests are given below:

Rorschach Test

Developed by a Swiss psychiatrist, Herman Rorschach, this ink blot test has 10 standard cards, 5 of the cards (I, IV, V, VI and VII) are achromatic, and 5 are chromatic (II and III have red as additional colour whereas VIII, IX and X are multicoloured cards). The test is administered in a standardized way in which the above set of ink blots in a variety of colours and shapes is presented to the subject, who is asked to describe what they perceive. Stages of test administration varies for different ages. Introduced as a test of imagination the responses are scored for location (whole, major or minor usual details, unusual detail areas or white space responses), determinants (form alone, colour, movement, shading, depth), and content categories (human, animal, anatomy, object, plant, fire, cloud, etc.) as well as for popular (occurring with higher than one in six responses), or original (occurring in less than 200 records). The quality of responses as positive form level is also seen as F^+, and percent of popular to total responses is seen as measure of touch with reality. There are also a number of scoring methods with Indian norms. While interpreting these ink blot designs, children tend to reveal their problems.

Children's Apperception Test (Indian Adaptation by Uma Chaudhury)

This test consists of ten animal pictures involved in activities such as eating, sleeping alone, toilet training and playing competitive games. The subject is required to narrate stories based on the animal pictures, describing the animals, what they were thinking and doing, and what led to the activities that they were performing; and what would happen at the end. While narrating these stories, children often reveal their own imagination, feelings, attitudes, needs, struggles, problems, aspirations and fears.

Draw-a-Person Test

In this test, the child is first asked to draw a person, describe whether the person is a boy or girl, and then asked to draw a figure of its opposite sex. The child is also required to describe these two figures in detail: Their sizes, and activities, and thoughts. The descriptions as well as the appearance of these figures are interpreted as reflecting a child's personality, its fears, anxieties, aspiration, etc. Usually, children draw figures of their own sex first but sometimes girls tend to draw male figures first. Emphasis on symmetry, buttons and pockets in the figures indicate dependency in a child; depressed subjects draw extremely small figures, and schizophrenics tend to draw mutilated body parts or internal anatomy as well.

Draw-a-Person Test (DAPT) Machover (1949)

This test was developed where the individual is directed to draw a person that related intimately to the impulses, anxiety, conflicts and psychological characteristics. DAPT is a projective test used in children to understand his/her inner mind, to uncover internal psychological motivations, deep seated emotions, self-concept, etc. which are otherwise inhibited or repressed from conscious expression. Kohli et al. (2006) have worked on the test in India.

Kohli et al. (2006) used the test on Indian children and reported comparative findings and differential profile of drawings in groups of internalizing versus externalizing disorders among them. It is possible to differentiate normal children form those with psychiatric disorder and also those with internalizing or externalizing disorder on the basis of drawings.

Rosenzweig Picture—Frustration Study (Child Form)

Pareek and his co-workers have adapted 24 pictures from this study to Indian conditions, depicting frustrating situations like:

a. *A lady telling a child who is looking at the cupboard:* 'The last thing that I had I have given to your brother. Now nothing is left';

b. *One child telling another:* 'You are an ass, 'etc. The child's responses to these frustrating situations are classified as follows: whether aggression is shown towards self, other significant family members, or on harmless things, the presence of sibling rivalry, negative attitude towards observance of general rules, appreciation of other people's difficulties and the degree to which such feelings are present or absent in the subject.

Play Observation

Children play out their problems: Through an analysis of the child behaviour (it should be one way screen, if possible) an attempt is made to understand why the child has behavioural problems. The way the child plays with some of the play materials, toys, clay, colours, objects, etc. reflects his/her attitude towards them. Sometimes aggression is manifested towards certain toys, at times the child may repeatedly touch all its toys for brief periods of time (as brain damaged children do), sometimes the child may prefer one type of play situation and/or talk while playing with certain toys all these responses reflect the child's world view, and his/her reaction to the world, thus providing useful data on the subject.

Almost all the projective tests are used as personality tests as well as to measure psychopathology in children. Perhaps this is due to the fact that their personality is still in the developmental stage, and is rightly called developmental psychopathology. Considerable work has been done in this area as is evident from the many tests that have just been mentioned.

SPECIFIC TESTS FOR THE HANDICAPPED

NIMHANS Index of Specific Learning Disabilities (Kapur M, John A, Rozario J, Oommen A 1991)

This is a comprehensive battery of tests to assess Specific Learning Disabilities comprising of assessment of general intellectual abilities using Malin's Intelligence Scale for Indian Children (MISIC) and separate battery of tests for younger age (5–7 years) children as Level I, and older children as level II. Level I includes tests, attention, visual discrimination, visual memory, auditory discrimination, auditory behaviour, auditory memory, speech and language (verbal expression), visuomotor and writing skills.

Level II includes tests of attention, reading, spellings, comprehension, perceptuomotor abilities, memory, arithmetic ability.

NIMHANS Index of Specific Learning Disabilities is an Indian scale, standardized on Indian children with adequate reliability (0.53) and criterion validity (0.75 and 0.61) for teacher's and clinician's assessments (Uma H, Oommen A and Kapur M, 2006, p121).

Some assessment tools have been specifically developed or adapted for the mentally and visually handicapped children in India at their respective national institute at Secunderabad in Andhra Pradesh and Dehradun in Uttarakhand. Information on these tests, including their standardization procedures and normative data are available from these centres. Detailed information is also available at their regional centres in India. Similarly, the All India Institute of Speech and Hearing, Mysore has developed informative data on selected tests for speech and hearing impaired children, and may be contacted directly or through the National Test Library in Delhi.

Home Observation for Measurement of Environment (HOME environment Inventory) Caldwell and Bradley (1984)

This scale assesses the quality of home environment through interview as well as observation of the child at home in natural setting. Three main probe areas deal with trips out of the home; visit to the home and toys that are available to the child; and the way family arranges daily routine and discipline. This scale has been translated, adapted and shortened in Hindi by Kohli et al. 2005, making it available for clinical population in Indian setting. The inventory has 8 sub scales namely:

1. Stimulation through toys, games and reading material
2. Language stimulation
3. Physical environment: Safe, clean and conducive
4. Pride, affection and warmth
5. Stimulation of academic behaviour
6. Modeling and encouraging of social maturity
7. Variety of stimulation
8. Physical punishment

How to Choose and Interpret a Test, and Communicate its Results?

Psychodiagnostics refers to the total process of psychological evaluation (with the help of standardized tests) of a person as a whole with diagnostic, prognostic and therapeutic implications (for qualitative and quantitative, and positive and negative mental health purposes). The purpose of a referral in clinical practice may be broad or narrow depending upon the reason for it. For example, a child may be referred to the clinical psychologist for an evaluation of his present cognitive functions. Here, the purpose of referral is much broader than when it is merely to rule out or confirm the presence of mental retardation. In the latter case, a detailed evaluation is uncalled for unless it is also required for purposes of counseling, rehabilitation, speech therapy, etc. Sometimes, IQ assessments are required for screening purposes at the time of admission to institutes for special education.

Psychodiagnostic tools have their uses, merits and limitations. The popularity of a test is not a reliable index of its validity. A test is said to be valid for a function with which it correlates. No test is valid for making all sorts of decisions. Usually, a test manual mentions (or ideally should mention) the uses and limitations of the test, warning about any possible misuse of misinterpretation. Under certain known conditions, standardized tests can give useful information and guidelines. While selecting a test, one has to look at its reliability, and validity; whether it has been properly standardized; and if it has been standardized on a relevant local population with meaningful local norms. Reliability is said to be high if the test shows high consistency (gives same scores over a brief period of time). Its validity cannot exceed the square root of its reliability. Though most of the tests have been developed in the developed countries in west, a large number of these tests are still being used in Indian clinics unchanged or with slight modifications (mostly it is lip service) to suit Indian conditions. It is often ignored that the effectiveness of diagnostic tests vary markedly between the developing and the developed countries due to enormous variations in subjects' education, socio-economic status and culture in two settings. The economic realities, pressure on the delivery of services and paucity of trained personnel in developing countries warrants the use of tests which are economical in terms of time, cost and effectiveness for the majority of its clinic population (children and their parents) located in a rural setting. Ignorant in the use of psychological tests, they often do not understand or appreciate the need to cooperate while undergoing the tests as necessary consideration in its administration and interpretation. Special care has to be taken while interpreting test results, and communicating them to the parents, patients or the team members treating a patient.

Ethics in Testing

Each person is unique in some ways and has a right to be treated as such. A person' right to refuse to undergo testing, confidentiality of test results, right to know one's own test results, should be respected.

Training in Psychodiagnostics

Due to the complexity in the standardized administration of some tests and dangers of misinterpretation of test scores, the need for intensive training in psychodiagnostics has often been emphasized for valid reasons. Untrained testers often forget the need for standardized administration of tests, proper scoring and their interpretation, despite the warnings in the test manuals. For example, response styles (tendency to choose socially desirable responses in place of true responses; tendency to agree or disagree; tendency to choose middle category of responses or to choose extreme responses, etc.) and poor motivation among children to take tests have to be considered a possible source of biases. Children sometimes have negativistic tendencies which stand in the way of reliable test results. Unfortunately, there are no standard guidelines for establishing good rapport with such subjects. Test administration is an art that has to be learned and cultivated. Even communication of test results has to be learned—what to tell, how much to tell, when to tell and whom to tell. Telling parents that their child is mentally retarded or autistic may require special communication skills. It would be necessary to prepare parents mentally as the news may come as a great shock to them. Although the information on a child's condition should not be withheld, the language, the tone, the manner in which unpleasant facts have to be communicated is a skill that has to be learned, it should never be too abrupt or, conveyed in an inhuman manner.

Conclusion

The above review shows that a considerable amount of reliable work has been done in India in the area of assessment in intelligence, memory, perceptuomotor and other cognitive functions in children as also in the assessment of their personality. Many tools have been developed and adapted in each of these areas. The lists of tools provided in this chapter are not complete. Further refinements are always possible and would be required as this is an ongoing process. At no point in time is it possible to claim that a perfect test has been developed in any of these areas, which is equally valid for all types of population and in different cultures. It is sufficient to say that the psychometric assessment of children has come of age in India.

ANNEXURE

List of firms dealing with psychological tests:

1. Mansayan, Aggarwal Complex, 5-524 School Block, Shakarpur, Delhi 110092
2. National Psychological Corporation, 4/230, Kacheri Ghat, Agra, 282004
3. Agra Psychological Research Cell, Tiwari Kothi, Belan Ganj, Agra, 282004
4. Psychoeducational Testing Centre, C2A/16/108, Janakpuri, New Delhi, 110058
5. Ankur Psychological Agency, 22/481, Indira Nagar, Lucknow, UP
6. Indian Psychological Corporation, Shanti Sadan, Rai Behari Lal Road, Lucknow, UP
7. Psycho-centre, T-22, Green Park, New Delhi, 110016
8. Rupa Psychological Centre, B 19/60B, Deariabir, Bhelupura, Varanasi, 221010
9. Swayam Siddha, 720, 16th Main, Saraswathipuram, Mysore, 570009
10. Psycho-Cum Services, B-4, 80/2, Safdarjung Enclave, New Delhi 110029

Notes

1. Details about individual tests, their prices etc. can be had directly from the publisher through their catalogues.
2. National test library instituted by the National Council of Educational Research and Training (NCERT), Delhi, may also be consulted for information about tests and their sources.

3. Specific tests for the mentally, speech, visually and hearing-impaired children can be had from respective centres or institutes *viz.* National Institute for the Mentally Handicapped, Manovikas Nagar, Secunderabad, 500011; National Institute for the Visually Handicapped, Dehradun; and the All India institute of Speech and Hearing Mysore.

BIBLIOGRAPHY

1. Achenbach, TM and Edelbrok CS. Manual for Child Behaviour Checklist an Revised Child Behaviour Profile, Queen City Printers Inc., USA, 1983.
2. Bagh D. Use of the Rorschach Inkblot Test among School Adolescents. Indian Journal of Psychology 1955;30:1–10.
3. Bakwin H and Bakwin RM. Clinical Management of Behaviour Disorders in Children. W.B. Saunders Co., Philadelphia, 1960.
4. Barna Das IP, Kapur M, Uma H, Sinha UK (2006) In Hirisave U, Oommen A, Kapur M (2006) Tests of Memory for Children. In Psychological Assessment of Children in the clinical setting. Publication no. 48, NIMHANS, Bangalore.
5. Bayley N. Manual for Bayley Scales of Infant Development, Psychological Corporation, New York, 1969.
6. Behrens ML, Meyor DI, Goldforb W, et al. The Henry Ittlson Centre Family Interaction Scales. Genetic Psychology Monograph, 1969;80.
7. Bender L. A Visual-motor-gestalt Test and its Clinical Use, American Orthopsychaitric Association, New York, 1938.
8. Benton AL. Revised Visual Retention Test, Psychological Corporation, Manual San Antario, TX, 1974.
9. Bharath Raj J. DST (Development Screening Test)', Swayamsiddha, Mysore, 1983.
10. Bhargava M and Sandhu R. Guidelines for Bender Visual Motor Gestalt Test, Ankur Psychological Agency, Lucknow, 1987.
11. Bhatia CM. Performance Tests of Intelligence under Indian Conditions. Oxford University Press, Bombay 1955.
12. Boll TJ. Right and Left Cerebral Hemisphere damage and tactile perception: Performance of the ipsilateral and contralateral sides of the body. Neuropsychologia, 1974;12: 235–38.
13. Burke HR. 'Ravens Progressive Matrices: Validity, reliability and Norms' Journal of Psychology, 1972;82:253–57.
14. Caldwell B, Bradley R (1984) Home Observation or measurement of the Environment (HOME) Revised Ed. Univ. of Arkansas, Little Rock USA.
15. Catell RB. Guide to Mental Testing, University of London Press, London, 1946.
16. Chaudhury U. The CAT- The Indian Adaptation, Book Land Pvt. Ltd., Calcutta, 1960.
17. Collarrusso RP and Hammill DD. Motor-Free Visual Perception Test. Academic Therapy Publications 1972.
18. D'Elia LF, Satz P, Uchiyama CL, and White T (1996). Colour trails test. Florida: Psychological Assessment Researcher, Inc. 1996.
19. De Renzi E, and Vignolo L. The token test: A sensitive test to detect receptive disturbances in aphasics, Brain, 1962;85:665–678.
20. Dhar V, Kohli S. Manual for Learned Helplessness Scale, Haryana Council of Psychological Research, Bhiwani, 1987.
21. Doll EA. Vineland social maturity scale: Manual of Directions (Ref. Ed.) American Guidance Services, USA, 1965.
22. Dwivedi, CB. Manual of Directions of Bender-Gestalt Test for Children, Rupa Psychological Centre, Vaanasi, 1987.
23. Frankenburg WK, Dodds J, Archer P, Shapiro H and Bronick B. 'A Major Revision and Standar-dization of the Denver Developmental Screening Test', Paediatrics, 1992;89:91–97.
24. Gessel A. Fessel Development Schedule, Psychological Corporation, New York, 1949.
25. Giel R. De Arango MD, Harding TW et al. Childhood Mental Disorders in Primary Health Care: Results and Observations in Four Developing Countries, Paediatrica, 1981;68:677–88.
26. Hathway AR, McMinley JC. The Minnesota Multiphasic Personality Inventory (Rev. ed.),

University of Minnesota Press, Minneapolis, 1943.

27. Heaton RK, Chelune GJ, Talley JL, Kay GG and Curtis G. Wisconsin Card Sorting test Manual. Odessa. Florida: Psychological Assessment Resources, Inc. 1993.

28. Jones-Gotman M, and Milner B. Design fluency: The invention of nonsense drawings after focal cortical lesions. Neuropsychologia, 15, 653–674.

29. Jones-Gotman M. Memory for designs: the lippocampal contrilention. Neuro-psychologia, 1986;24:193–203.

30. Kapoor M., "Developmental Checklist for Children (DPCL)—A Preliminary Report, NIMHANS Journal, 1995;13:1–19.

31. Kapur M (1974). Colour Cancellation Test in Measurement of Organic Brain Dysfunction. Doctoral Thesis, Bangalore University, Bangalore.

32. Kapur M, Barna Das IP, Reddy MV, Rozario J and Uma H (2006) in Uma H, Oomen A and Kapur M (Eds.) Developmental Psychopathology Checklist for Children (DPCL). In Psychological Assessment of Children in the Clinical Setting a Publication no. 48, NIMHANS, Bangalore.

33. Kapur M, John A, Rozario J, Oomen A (1992). NIMHANS Index of Specific Learning Disabilities. Department of Mental Health and Social Psychology, NIMHANS, Bangalore.

34. Kapur M., Mental Health of Indian Children, Sage Publications, New Delhi, 1995.

35. Kar BR, Rao SL, Chandramouli BA and Thennarasu K. NIMHANS Neuropsychological Battery for Children—Manual Publication No. 61, 2004 NIMHANS, Bangalore.

36. Kaufman AS, Kaufman ML, Kaufman-ABC: Kaufman Assessment battery for Children, Circle Pines MN: American Guidance Service, 1983.

37. Kazadin AE, Evaluation of Pleasure Scale in the Assessment of Anhedonia in Children, Journal of American Academy of Childand Adoelscent Psychiatry 1989; 364–72.

38. Kohli A, Kaur M, Malhotra R (2006) Draw-a-Person Practice Manual: Normative and Clinical data. Prasad Psycho Corporation, J 1/58 Daranagar, Varanasi, India.

39. Kohli A, Mohanty M, Kaur RP. (2005) Adaptation of HOME Inventory in simple Hindi. E-Journal Indian Association of Child and Adolescent Mental Health Oct. 1 (4):2

40. Kohli A, Mohanty M, Malhotra R, Verma SK (1998). Measurement of memory in children: Construction of a simple clinical tool in Hindi. Behavioural Medicine Journal 1(2) 34–42.

41. Koppitz EM. The Bender-Gestalt Test for Young Children, Grunne and Stratton. Orlando, FL, 1964.

42. Kulshreshtha SM. Manual of Standford-Binet Intelligence Scale—Hindi Adaptation of Third Revision', Manas Sewa Sansthan Prakashan, Form L-M Allahabad, 1971.

43. Kulshreshtha SP and Rahniwal DN. Trends and Status of Psychological and Educational Testing in India, Jugal Kisore and Co., Dehradun, 1984.

44. Lezak MD. Neuropsychological Assessment (3rd ed.) New York: Oxford University Press. 1995.

45. Long L and Mehta PH (eds). The First Mental Measurement Handbook for India, NCERT, Delhi, 1966.

46. Luria A. Higher Cortical Functions in Man. Ldonon: Tavistock. 1966.

47. Luria A. The Working Brain. New York: Basic books. 1973.

48. Maj M, D'Elia L, Satz P, and Janssen R. Evaluation of two new neuropsychological tests designed to minimize cultural bias in the assessment of HIV- I seropositive persons: A WHO study. Archives of Clinical Neuropsychology, 8, 123–135.

49. Malhotra S and Malhotra A. Manual for Malhotra Temperament Schedule, National Psychological Corporation, Agra, 1988.

50. Malhotra S, Malhotra A, Varma VK. Child Mental Health in India, Macmillan India Ltd., Delhi, 1992.

51. Malin AJ, Vineland Social Maturity Scale-Nagpur Adaptation, Indian Psychological Corporation, Lucknow, 1972.

52. Malin AJ. Malin's Intelligence Scale for Indian Children (MISIC). Indian Journal of Mental Retardation, 1969;4:15–25.

53. Malin AJ. Manual for Malin's Intelligence Scale for Children, Nagpur Child Guidance Centre, 1969.

54. Millon T, Green CT, Meagher RB. Millon's Adolescent Personality Inventory: Manual, National Computer Systems, Minneapolis, 1982.

55. Murthy HN. 'A Short Scale of the Bhatia's Performance tests', Indian Psychological review, 1966;2:133–34.

56. Neki JS and Prabhu GG. Personality Development and Personal Illness. All India Institute of Medical Sciences, Mental Health Monograph Series No. 2, New Delhi, 1974.

57. Nijhawan HK. Anxiety in School Children, Wiley Eastern PVT. Ltd., New Delhi, 1971.

58. Oakland T and US. 'International Perspectives on Tests used with Children and Youths', Journal of School Psychology, 1993;31:501–17.

59. Pareek U and Rao TV. Handbook of Psychological and Social Instruments, Samasthi, Baroda, 1974.

60. Pareek U, Rao TV, Ramalingaswamy P and Sharma BR. A Manual for Battery of Preadolescent Personality Tests, Rupa Psychological Centre, Varanasi, 1976.

61. Pareek U. Behavioural Science research in India—A Directory, Behavioural Science centre, Delhi, 1966.

62. Pareek V and Rao TV. Handbook of Psychological and Social Instruments, Samasthi, Baroda, 1974.

63. Pareek V. Reliability of the Indian Adaptation of the Rosenzweig Picture Frustration Study', Journal of Psychological Researches, 1958;2:18–27.

64. Pershad D and Verma SK (eds). The Concept and Assessment of Intelligence Indian Perspective, National Psychological Corporation, Agra, 1988.

65. Pestonjee DM. Third Handbook of Psychological and Social Instruments, 1997.

66. Phatak P 'Motor and Mental Development of Indian Babies from One Month to Thirty Months', Indian Paediatrics, 1969;6:18–22.

67. Phatak P 'Revision and Extension of Phatak Draw-a-Man Scale for Indian Children of Age Groups 2 and ½ to 16 years', Psychological Bulletin, 1984;29:34–46.

68. Porter RB and Catell RB. Handbook for Children's Personality Questionnaire; 1972.

69. Porteus SD. Porteus Maze Test, George H. Harap and Co. Ltd., London, 1962.

70. Porteus SD. The Porteus Maze Test. London: George G. Harrap and Co. Ltd. 1965.

71. Prabhu GG, 'Personality Assessment in the Clinical Setting', JS Neki and GG Prabhu (eds). Personality Development and Personal Illness, AIIMS Mental Health Monograph Series No. 2, 1974, pp. 75–96.

72. Puri A, Pershad D, Singhi P and Verma SK. 'Extending Utility of Developmental Screening Test', Creative Psychologist, 1995;7:14–45.

73. Puri A, Singhi P, Pershad D, Walia BNS and Verma SK. Manual for Indian development Screening Schedule, Unpublished Manuscript, Dept of Paediatrics, PGI, Chandigarh, 1994.

74. Ramachandran KV. A Survey of School Children in Bombay City with Special Reference to Their Physical efficiency, Mental and Nutritional Status, Asia Publishing House, Bombay, 1968.

75. Raven J, Raven JC and Court JH. Standard Progressive Matrices. Oxford; Oxford Psychologists Press, 2000.

76. Ravens JC. Guide to Using the Coloured Progre-ssive Matrices, HK Lewis and Co. Ltd., London, 1965.

77. Reitan RM. Sensorymotor functions, intelligence and cognition, and emotional status in subjects with cerebral lesions. Perceptual and Motor skills, 1970;31:275–284.

78. Remmers, HH and Baurnfiend H, SRA, Junior Inventory Form A., Science Research Associates, Illinois, 1951.

79. Rutter M. A Child's Bheaviour Questionnaire for Completion by Teachers', Journal of Child Psychology and Psychiatry, 1967;8:1–26.

80. Smith EE and Jonides J. Working memory in Humans: Neuropsychological Evidence. In MS Gazzaniga (Ed.), Cognitive Neurosciences (pp. 1009–1020). Cambridge, MA: MIT Press 1995.

81. Sparrow SS, Balla DB, Cicchetti DV. The Vineland Adaptive Behaviour Scales, American Guidance Service, USA 1984.

82. Tests in Print, Published by the NCERT, Delhi.

83. Thakur GP and Thakur M, Thakur Death Anxiety Scale, Rupa psychological Centre, Varanasi, 1984.

84. Thomas A and Chess S. Temperament and Development, Brunner/Mazel, New York, 1977.

85. Uma H, Oomen A and Kapur M (2006). In Hirisave U, Oommen A, Kapur M (Eds.) Psychological Assessment of Children in the clinical setting. Publication no. 48, p 121, NIMHANS, Bangalore.

86. Venkatesh S, et al. 'Neuropsychological Assessment in Organic Brain Pathology: An Overview', Psychological Studies, 1993;38;125–31.

87. Verma SK 'Development of Psychological tests: 10 Years Experience', Journal of Rajasthan Psychaitric Society, 1978;1:43–56.

88. Verma SK and Nehra A, 'Psychodiagnostics', Psychiatry Today, 1997;81–84.

89. Verma SK and Pershad D, 'Psychometric Assessment in India: An Overview of the literature in the Last Decade with particular Emphasis on Cultural and Methodological Problems', in SP Kulshreshtha (ed.). Trends an Status of Psychological and Educational testing in India, 1984,1–25

90. Verma SK, 'Assessment', in MS Bhatia and NK Dhar (eds.) A Comprehensive Textbook of Child and Adolescent Psychiatry, CBS Pub. & Dist, 1996, pp. 2.1–2.19.

91. Verma SK, 'Intelligence assessment in the Mentally Retarded: Some Experiences, Indian Journal of Mental Retardation, 1971;10–14.

92. Verma SK, 'Measurement in Psychiatry', JN Vyas and N. Ahuja (eds.) BI Churchill Linvingstone Pvt. Ltd. Delhi, 1992;353–67.

93. Verma SK, Pershad D and Kaushal P. Gessel Drawing Tests as a Measure of Intelligence in the mentally Retarded Children. Indian Journal of Mental Retardation, 1972;5:64–68.

94. Verma SK, Pershad D and Randhawa A, 'Are Indian Children Slow? Report of an Enquiry with a Speed Measure of Intelligence', Child Psychiatry Quarterly, 1980;13:67–71.

95. Verma SK, Psychodiagnostics an Evaluation', Psychological Studies, 1993;38:101–13.

96. Verma SK. 'Brain Damaged Child: Psychometric Aspects', Indian Journal of Mental Retardation, 1970;3:87–121.

97. Wechsler D., Manual for Wechsler Intelligence Scale for Children (Revised), The Psychological Corporation, New York, 1974.

98. Wig NN. Development of Psychological tests in India: An Over view of the Current Situation', Indian Journal of Clinical psychology, 1983;10:42.

Structured Assessment and Some Indian Scales

Psychiatric diagnosis depends almost entirely on psychiatric interview. However, there are several possible sources of bias in interviewing which may yield erroneous data and ultimately an erroneous diagnosis. The bias may come from the interviewer who may differ in the level of training and expertise; in amount of time spent with patient; in the degree of probing used to elicit information; in degree of familiarity with language and sociocultural background of the patient. Bias may also come from the interview method, i.e., the type and format of questions such as open ended vs forced choice; language used for interview if different from the language of the patient; degree of completeness and comprehensiveness of interviewing; in interpretation of the observations and so on. Individuals differ in the manner in which they express their inner feelings, thoughts and other psychic experiences. There is major difference in the use of words to denote psychological experiences, for example, Indian patients more often use somatic expressions to describe their emotional states. People in India more often involve external attributions such as diet, weather, magicoreligious influences and so to explain disorders. Another difficulty that is often faced while interviewing patients in India is that they are unable to date the events or happenings making it difficult to establish a clear chronology. It requires extra effort and indirect probing of events around the events to understand the correct dates or at times one has to contend with the approximate dates.

To overcome such difficulties in interviewing and to avoid biases, methods of interviewing became more and more structured and standardized. Also, with increasing advancements and refinements in diagnostic criteria and classifications, structured interviewing became a necessity. In order to elicit and document psychopathology in a most reliable manner, it is necessary that the concerned phenomenon is clearly defined and guidelines for eliciting it are clearly laid. Among the reasons for poor reliability of psychiatric diagnosis in children, lack of structured instruments for measuring psychopathology has been a major factor. Structured interviewing method involves predetermining the content, format, and sequence of questions; defining the responses, assigning scores or weightage to responses; laying rules for collating scores. There can be variations in the extent of structure provided which may be totally fixed or flexible to some extent. Overall, there are set rules for interviewing and interpretation of responses. The advantage of structured interview format is high reliability and absence of bias which is desirable whereas the disadvantage is lack of flexibility which is needed for clinical work. Therefore, semistructured interview is relatively preferred for clinical work. Structured assessment is also useful for teaching purposes where the format and the content of questions can be used as a guide or an aid to interviewing by trainees or by less experienced professionals.

In practice, structured assessment of psychopathology can be used for:
i. Differentiating children with psychiatric disorder from those who are normal;
ii. Quantifying the severity of disorder;
iii. Determining the nature or type of disorder; or
iv. For diagnosing a particular or several diagnostic categories that are intended. Characteristics of the instruments are different according to intended purposes.

There can be structured instruments to measure other specific areas such as level of functioning, degree of disability, life events and stress, temperament, coping, parental handling, etc.

Adequate standardization of the structured measurement tools is necessary before they can be put to use. Process of standardization involves study of its reliability, validity and population norms.

Reliability is a measure of the extent to which the instrument is likely to yield same or consistent scores for a given case when administered by different persons, or at different times interval provided the condition of the case has not changed. Validity is a measure of the extent to which the instrument measures what it purports to measure. Population norms are the distribution of scores, depicted as mean and standard deviation, in the population for which the instrument has been designed. Reliability, validity and norms, also termed as the psychometric properties of the test, must be satisfactory before a test can be put the wider use. Each test can be used, ideally for only that population, for which it has been designed and on which it has been standardized. Any standard test when needed for use on another population should be subjected to a process of re-standardization on that population which is called as adaptation. It may require change in items, addition or deletion of items, as may be necessary, change in the wording or language, change in the overall length of the questionnaire making it shorter or longer and so on. Adaptation is needed when the age range of the instrument's application has to be expanded or changed; when it is to be used on a population that differs in cultural or geographical or linguistic characteristics; or when the scope of coverage of disorders needs to be changed and so on.

Various types of available mental health assessment tools are:
- Behavioral rating scales
- Standardized clinical interviews
- Psychological and cognitive assessments Projective assessments
- Self-report questionnaires

There are numerous assessment tools developed for different purposes that one can choose from. It is not possible to describe all of them. Some of structured instruments commonly used in children and adolescents are listed below.

Screening Instruments

1. Rutter's A scale for completion by parent (Rutter, Tizard and Whitmore 1970).
2. Rutter's B Scale for Completion by Teachers (Rutter 1967).
3. Child Behaviour Checklist (CBCL) (Achenbach and Edelbrock 1983)
4. Reporting Questionnaire for Children (RQC) (Giel et al. 1980)
5. Preschool Behaviour Questionnaire (Behar 1977)
6. Behavioural Screening Questionnaire (Richman and Graham 1971)
7. Strengths and Difficulties Questionnaire (SDQ) (Goodman 1997)
8. Youth Survey Report (YSR) (Achenbach, 1991)
9. Childhood Psychopathology Measurement Schedule (CPMS) (Malhotra et al. 1988).
10. Developmental Psychopathology Checklist for Children (DPCL) (Kapur et al. 2006).

11. Patient Health Questionnaire (PHQ) Screeners—Child Screening Tests (Johnson et al 2002)
12. Pediatric Symptom Checklist (PSC) (Jellinek et al 1988)

Child Behaviour Checklist (CBCL)

CBCL (Achenbach, Edelbrock 1983, 1991 a, b, c) is a screening-cum-diagnostic instrument applicable to children aged 4–18 years (Achenbach 1991 a) which has been most widely used all over the world. It provides on two scales: Behaviour problem scale and social competence scale, it takes about 20–25 minutes for administration and has been found to be highly reliable. There are separate versions for teachers (Achenbach 1991c); for adolescents aged 11–18 years which is named as youth self-report (Achenbach 1991b) and for two males and females. Recently there is another version for preschool children aged 2–3 years (Achenbach and Edelbrock 1987) higher order factor analysis of CBCL has yielded factors called as "broad band" syndromes. Two broad band syndromes are "externalising" and "internalising" disorders which subsume several narrow band syndromes respectively. CBCL in various forms has very high reliability as well as validity. Norms are available for separate age and sex groups. The scale has been translated in several languages and has been used in many cross-cultural studies. The Indian adaptation of CBCL (called Childhood Psychopathology Measurement Schedule) in Hindi and English languages has been done and is described in detail in the following section (Malhotra et al. 1988).

Rutter A and B Scales

Rutter A scale for completion by parents (Rutter et al. 1970) and Rutter B scale for completion by teachers (Rutter 1967) have been the earliest screening tests devised for epidemiological studies on children which have been extensively used over three decades. However, there are several recent reports that have highlighted the shortcomings of these scales such as being outdated in coverage (Goodman 1997), having low specificity and sensitivity (Malhotra et al. 1998). These are used at first stage of screening of population and those scoring above the cut-off score are required to be subjected to a psychiatric evaluation. In a large epidemiology study on school children in Chandigarh, India, (Malhotra et al. 1995) Rutter B Scale for teachers identified 66% children as false positive (i.e. specificity 34%) and left out 48% children with psychiatric disorder as false negative (i.e. sensitivity approx. 52%), at the recommended score of 9 or above. In this study, confirmation of diagnosis was done by parent interview and detailed psychiatric assessment. This is the first study examining the applicability of this scale on Indian children.

Reporting Questionnaire for Children (RQC)

This is a 10-item questionnaire that enquires into the presence of gross and major neuropsychiatric disorders such as mental retardation, epilepsy, enuresis, speech problems in large epidemiological surveys. (Giel et al. 1980). Presence of a single 'yes' response indicates presence of the disorder. RQC has been used in some WHO surveys.

Strengths and Difficulties Questionnaire (SDQ)

The SDQ (Goodman 1997) is a new behavioural screening questionnaire, designed to assess the behaviour, emotions and relationships in children aged 4–16 years. It is a brief questionnaire (25 items) that can be completed by parents or teachers in five minutes. There is a self-report version of SDQ for children aged 11–16 years. It measures both the strengths as well as the difficulties and yields scores on five scales namely emotional symptoms, conduct problems, inattention-hyperactivity, peer problem and prosocial behaviour; and a total difficulties score. It is a well standardized test and signifies an advancement over Rutter A and B scales.

Preschool Behaviour Questionnaire

This scale (Behar 1977) is an adaptation of Rutter A scale, making it suitable for preschool children. This is a brief scale with rather limited utility, which did not gain much popularity.

Behaviour Screening Questionnaire (BSQ)

This is a structured interview for preschool children (Richman and Graham 1971) that assesses a wide range of behaviour/emotional problems occurring in a variety of everyday life situations of children. It requires some training for conduct of interview and direct observation of the setting in certain situations. BSQ has remained a good instrument for this age.

Developmental Psychopathology Checklist for Children (DPCL):

DPCL is 124 item scales that have six subsections, i.e.:
  i. Developmental history (items 1–10)
  ii. Developmental problems (items 11–28)
  iii. Psychopathology (items 29–78)
  iv. Psychosocial factors (items 79–101)
  v. Temperament (items 102–118)
  vi. Social support and assets of the child (items 119–124)

Items are rated as 'yes' or 'no' for present and absent for all subsections except temperament which is rated on four-point scale to match with Satvik, Rajasik and Tamasik descriptions of temperament. The scale has been tried on 221 children and led to seven clusters of psychopathology namely hyperkinesis, autism, conduct disorder, learning disorder, hysteria, emotional disorder and psychoses.

The scale has adequate reliability and validity. The scale is still at a preliminary stage of development and the authors consider this as a brief, simple and comprehensive

tool that can be used across disorders, age and gender.

Patient Health Questionnaire (PHQ)

PHQ offers screening tools ranging from 2–83 questions that assess mood problems, anxiety, eating disorders, alcohol use, somatoform disorders. It has various versions *viz.* PHQ 4: 4 questions designed to assess anxiety and depression in 11 yrs + in general population; PHQ-SADS: 38 questions to assess anxiety, panic, depression and somatoform disorders; Brief PHQ: 34 questions to screen for anxiety, depression, eating disorders, alcohol use, somatoform disorders in general population.

Pediatric Symptom Checklist (PSC)

PSC is a tool to screen for psychological, behavioural and emotional symptoms in children and adolescents. PSC-17 is a 17-item version for quick screening and there is a 55 item version for in depth assessment in children aged 4–17 yrs. There is youth version PSC-Y for adolescents 12–18.

Diagnostic Instruments

1. Child Behaviour Checklist (CBCL) (Achenbech and Edelbrock 1983).
2. Diagnostic Interview for Children and Adolescents (DICA) (Herjanic and Campbell 1977).
3. Diagnostic Interview Schedule for Children (DISC) (Costello et al. 1984a).
4. Kiddie Schedule for Affective Disorders and Schizophrenia (K-SADS) (Puig-Antich and Chambers 1978).
5. Interview Schedule for Children (ISC) (Kovacs 1983).
6. Child Assessment Schedule (CAS) (Hodges et al. 1982, 87)
7. Childhood Psychopathology Measurement Schedule (Malhotra et al. 1988).
8. Connors Rating Scales (Connors 1973).
9. Mini international neuropsychiatric interview (MINI) (Sheehan et al. 1998) is a short structured clinical interview

which enables researchers to make diagnoses of psychiatric disorders according to DSM-IV or ICD-10. The administration time of the interview is approximately 15 minutes and was designed for epidemiological studies and multicenter clinical trials.

Diagnostic Interview Schedule for Children (DISC)

DISC (Costello et al. 1984) is a highly structured interview in which the wording of questions, the sequence and manner of asking and scoring are predetermined. It elicits information during the last one year but timeframe could be changed to 1 month or 6 months, and is applicable to children aged 6–18 years. There are both parent and the child version which takes about 60–70 mts (parent version) to 45–60 mts (child version). Symptoms are coded for its presence/absence as well as for its severity. Diagnosis is generated by computer algorithms. Extensive data on reliability and validity studies are available. DISC is the only instrument designed solely and specifically for epidemiological studies.

Diagnostic Interview with Children and Adolescents (DICA)

It is a highly structured diagnostic instrument (Herjanic and Campbell 1977), for children 6–17 years old. The questions are framed around syndromes and elicit 'present' or 'absent' responses. The interview brings out information on the onset, duration and severity of symptoms, and the summary scores are compatible with ICD-9, and DSM III and DSM-III-R diagnoses. It takes about 60–90 minutes for administration and both parent and child versions are available. Reliability and validity are satisfactory. This instrument has been extensively used in many studies.

Child Assessment Schedule (CAS)

CAS (Hodges, et al. 1982) is a semi-structured interview covering most of the childhood

psychiatric disorders and generates DSM-III diagnoses. It is applicable to children 7–16 years and covers symptoms during the last 6 months. There are separate parent and child versions, each takes 45–60 mts. It is relatively easy to administer score, and has shown adequate reliability and validity.

Interview Schedule for Children (ISC)

This was developed by Kovacs (1983) for longitudinal studies on depression. It is semi-structured interview and requires highly trained clinicians to do it. It generates DSM-III diagnoses in children 8–17 years. It takes 90–120 mts interview with the parent first, followed by 45–60 mts interview with the child. ISC has not been used by many other workers but appears to be a useful instrument for studies on depression in children.

Kiddie Schedule for Affective Disorders and Schizophrenia (K-SADS)

K-SADS (Puig-Antich and Chambers 1978) is a semi-structured, diagnostic interview schedule for 6–17 years old children. The revised version by Orvaschel and Puig-Antich in 1987 brings out DSM-III-R diagnoses. It requires a trained clinician to do the interview. The format of interviewing like a clinical interview where history of presenting symptoms and current illness is taken in detail. There is a section on symptomatology specific to the diagnosis and on Global Assessment of functioning in the child. Diagnoses of affective disorders, anxiety and schizophrenias are emphasized. Epidemiological version of K-SADS (E) is also available. The interview is more specific for selecting children with affective disorders and has been used in several drug studies. However, its usefulness as in epidemiological studies or as a wider diagnostic instrument is limited.

Connor's Rating Scales (Connors 1973)

Connor's scale was originally designed for drug studies and for measuring treatment effects. The parent form, i.e. the Connors Parent Rating Scale (Goyette et al. 1978) is a 48 item scale, covers a wide range of symptoms particularly those that are seen in ADHD and conduct disorders. This is one of the most widely used scales. There is a teacher version (Goyette et al. 1978) and an abbreviated symptom questionnaire of 10 most frequently endorsed items (Goyette et al. 1978) which measures change with treatment.

Childhood Psychopathology Measurement Schedule (CPMS)

This is an adaptation of CBCL for using it on the Indian population. This is the only one scale that has been systematically standardized studied and reported in India and also has been extensively used in numerous studies in India. Being the only one Indian scale it has been described in detail.

This scale can be used both as a screening instrument in the epidemiological studies for measuring psychopathology and for arriving at eight factorially derived diagnoses. It is applicable to children 4–14 years old. The details on its development and standardization and applicability are given in section 7.2 (pp 98–100) and the scale is given in the Appendix 2.

Mini-international Neuropsychiatric Interview (MINI)

This is a short structured clinical interview which enables researchers to make diagnoses of psychiatric disorders according to DSM-IV or ICD-10. The administration time of the interview is approximately 15 minutes and was designed for epidemiological studies and multicenter clinical trials.

Scales to Measure Specific Psychopathologies

Listed below are some scales designed to measure specific psychopathology which have reasonable psychometric properties and have been used in important studies.

- **Depression**
  - Children's Depression Inventory (Kovacs and Beck 1977)
  - Beck's Depression Inventory for Adolescents (Chiles et al. 1980)
  - Children's Depression Rating Scale (Poznanski et al. 1979)
  - John Hopkins Depression Scale (Joshi et al. 1990)
- **Mania**
  - Young Mania Rating Scale Parent Version (P-YMRS) (Gracious et al 2002)
- **Anxiety**
  - State-Trait Anxiety Inventory for Children (STAIC) (Spieberger 1973)
  - Child Assessment Schedule (Hodges et al. 1982)
  - Children's Manifest Anxiety Scale (Castenada et al. 1956)
  - Visual Analogue Scale for Anxiety (Bernstein et al. 1986)
  - Anxiety Rating Scale for Children (Erbangh 1984, 86)
- **Phobia**
  - Fear Survey Schedule for Children (Scherer and Nakamura 1968)
  - Revised Fear Survey Schedule for Children (King et al. 1989)
- **Obsessive compulsive disorder**
  - Leyton Obsessional Inventory—Child Version (Berg, et al. 1986)
  - The Yale-Brown Obsession Compulsive Scale (Goodman et al. 1989 a and b)
  - Yale Global Tice Severity Scale (Leckman et al. 1989)
- **ADHD, conduct and behaviour disorders**
  - Eyberg Child Behaviour Inventory (Eyberg and Robinson 1983)
  - The Self Control Rating Scale (Kendall and Wilcox 1979)
  - Self Reported Delinquency Scale (Elliott and Ageton 1980)
  - The Child Behaviour Rating form (Edel-brock 1985)
  - Connors Parent Rating Scale (Goyette et al. 1978)
  - Vanderbilt ADHD Diagnostic Rating Scale (Wolraich ML 2003)

- **Pervasive developmental disorders**
  - The Behaviour Rating Instrument for Autistic and Atypical Children (Rutterberg et al. 1977)
  - The Behaviour Observation Scale for Autism (Freeman et al. 1978)
  - The Childhood Autism Rating Scale (Schopler et al. 1980)
  - The Autism Diagnostic Interview (Le Couteur et al. 1989)
  - The Interview for Childhood Disorders and Schizophrenia (Russell et al. 1989)
  - Kiddie Formal Thought Disorder Rating Scale (Caplan et al. 1989).
  - Modified Checklist for Autism in Toddlers (M-CHAT R/F) (Robins, Barton and Fein 2014)
- Eating disorders
  - Eating Disorders Inventory (Garner et al. 1983)
  - Eating Attitudes Test (Garner and Garfinkel 1979)
  - Slade Anorexic Behaviour Scale (Slade 1973)
  - Anorexic Attitudes Questionnaire (Gold-berg et al. 1979)

Bayley Scales of Infant and Toddler Development Version 4 (2019) (P Balasundaram)

BSID primarily assesses the development of infants and toddlers, ages 1–42 months. Measures consist of a series of developmental play tasks and takes between 45–60 minutes to administer and derives a developmental quotient (DQ) rather than an intelligence quotient (IQ). This is an extensive formal developmental assessment tool for diagnosing developmental delays in early childhood. It assesses development in 5 domains—cognition, motor, language, socio-emotional, and adaptive behavior. BSID helps in early identification of intellectual delay and monitor progress over time.

Apart from evaluation of psychopathology, diagnosis, developmental level, a structured approach to assessment is useful for several other domains of functioning and interactions. One such important area is the degree of functional impairment due to illness, affecting school performance, peer relationships, relationships with parents and family members, social activities, etc. Assessment of functioning impairment is necessary to determine whether a set of problems constitutes a clinical condition requiring intervention and also to determine the severity of illness and its impact on child's life. Certain problems, if not associated with functioning impairment, or construed as not reaching the threshold for diagnosis can be left alone. Structured instruments to measure impairment in psychosocial functioning are available which can be used as an aid to clinical assessment and for research.

Psychosocial Functioning

Social Adjustment Inventory for Children and Adolescents (SAICA): (John et al. 1987)

This scale provides ratings for psychosocial problems of children and adolescents. It takes only 20 minutes for administration.

Children's Global Assessment Scale (CGAS) (Shaffer et al. 1983)

CGAS is a simple and reliable scale of assessment of overall functioning of a child, taking into account symptoms and psychosocial impairments. This is based on axis V of the DSM-III-R and provides a single score of global functioning. This scale is very useful and has been widely used in research.

There is one serious limitation to the use of all the above-mentioned scales, that most of these are not developed or adapted for use in India. Direct applicability of these scales to Indian population cannot be presumed and for any methodologically sound work, a preliminary testing of these scales to local population will be necessary.

While development of indigenous instruments is desirable and ideal but it is time-consuming and tedious. Therefore, one may go in for adaptation. Adaptation process includes translation, testing of reliability, validity and providing norms as the minimum requirement. Apart from CPMS which is an Indian adaptation of CBCL, no scale for assessment of psychopathology or diagnosis has been developed in India.

Recognizing this lack of indigenous instruments as a serious issue, that hampered research in child psychiatry in India, we set out to develop and adapt a minimum set of instruments for measuring broad areas such as psychopathology, temperament, parental handling and life events. These were considered as important for understanding of the common causes and correlates of psychiatric disorders in children and also suggested domains for intervention. Details of the process of development and standardization are given for each of these scales. Over the years, all the four scales namely Childhood Psychopathology Measurement Schedule (CPMS), Temperament Measurement Schedule (TMS), Parental Handling Questionnaire (PHQ), Life Events Scale for Indian Children (LESIC) have been widely used in several research projects by several authors all over the country. The norms have been revised on a large-scale epidemiological study and new norms have been provided. Details of these scales along with standardization procedure and data are included here (sub chapters 7.1, 7.2, 7.3, 7.4) for a comprehensive reference.

BIBLIOGRAPHY

1. Achenbach TM (1991a): Manual for Child Behaviour Checklist/4–18 and 1991 Profile Burlington VT: University of Vermont. Dept. of Psychiatry.
2. Achenbach TM (1991b): Manual for youth self-report. Burlington VT. University of Vermon. Dept. of Psychiatry.
3. Achenbach TM (1991c): Manual for Teacher's Report Form and 1991 Profile Burlington VT: University of Vermont. Dept of Psychiatry.
4. Achenbach TM, Edelbrock CS (1983): Manual for child behaviour checklist and revised child behaviour profile- Burlington VT, University of Vermont.
5. Achenbach TM, Edlebrock C, Howell CT (1987): Empirically based assessment of the behavioural/emotional problems of 2 and 3 years old children. Journal of Abnormal Child Psychology, 15:629–650.
6. Behar L (1977): The Preschool Behaviour Questionnaire—Journal of Abnormal Child Psychology. 5:265–275.
7. Berg CJ, Rapoport JL, Flament M (1986): The Leyton Obsessional Inventory—Child version: Journral of American Acad of Child Adolescent Psychiatry, 25:84–91.
8. Bernstein GA, Garfinkel BD, Argust GJ (1986): Visual Analogue Scale for Anxiety—Revised Presented at the Annual Meeting of the American Academy of Child and Adolescent Psychiatry. Los Angeles, CA, Oct. 1986.
9. Caplan R, Guthrie D, Fish B, et al. (1989): The Kiddie Thought Disorder Rating Scale: Clinical Assessment, reliability and validity. Journal of Amer Academy of Child and Adolescent Psychiatry. 28:408–416.
10. Castenada A, Mccandless B, Palermo D (1956): The children's form of the Manifest Anxiety Scale Child Development. 27: 317–326.
11. Chiles JA, Miller MI, Cox GB (1980): Depression in adolescent delinquent population: Archives of General Psychiatry 37, 1179–1184.
12. Connor's CK (1973): Rating scales for use in drug studies with children. Psychophaarmacol. Bull (special issue: Pharmacotherapy with children), pp 24–84.
13. Cosello AJ, Edelbrock C, Dulcan MK, et al. (1984): Development and testing of the NIMH Diagnostic Interview for Children in a clinic population. Final Report. Rockville MD, Centre for Epidemiological Studies, National Institute of Mental Health.
14. Edelbrock C (1985): Child Behaviour Rating Form: Psychopharmacology Bull 21:835–838.
15. Elliott DS, Ageton SS (1980): Reconciling Race and Class differences in self-reported and official estimates of delinquency. American Sociological Review: 45:95–110.
16. Erbangh SE (1984). Anxiety Rating for Children. Cited in Bernstein GA, Garfinkel

BD: School phobia: overlap of affective and anxiety disorders. Journal of American Academy of Child Psychiatry 1986;25: 235–241.

17. Eyeberg SM, Robinson EA (1983): Conduct problem behaviour; standardisation of a behaviour rating scale with adolescents. Journal of clinical child psychology. 12:347–354.

18. Freeman BI, Rituo ER, Guthrei D, et al. (1978). The Behaviour Observation Scale for Autism. Initial methodology data, analysis and preliminary findings on 89 children. Journal of American Academy of Child and Adolescents Psychiatry. 17:576–588.

19. Garner DM, Garfinkel PE (1979): The Eating Attitudes Test: An index of symptoms of anorexia nervosa. Psychological Medicine. 9:273–279.

20. Garner DM, Olmstead Mp, Pollivy J (1983): Development and validation of a multi-dimensional eating disorder inventory for anorexia nervosa and bulinna. International Journal of Eating Disorders. 2:15–34.

21. Goldberg SC, Halmi Ka, Eckert ED (1979): Attitudinal dimensions in anorexia nervosa. Journal of Psychiatric Research. 15:239–251.

22. Goodman R (1997): Strengths and difficulties Questionnaire (SDQ): A Research note. Journal Child Psychology. Psychiat. 38:581–586.

23. Goodman WK, Pdice LH, Rasmussen SA, et al. (1989a). The Yale-Brown Obsessive Compulsive Scale I: Development, use and reliability. Archives of General Psychiatry. 46:1006–1011.

24. Goodman WK, Price LH, Rasmussen SA, et al. I2989b). The Yale Brown Obsessive Compulsive Scale II: Validity, Archives of General Psychiatry. 46:1012–1016.

25. Goyette CH, Cvomors CK, Ulrich RF (1978): Normative data on Revised Connors Parent and Teacher Rating Scales. Journal of Abnormal Child Psychology. 6:221–236.

26. Gracious BL, Youngstrom EA, Findling RL, Calabrese JR (2002). "Discriminative validity of a parent version of the Young Mania Rating Scale". Journal of the American Academy of Child and Adolescent Psychiatry. 41 (11):1350–9. CiteSeerX 10.1.1.198.9176. doi:10.1097/00004583-200211000-00017. PMID 12410078

27. Herjanic B, Campbell N (1977): Differentiating psychiatrically disturbed children on the basis of a structured interview. Journal of Abnormal Child Psychology 5:127–134.

28. Hodges K, Kline J, Stern L, et al. (1982). The development of child assessment interview for research and clinical use. Journal of Abnormal Child Psychology 10:173–189.

29. Jellinek, M. S.; Murphy, J. M.; Robinson, J.; Feins, A.; Lamb, S.; Fenton, T. (1988). "Pediatric symptom checklist: Screening school-age children for psychosocial dysfunction". Journal of Pediatrics. 112(2): 201–209. doi:10.1016/S0022-3476(88)80056-8. PMID 3339501.

30. John K, Gammon GD, Prnsoff Ba, et al. (1987). The Social Readjustment Inventory for Children and Adolescents (SAICA): Testing of a new semi-structured interview. Journal of Amer Academy of Child and Adolescent Psychiatry. 26: 898–911.

31. Johnson JG, Harris ES, Spitzer RL, Williams JBW: The Patient Health Questionnaire for Adolescents: Validation of an instrument for the assessment of mental disorders among adolescent primary care patients. J Adolescent Health 30:196–204, 2002.

32. Joshi PTI, Cpozzoli JA, Coyle JT (1990). The John Hopkins Depression Scale: Normative data and validation in child psychiatry patients. J. American Academy of Child and Adolescent Psychiatry. 29;283–288.

33. Kapur M, Barna Das I.P., Reddy MV, Rozario J, and Uma H (2006) In Psychological assessment of children in the clinical setting U. Hirisave, A Oomen and M Kapur Eds. Publication no. 48, NIMHANS, Bangalore.

34. Kendall PC, Wilcox LE (1979). Self-control in children: Development of a rating scale. Journal of a consulting and clinical psychology. 47:1020–1029.

35. King NJ, Ollier K, Iacuone R, et al. (1989): fears of children and adolescents: a cross-sectional austiatiion study using Revised Fear Survey Schedule for Children. J Child Psychology Psychiatry, 30:775–784.

36. Kovacs M (1980). Rating scales to assess depression in school aged children. Acta Pedopsychiarica. 46:305–315.

37. Kovacs M (1985). The Interview Schedule for Children (ISC): Psychopharmacology Bull. 21:991–994.

38. Kovacs M, Beck AT (1977). An empirical clinical approach towards a definition of childhood depression. In Depression in Children. Diagnosis, Treatment and Conceptual Modesl. Eds. School terbrandt JG, Raskin A. pp 26. Raven, New York.

39. Le Conteur A, Rutter M, Lord C, et al. (1989). Autism Diagnostic Interview: A standardized investigation based instrument. Journal of Autism and Developmental Disorders. 19:363–388.

40. Leckman JF, Riddle MA, Hardin MT, et al. (1989). The Yale Global Tic Severity Scale: Initial testing of a clinician-rated scale of tic severity. J. American Academy of Child and Adolescent Psychiatry. 28:566–573.

41. Poznanski EO, Cook SC, Caroll BJ (1970). A depression rating scale for children. Pediatrics 64:442–450.

42. Palanikumar Balasundaram; Indirapriya Darshini Avulakunta (November 21, 2022). "Bayley Scales Of Infant and Toddler Development". StatPearls.

43. Richman N, Graham P (1971). A Behavioural Screening Questionnaire for use with three year old children: Preliminary findings. Journal of Child Psychology and Psychiatry. 12:5–33.

44. Robins, D. L.; Casagrande, K.; Barton, M.; Chen, C. M. A.; Dumont-Mathieu, T.; Fein, D. (2014). "Validation of the modified checklist for autism in toddlers, revised with follow-up (M-CHAT-R/F)". Pediatrics. 133 (1): 37–45. doi:10.1542/peds.2013-1813. PMC 3876182. PMID 24366990.

45. Rutter M (1967). A children's behaviour questionnaire for completion by teachers: Preliminary findings. J. Child Psychology and Psychiatry and allied professions. 8:1–1.

46. Rutter M, Tizard J and Whirmora K (1970). Education, health and behaviour. London.

47. Rutterberg BA, Kalish BI, Wenar C, et al. (1977). Behaviour Rating Instrument for Autistic and other Atypical Children (BRIAC0-Revised Edition. Philadelphia PA. Developmental Centre for Autistic Children.

48. Ryaawk AT, Bott L, Sammons C (1989). The phenomenology of schizophrenia occurring in childhood. Journal of Amer Academy of Child and Adolescent Psychiatry. 28:399–407.

49. Scherer Mw, Nakamura CY (1968). A fear survey schedule for children 9FSS-FC): a factor analytic comparison with manifest anxiety (CMAS). Behaviour Research and Therapy. 6:173–182.

50. Schopler E, Reichler RJ, De Vallis RF, et al. (1980). Towards objective classification of childhood autism: Childhood Autism Rating Scale (CARS). Journal Autism and Developmental Disorders. 10: 91–103.

51. Shaffer D, Gould MS, Busic J, et al. (1983). A Children's Global Assessment Scale (CGAS). Archives of General Psychiatry 40, 1228–1231.

52. Sheehan DV, Lecrubier Y, Sheehan KH, et al. (1998). "The Mini-International Neuropsychiatric Interview (M.I.N.I.): The development and validation of a structured diagnostic psychiatric interview for DSM-IV and ICD-10". J Clin Psychiatry. 59 (Suppl 20): 22–33. PMID 9881538

53. Speilberger CD (1973): manual for state-Trait Anxiety Inventory for children. Pale Alto CA. Consulting Psychologists Press.

54. M Wolraich, W Lambert, M Doffing, L Bickman, T Simmons, K Worley. Psychometric Properties of the Vanderbilt ADHD Diagnostic Parent Rating Scale in a Referred Population. Journal of Pediatric Psychology. 28(8): 559–568 (2003).

7.1 TEMPERAMENT MEASUREMENT SCHEDULE

CONCEPT

The general concept of temperament goes back to at least mediaeval times when it referred to a person's mental disposition based on the humoral theory of personality that linked four cardinal 'humors' to distinctive personality attributes. Hippocrates in 370 BCE theorized that there are four separate temperaments associated with four fluids (humors) of the body: Choleric temperament (yellow bile from the liver), melancholic temperament (black bile from the kidneys), sanguine temperament (red blood from the heart), and phlegmatic temperament (white phlegm from the lungs), that characterize personality traits and human behaviors.

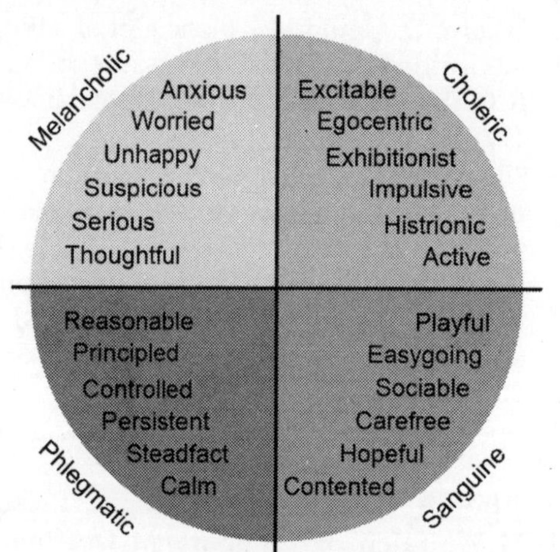

Although this humoral theory has been put to rest, the concept of temperament to day retains much of that emphasis.

Temperament is an ancient psychobiological concept with a long history but with a short scientific past. Gasell's (1937) assessed certain characteristics in children such as activity level or energy output, adaptability and liveliness of emotional texpression, and concluded that "certain fundamental traits of individuality, whatever their origin, exist early, persist late and assert themselves under varying environmental conditions".

"Temperament refers to the characteristic phenomenon of an individual's nature, including his susceptibilities to emotional stimulation, his customary strength and speed of response, the quality of his prevailing mood, and all the peculiarities of fluctuation and intensity of mood, these being phenomenon regarded as dependent on constitutional make-up, and therefore largely hereditary in origin" (Allport 1961). Temperament has been conceptualized to be broad personality dispositions rather than specific traits that one expected to differentiate during development much like intelligence.

Major credit in temperament research goes to the pioneering work of Alexander Thomas and Stella Chess who launched the famous New York Longitudinal Study (NYLS) in 1956, in order to explore in a systematic manner, the individual differences in children and their significance for the developmental process. In one of their early papers (Chess et al. 1959), they mentioned that "we believe that the data indicate that the individual specific reaction pattern appears in the first few months of life, persists in a stable form thereafter, and significantly influences the nature of the child's response to all environmental events, including child care practices."

According to Buss and Plomin (1975), temperament begins as inborn dispositions, subsequent course of which is determined by a complex interaction with the environment but the environment, in turn, is also affected by the dispositions. The social environment may be shaped by temperament initially or through feedback. There are limits to the impact of the environment, and temperament–environment mismatches can lead to strain. Thomas and Chess (1977) also emphasized on the interactionist concept of the developmental process, where temperament and environment reinforce to modify each other through a constantly evolving process of development. "Goodness of fit" results when the properties of the environment and its expectations and demands are in accord with the organism's own capacities, characteristics and style of behaving. When this consonance between organism and environment is present, optimal development in a progressive direction is possible. Conversely, poorness of fit involves discrepancies and dissonances between environmental opportunities and demands and the capacities and characteristics of the organism so that distorted development and maladaptive functioning occurs.

There is extensive and consistent data showing that infants and young children differ strikingly in their behavioural characteristics (Buss and Plomin 1975: Rutter 1977; Bates 1980; Dunn 1980; Keogh and Pullis 1980; Korner 1973). These individual characteristics influence and are influenced by caregiver behaviour in the form of interacting variables during the course of development. There is also evidence to suggest that there is a substantial temporal consistency in temperament over period of several months up to a year or so but the correlations extending over several years are generally low. Thomas and Chess (1977) concluded that temperament does not necessarily follow a consistent and linear course. It is possible that certain characteristics are more stable than others; more global levels of analysis such as measuring general difficultness, stubbornness, might capture the essence of temperament better than molecular behavioural measures (Bates 1980). Moreover, behavioural repertoire of the individual increases with development and so do the temperamental vissicitudes. Empirical findings from twin studies (Buss and Plomin 1975, Torgersen and Kringlen 1976, Matheny 1980, Goldsmith and Gottesman 1981), are reasonably consistent in showing that genetic factors play a significant part in individual variability for at least some temperamental features.

Genetic influence in no way implies fixed predetermination and immutability of temperament. Phenotypic characteristics are always a final product of the continuously evolving interaction between genes and the environment.

MEASUREMENT OF TEMPERAMENT

Recent research on temperament measurement has largely followed from the NYLS study (Thomas et al. 1963, 1968, 1970) which began with nine dimensions of temperament, derived from parental interview data described as follows:

1. *Activity level:* The extent to which a motor component exists in the child's functioning.
2. *Rhythmicity:* The predictability and/ or unpredictability in time of such functions as the sleep–wake cycle, hunger, feeding, elimination, etc.
3. *Approach or withdrawal:* The nature of response to a new stimulus (food, person, toy, etc. whether of approach or of withdrawal.
4. *Adaptability:* The ease with which the response is modified in the desired direction.
5. *Threshold of responsiveness:* The intensity level of stimulus that is necessary to evoke a discernible response, e.g. reaction to sensory stimulus, environmental object, etc.
6. *Intensity of reaction:* The energy level of response, irrespective of its quality or direction.
7. *Quality of mood:* The amount of pleasant, joyful behaviour as contrasted with unpleasant, crying, unfriendly behaviour.
8. *Distractibility:* The effectiveness of extraneous environmental stimuli in interfering with or in altering the direction of the ongoing behaviour.
9. *Attention span and persistence:* Attention span concerns the length of time a particular activity is pursued and persistence refers to the continuation of an activity in the face of obstacles.

The interview focused on the details of daily living like feeding, play, sleep, etc. and the behavioural characteristics of the child during these routine functions. Behaviour was described in factual descriptive terms with a concern not only for what the child did but how he did it. It is only by taking multiple samples of behaviour in various situations that the chance of obtaining a valid appraisal of general response dispositions or temperament attributes can be maximized (Epstein 1979). Thomas et al. (1968) found significantly high correlation between parent interview ratings and direct observation ratings.

Carey (1970, 1972); McDevitt and Carey (1978); Persson Blennow and McNeil (1979, 1980); Graham et al. (1973); Garside et al. (1975), have devised temperament measurement instrument based primarily on the 9 dimensions of Thomas and Chess which have been found to be reliable, valid as well as economical to administer and score.

Thomas and Chess (1977) themselves have developed a short questionnaire separately for parents and teachers for three to seven years age period. The final questionnaire consists of 72 items with eight for each of the nine categories on a five-point scale and is recommended for both sexes.

Most of these instruments described above have been developed for infancy, preschool and early school-age periods. Although temperament measurement for research can be done through these instruments, in the clinical practice it can be done through flexible, semi-structured parent interviews. The information thus gathered is qualitative and impressionistic but extremely useful in clinical practice.

Study of temperament in infancy and preschool period is important for studying development longitudinally and for identifying children at risk. In actual clinical practice when the children have developed psychiatric disorder, an analysis of the pathogenesis of the disorder will necessitate the study of their temperament as well. An understanding of temperamental attributes and of the parental handling patterns help in devising the intervention strategy. Therefore, it was of paramount importance that a temperament measurement tool for use in the clinical population should be developed. None of the instruments described above have been developed for use specially in the psychiatrically sick population of children. Moreover, the maximum age limit to which these can be used is 7 years and that too only for two of the questionnaires (McDevitt and Carey 1978, Thomas and Chess 1977).

All these questionnaires were developed in different language and cultural contexts. Main problems in the cross-cultural application of the questionnaires lie in:
a. The situations that are used to measure various temperament variables are often not identical;
b. Functional equivalence of concepts and language is to be kept in mind as norms are not applicable across cultures.

With regard to the cross-cultural applicability, Persson-Blennow and McNeil (1979) commenting on their questionnaire for measurement of temperament in six-month old infants emphasized that "the questionnaire and its norms were developed within the current language and child rearing contexts. A translated form of a questionnaire and its norms are thus not necessarily automatically appropriate for use outside Sweden and their applicability must be determined before eventual use in other cultural or language contexts".

Therefore, the need for development of a temperament measurement tool for use in India was evident because none such instrument existed in the country and the other tools neither in their existing form nor their translated versions could be applicable to Indian population. Moreover, self-administered questionnaires of Carey (1970), McDevitt and Carey (1978), Thomas and Chess (1977), Persson-Blennow and McNeil

(1979, 1980) could not be administered to the illiterate segments of Indian population. It was necessary to develop a temperament measurement tool in the local language to be administered in the form of an interview schedule, keeping in mind the relevant situations of measurement applicable to the Indian culture.

TEMPERAMENT MEASUREMENT SCHEDULE

Development and Standardization

A temperament measurement schedule for children was developed and standardized for use in India. Questions in simple Hindi and English were devised from the published descriptions of behaviour associated with each of the nine dimensions of Thomas et al. (1963, 1968) and also with some help from Temperament Characteristics Schedule of Graham et al. (1973) and from authors own clinical experience taking behavioural items considered logically consistent with the category definitions. Since the direct and rigid translation in Hindi of the scales/ questionnaires available would not be applicable, the questions were framed in simple Hindi keeping the basic concepts in mind. Standardization method has been reported in detail elsewhere (Malhotra and Randhawa 1982).

The final form of the temperament measurement schedule comprises 45 items (five items in each of the nine variables) rated on a five-point scale. Definitions were provided for the two extreme scores 1 and 5, with a midpoint at 3. Scores lesser than 3 were in the negative direction and greater than 3 on the positive direction for the intensity and the frequency of the behaviour measured by each item, e.g. low score on activity level meant a less active child and vice versa. Mean scores for each of the variables were computed by dividing the total score by 5. The TMS is a bilingual scale with items in both Hindi and English with the scoring instructions, devised for children between 4 and 14 years of age, and for both sexes. The data was obtained on emotionally disturbed children attending the child guidance clinic for the measurement of their temperament before the onset of symptoms and on the normal children.

As part of standardization procedure, reliability exercise was carried out and the correlation values for test-retest and inter-rater reliability were +0.61 to +0.86 for various items (Malhotra 1982).

Factor analysis was carried out on the data for the separate for two groups of emotionally disturbed and normal children. Factors with eigen value greater than one were extracted using varimax rotation. Factor loading of ±0.4 or greater were taken as significant. Four factors emerged accounting for 74.47% of the total variance in the normal group and 72.14% of variance in the sick group and the two factors matrices showed similarities. All the variables had significant loading on only one factor each except rhythmicity which loaded on factor I in the normal group and on factor II in the disturbed group. All other variables loaded on the same factor in both the groups. Therefore, rhythmicity was kept as a separate independent variable in order to retain the similarity of the two-factor matrices.

As we can see from Table 7.1, the nine temperament variables were reduced to five 5 dimensions. Each of the dimension along with the assigned names have been described below. The mean scores on the constituting temperament variables are to be added to arrive at the factor scores.

Factor I: It comprises three variables: approach-withdrawal, adaptability and threshold. As each of the three variables can be scored ranging from 1 to 5, the total range of possible scores for Factor I would be 3–15 (sum total of the mean scores on the 3 variables). This factor has been named as the Sociability factor and high scores on this shows that the child is quite responsive to the environment, adjustable, adaptable, un-inhibited.

Table 7.1: Factor structure in the two groups			
Factor	**Variable**	**Factor loading emotionally disturbed**	**Factor loading normal**
1. Sociability	Approach-withdrawl	0.73	0.84
	Adaptabilty	0.85	0.85
	Threshold	0.77	0.66
2. Rhythmicity	Rhythmicity	−0.26	0.75
3. Emotionality	Mood	0.58	−0.89
	Persistence	0.64	−0.40
4. Energy	Activity	−0.79	0.68
Intensity		−0.82	0.84
5. Distractibility	Distractibility	−0.92	0.88

Factor II: This is constituted by two temperament variables, i.e. mood and persistence. The possible range of score on this factor would be 2–10. This factor has been named as emotionality. High score on this will indicate generally positive, happy mood and low score will show that the child has predominantly negative mood or variable but mostly negative mood.

Factor III: This factor has two constituent variables, i.e. activity and intensity, giving a possible range of score as 2–10. It has been named as energy. High score means more of physical as well as psychological energy exhibited in the child's behaviour and reactions and vice versa.

Factor IV: It comprises only one temperament variable, i.e. distractibility. Thus, the range of score would be 1–5. It basically denotes attention span and distractibility. High score on this variable indicates fleeting attention and high distractibility and low score points towards low distractibility and high attention.

Factor V: Rhythmicity has been retained as an independent variable. High score indicates a well-regulated child and vice versa if the score is low.

Thus finally these 5 temperament factors have been taken and treated as the independent temperament dimensions.

Two measures of validity were studied, construct validity and factorial validity

reported separately in two papers (Malhotra and Randhawa 1983 a and b), respectively.

Temperament has been found to be a valid concept applicable to Indian populations that could discriminate between the emotionally disturbed and healthy groups of children (Malhotra and Randhawa 1983 a; Malhotra, Malhotra and Randhawa 1983 b, c). Since its standardization, temperament measurement schedule (Appendix II) has been used extensively in studies on children in Indian in several centres. Temperament factors that constitute risk for Indian children differ to some extent from those described for Western children (Malhotra 1989 a) and moreover, our studies have shown that temperament is not merely a general risk factor, it poses specific risk for certain specific disorders (Malhotra 1984, Malhotra 1989 b).

Norms for the variables were revised after its application on a large representative sample of school children, of 4–14 yrs age, in the Chandigarh in 2015 and are given in Table 7.2.

Temperament measurement schedule has been used extensively in India in various researches, primarily to characterize normal children, identify children at risk for developing psychiatric disorders, or to segregate children who have disorders from those who do not. It has been found that temperament can discriminate between

Table 7.2: Population norms on temperament measurement schedule			
Temperament variable	**Mean**	**SD**	**% within ± 1SD**
Activity	3.16	0.31	10–85
Approach-withdrawal	3.31	0.39	13–85
Adaptability	3.17	0.39	10–85
Mood	3.13	0.27	13–90
Persistence	3.20	0.46	13–87
Intensity	3.16	0.44	14–89
Threshold of responsiveness	3.01	0.46	13–89
Rhythmicity	2.79	0.31	15–93
Distractibility	3.22	0.39	18–85
Temperament factors			
Emotionality	6.32	0.57	16–93
Energy	6.31	0.59	16–92
Sociability	9.45	0.94	15–88
Rhythmicity	2.79	0.31	15–93
Distractibility	3.22	0.39	18–85

emotionally disturbed and normal children (Malhotra et al. 1983 c) and based on temperament risk of developing emotional disorder can be predicted. In another study temperament was found to be a significant discriminant variable in determining the phenomenology of psychiatric disorders in children, where children with conduct disorder were found to have high energy, those with low intelligence and behaviour problems had negative emotionality and those with somatization disorders showed low distractibility (Malhotra, Varma and Verma 1986). In another study, children with conduct disorders were found to have high activity and intensity of emotional reactions, and negative mood, whereas, those with conversion disorders exhibited low distractibility (Malhotra et al. 1989 b). In a study of temperament of children with mental retardation as compared to those with normal intelligence. It was found that children with mental retardation had excess of psychopathology in them and also signs of difficult temperament in terms of low sociability, low attentivity and negative mood as compared to those

of normal IQ children, and there was positive relationship with intelligence level and positive mood (Malhotra 1990). Temperament is a significant intervening variable in determining the psychological adjustment of children with physical illness where it was found that physically sick children were psychologically maladjusted and temperament of low distractibility contributed significantly to variance in maladjustment (Malhotra and Malhotra 1990). Further, it has been found that temperament of children of addicts differed from those of normal parents in terms of being low in rhythmicity, adaptability and distractibility, also differed from general population in showing negative emotionality, withdrawal and low threshold of responsiveness (Malhotra et al 1993). Similarly, studies showed that temperament of children of mentally ill parents is differs from those of normal parents (Malhotra and Kaur 1997); and temperament of children of alcoholic fathers differs from that of non-alcoholic fathers (Sharma et al. 1997). Assessing temperament of children in routine psychiatric practice has a very significant clinical relevance as it provides an explanatory framework to understanding the risk and pathogenetic mechanisms, so relevant for planning interventions and prevention.

BIBLIOGRAPHY

1. Allport GW. (1961). European and American Theories of Personality. In David HP, Von Bracken H (Eds.) Perspectives in Personality theory, pp324, Basic Books, New York.

2. Bates JE (1980). The concept of difficult temperament. Merril-Palmer Quarterly, 26 (4), 299–319.

3. Buss AH, Pulmin, R. (1975). A temperament theory of personality development. New York, John Wiley and sons.

4. Carey WB, (1970). A simplified method for measuring infant temperament. Jr. Pediatrics, 77, (2) 188–194.

5. Carey WB, (1972). Clinical Applications of Infant Temperament Measurements. Jr. Pediatrics, 81, 756–758.

6. Chess S, Thomas, A., Birch, H.H. (1959). Characteristics of Individual Child's behavioural responses to environment. Am. J. Orthopsychiat, 29, 791–802.

7. Dunn J, (1980). Individual differences in temperament in Rutter, M ((Ed). Scientific foundations of developmental Psychiatry, pp 101–109. London, Heinemann Medical.

8. Epstein S, (1979). The stability of behaviour, I: On predicting most of the people much of the time. J. Pers Soc. Pstcgik. 37, 1097–1126.

9. Garside RF, Berch, H. Mcl., Scott D Chambers, S, Kolvin, I., Tweddle, EG and Barber, L.M. (1975). Dimensions of temperament in infant school children. J Child Psychol Psychiat, 16, 219–231.

10. Gessel A, (1937). Early evidences of Individuality in the Human infant. Sci Monthly 45, 217–225.

11. Goldsmith HH, Gottesman, I.I. (1981). Origins of variation in behavioural style: A longitudinal study of temperament in young twins. Child Development 52, 91–103.

12. Graham P, Rutter M, George S. (1973). Temperamental characteristics as predictors of Behaviour disorders in children. Amer. J. Orthopsychiat 43 (3), 328–339.

13. Keogh BK, Pullis ME (1980). Temperament Influences on the development of exceptional children. Adv. Spec Educ 1: 239–276.

14. Korner AF. (1973). Individual differences at birth: Implications for early experience and later development. In J.C. Westman (Ed) Individual differences in children, Wiley, New York.

15. Malhotra S, Randhawa A. (1982). A schedule for measuring temperament in children: Preliminary date on development and standardization. Indian J. Clini Psychol 9, 203–210.

16. Malhotra S, Randhawa A. (1983a). Temperament and emotional disorders of childhood; Applicability in Indian population. Child Psychiatry Quarterly 16 (2), 59–67.

17. Malhotra S, Malhotra A, Randhawa A. (1983b). Children's temperament: Factorial validity. Indian J Clini Psychol 10, 399–406.

18. Malhotra S, Malhotra A, Randhawa A. (1983c). Temperament as a discriminating variable between emotionally disturbed and normal children. Indian J Clini Psychol 10, 79–84.

19. Malhotra S. (1984). Study of temperament and its relationship with the phenomenology of childhood psychiatric disorders. Ph.D thesis submitted to Postgraduate Institute of Medical Education and Research, Chandigarh.

20. Malhotra S, Varma VK, Verma SK (1986). Temperament as determinant of phenomenology of childhood psychiatric disorders. Ind.J.Psychiat. 28(4) 263 276.

21. Malhotra S. (1990) Temperament characteristics of mentally retarded Children. Ind. J. Pediatrics 57, 213 218.

22. Malhotra S, Malhotra A. (1990) Psychological adjustment of physically sick children: relationship with temperament. Ind. Pediatrics 27 (6) 577 584.

23. Malhotra S, Basu D, Bhagat A, Malhotra A (1993). Temperament of children of addicts: A preliminary report. Journal of Hongkong College of Psychiatrists 3, 5 8.

24. Malhotra S, Kaur, R. (1997) Temperament study of children of mentally ill parents. Journal of Hongkong College of Psychiatrists 7(1). 39–45

25. Malhotra S (1988). Stability of temperament characteristics overtime. Child Psychiatry Quarterly. 21 (2), 43–49.

26. Malhotra S (1989 a). Varying risk factors and outcomes an Indian perspective. In Clinical and educational applications of temperament research. Eds. W.B. Carey and S.C. McDevitt. Pub Swets and Zeitlinger.

27. Malhotra S (1989 b). Temperament characteristics of children with conduct and conversion disorders. Indian Journal of Psychiatry 31 (2), 168–172.

28. Matheny AP. (1980). Assessment of temperament in twin children: A reconciliation between structured and naturalistic observations. In Gedda, L, et al (Eds.) Twin Research, 3, Part B. Intelligence, Personality and Development, pp 279–282. Alan, R. Liss, New York.

29. McDevitt, SC and Carey, W.B. (1978). The measurement of temperament in 3–7 year old children. Jr. Child Psychol Psychiat 19, 245-253.

30. Persson-Blennow, l, McNeil, TF (1979). A questionnaire for measurement of temperament in 6 month old infants: Development and standardization. Jr. Child Psychol Psychiat 20, 1–13.

31. Persson-Blennow L, McNeil, TF (1981). Questionnaire for measurement of temperament in 1 and 2 years old children. Development and standardisation. J Child Psychol Psychiat, 21, 37–46.

32. Rutter M (1977). Individual differences. In Rutter, M. Harsov, l (Eds.). Child Psychiatry: Modern Approaches, pp. 3–21. Oxford, Blackwell Scientific Publications.

33. Sharma, A., Malhotra, S., Raghunathan, M., Malhotra, A. (1997) A study of Event Related Potential P300 Characteristics in Children of alcoholics. Addiction Biology. 2: 431–438.

34. Thomas A. Brich, HG Hertzig, ME and Korn, S (1963). Behavioural individuality in early childhood. New York, New York University Press.

35. Thomas A, Chess A, Birch HG (1968). Temperament and Behaviour disorders in children, New York. New York University Press.

36. Thomas A, Chess S, Birch HG. (1970). The origin of personality. Scient. AM., 223, 102–109.

37. Thomas A and Chess S. (1977). Temperament and Development, New York: Brunner/Mazel.

38. Torgersen AM, Kringlen E. (1978). Genetic Aspects of temperamental differences in Infants: A study of same-sexed twins. J. American Academy of Child Psychiatry 17, 433–444.

7.2 CHILDHOOD PSYCHOPATHOLOGY MEASUREMENT SCHEDULE

One of the greatest obstacles to research in child psychiatry, addressing various issues of epidemiology, classification, etiology and treatments in India, has been the lack of well standardized reliable, culturally appropriate and valid instruments to measure psychopathology in children. Instruments available from the west are not directly applicable due to several reasons.

Assessment of child psychopathology has been approached in several different theoretical models such as projective approach, dimensional approach and target analysis approach. In keeping with the long tradition of psychoanalytic framework of child psychiatry, projective approaches were used. In addition to it being time consuming, it was found to have low validity and poor reliability in scoring and interpretation. Dimensional approach utilizing multivariate statistical analytic techniques such as factor analysis has been advocated to arrive at relatively independent, reliable and objective dimensions of behaviours from the symptom checklists. Over the years, the statistical dimensional approach has aided greatly the development of taxonomies of childhood psychiatric disorders. Moreover, lack of sufficient data on descriptions of psychopathology in children based on close clinical observations, encouraged greater reliance on statistical models. The target analysis approach, that focuses directly on target behaviour lacks conceptual basis and does not lend itself to interpretation and understanding of a vast variety of behaviours nor does it provide a classificatory scheme.

Child behaviour checklist (CBCL) by Achenbach and Edelbrock (1978, 79) has been the most extensively studied and widely used instrument all over the world. CBCL consists of 118 behaviour problem items and 20 social competence items. Behaviour problems items, on first order factor analysis yielded several factors, namely aggressive, delinquent, hyperactive, schizoid, anxious, depressed, somatic complaints and social withdrawal. These were called narrow band syndromes. On second order principal–component varimax analysis, it yielded two broad band factors labelled as internalizing and externalizing syndromes derived from all three sources of data obtained from parents, teachers and health workers.

Review of literature reveals that factor analysis has been the most popular multi-variate statistical method used to arrive at empirical classification. Despite great diversity of instruments, subjects, raters and statistical methods, empirical research have produced a number of syndromes with considerable consistency and reliability. These empirical syndromes may have been given different names by different authors but there are considerable similarities in their constellation and structures.

A comprehensive reliable and valid instrument to measure psychopathology in Indian children did not exist and was needed.

Since CBCL was found to be most comprehensive, well standardized, reliable and valid for clinic samples, CBCL was chosen for adaptation to make it suitable for Indian population in terms of language, relevance and applicability of items/symptoms, norms and cut-off scores. There was need for an interview schedule rather than for a self-administered questionnaire in order to use it on the illiterate segments of population.

ADAPTATION

Detailed procedure of adaptation and standardization has been already reported (Malhotra et al. 1988). Items from behaviour problems scale of CBCL were translated into Hindi language. Social competence scale was not used since in most parts, it was not relevant to Indian social system and moreover we were interested in assessment of psychopathology alone rather than the total evaluation of competencies or impairments. Items were recorded in a question form to make it a semi-structured interview which could be used as a guide to clinical interviews or as a self-administered questionnaire. Minor elaboration/probes can be used to elicit desired information. Some of the items that did not apply or did not score positive on initial try-outs (e.g. behaves like opposite sex, bragging and boasting) were dropped. Items (N = 75) that were marked positive in 5–95% of trial samples were retained. Scoring was done in 'yes' (score 1) or 'no' (score 0) responses.

Second order factorization of 75 items finalized after item analysis was done using varimax rotation. Eight factors emerged with eigen value greater than one and were retained, accounting for 65.11% of total variance.

Item constellation of each factor and complete scale named as Childhood Psychopathology Measurement Schedule (CPMS) is given in the appendix II.

Reliability

Test-retest and inter-rater reliability was studied. Correlation values for test-retest reliability after two weeks interval were +0.78 to +0.91, and for inter-rater reliability were +0.88 to +0.96 for various items, which were highly significant.

Validity

Two measures of validity; construct and criterion validity were studied. A group of 100 emotionally disturbed children compared with a matched control group of 100 normal healthy children had significantly higher scores on all the factors. CPMS factor scores were significantly higher than the means in the corresponding ICD-9 diagnostic categories.

There was significantly higher concordance between ICD-9 diagnostic categories

and mean scores on corresponding CPMS factors, indicating that CPMS factors had good correspondence with ICD 9 diagnoses (Malhotra et al. 1988).

A cut off score of 10 on the total CPMS gave a sensitivity rate of 82% and specificity rate of 87%.

Revised norms were derived on a much larger sample of school children, between 4–14 years of age, from the population in the city of Chandigarh and UT in 2015 and are given below.

Population Norms for Childhood Psychopathology Measurement Schedule

	Mean	SD	% within ±1 SD
Total CPMS Score	4.49	4.36	91
Factor I Low intelligence with behaviour problems	0.84	1.24	91
Factor II conduct disorder	1.48	2.28	91
Factor III Anxiety	0.49	0.79	90
Factor IV Depression	0.79	1.24	92
Factor V Psychotic symptoms	0.20	0.55	97
Factor VI Special symptoms	0.23	0.48	97
Factor VII Physical illness with emotional problems	0.31	0.56	96
Factor VIII somatization	0.53	0.78	88

In its final form, CPMS is a bilingual scale, both in Hindi and English comprises 75 items, to be rated as 'yes' (score) or 'no' (score 1), which can be used as an interview schedule or as a self-administered questionnaire or as a guide to clinical interviewing; applicable to children of both sexes in the age range of 4–14 years. Taking the cut-off score at 10 or more, CPMS can be used as a screening instrument in epidemiological studies. Total and specific factor scores can be used to quantify or categorize psychopathology as well as to measure change in clinical condition after intervention. Information can be obtained on whether the symptoms listed in CPMS were present during the past one month, or six months or any time or the most part of illness depending upon the purpose for which it is used. Informant should be parent, preferably mother or a parent surrogate.

Advantages of CPMS over CBCL include ease of administration; simplicity of scoring; applicability to a wide age range and local cultural context; availability of local norms; wider application such as for screening purpose, quantification of psychopathology and measurement of change. CPMS has been extensively used in studies in India with satisfactory results.

BIBLIOGRAPHY

1. Achenbach TM, and Edelbrock CS. (1978). The Classification of Child Psychopathology: A review and analysis of empirical efforts. Psychological Bulletin, 85 (6), 1975–1301.
2. Achenbach TM. (1979). The Child Behaviour Profile: An empirically based system for assessing children's behavioural problems and competencies. International Jr Mental Health, 7 (3–4), 24–42.
3. Achenbach TM. and Edelbrock CS (1981). Behavioural problems and competencies reported by parents or normal and disturbed children age 4 through 16. Monographs of the Society for Research in Child Development. 46, Serial No 118, Chicago, University of Chicago Press.
4. Malhotra S, Varma VK, Verma SK, Malhotra A. (1988). Childhood Psychopathology Measurement Schedule: development and standardization. Indian Journal of Psychiatry 30 (4); 325–331.

7.3 LIFE EVENTS SCALE FOR INDIAN CHILDREN

INTRODUCTION

Literature concerning life events and stress in childhood is sparse in contrast to that in adults. Classical life events approach of Holmes and Rahe (1967) was used in Coddington's Social Readjustment Rating Scale (Coddington, 1972 a and b, 1984), mainly extrapolating from relevant literature on adults. Several limitations of the life events checklist approach to study of stress in childhood have been discussed (Goodyer 1990 a and b, Rutter and Sandberg 1992). However, Coddington's Social Readjustment Rating Scale (SRRS) or its modifications (Monaghan, Robinson and Dodge 1979, Jensen et al. 1991) have been widely used.

Psychopathology in childhood has been found to be associated with many environmental factors and life events such as adverse family circumstances, maternal separation or deprivation, birth of a sibling, parental divorce, physical handicap, maternal depression. However, the impact of these events, needs to be interpreted in a particular socio-cultural context. Cultural relativity of stressful events needs to be kept in mind. The degree to which presence of these events may have affected the child's psychological functioning and behaviour may depend upon the overall or other circumstances and conditions of child's life.

Since no studies had been reported in India on stress and psychiatric disorders in children and there was no assessment measure developed for Indian population, to develop a measure of stress applicable to Indian population was considered necessary. Life Events Scale for Indian Children (LESIC) was developed and standardized by the author (Malhotra 1993). The method of adaptation is briefly described below.

Considering the cultural variations in the situations considered stressful and linguistic equivalence of items (Brown and Harris, 1986, pp 163–165), events considered stressful in Indian setting were identified and listed. Holm's and Rahe's (1967) approach of assigning weighted stress scores to events was followed. Rende and Plomin (1991) reported that parent's rating of stress is significantly higher than the child's rating of specific events and of composite stress measure.

Whether it is desirable to take children's perception or parent's perception in assessing stressfulness of events is yet unresolved. Malhotra et al (1992) did a study on the nature and extent of stress associated with psychiatric disorders in children as compared to normal children. The findings revealed that disordered children experienced as many life events in the last one year as normal children but these were of more serious nature because the corresponding stress score was significantly higher in the sick group. The finding supports the view that the nature and seriousness of events is more relevant to occurrence of psychiatric disorders rather than just the number of life events. It was also found that the sick children did not differ from normal children in terms of their stress experience prior to last one year. It supports the view that more recent happenings are more relevant than the remote ones.

ADAPTATION

Life Events Scale for Indian Children (LESIC) was developed and standardized by the author (Malhotra 1993).

British Life Event Inventory (Monaghan, Robinson and Dodge 1979), an adaptation of Coddington's SRRS (Coddington, 1972) was adapted for use on Indian population. The process of adaptation involved evaluation of the British Inventory by experienced professionals in terms of relevance of items and appropriateness of stress score, keeping in mind the Indian socio-cultural context. Few items considered not relevant were deleted (e.g. becoming a full-fledged member of a church, fathering an unwed pregnancy, pregnancy of unwed teenage sister), 15 new items were added (e.g. not being sent to school against child's wish, acquisition of television by family, physical punishment by parents, visit of relatives, etc.). Each event was assigned a stress score between 0–100 indicating the stressfulness of the event. Test-retest reliability after 3 months (0.89) and inter-rater reliability (0.99) of stress scores were very high. Rank order correlation between assigned scores and actual scores of original British Life Event Inventory items and between random scores of the modified version of the inventory at three months interval was very high (0.81 and 0.82, respectively). Final form of the scale has been called Life Events Scale for Indian Children (LESIC), given as appendix IV.

Parents of children, preferably mothers, is to be interviewed using LESIC. All the events listed in the scale are asked whether these occurred in the one year prior to the onset of psychiatric symptoms in the sick group, or any time before that. In the normal group of children, it is asked whether the event occurred during one year prior to assessment or any time before that. Care was taken to include only those events which were independent of the psychiatric disorder in them.

Total number of events (LE) and total stress score for each child was worked out. There are two time frames:

i. One year before onset of illness in sick children or one year before the assessment in healthy children; and

ii. Ever before that.

Stress scores of each event which occurred were summated to give an overall stress score (SS).

The child was further asked to qualitatively rate each event that occurred on perceived stressfulness on a 3-point scale (0-not stressful, 1-somewhat stressful, 2-very much stressful) to arrive at subjective valuation. This is called subjective stressfulness score. In addition, information regarding the age, sex, education of the child and clinical diagnosis as applicable is recorded.

In a comparative study of stress and life events in 80 psychiatrically ill and 100 normal children, it was found that sick children had higher number of life events and greater stress score. Sick children had encountered more serious life events and those in younger age range (4–7 years) had more stress and undesirable events than normal children of comparable age. Most common undesirable events in the sick group related to death, divorce, parental absence from home, serious physical illness in the child, child abuse or physical punishment, and problems related to school (Malhotra 1993). On the other hand, undesirable events in normal group of children included illness of sib or parent, not being sent to school against child's wish, which are obviously much less stressful. The findings also show that stress events have greater impact on children in younger age.

Norms for life events and stress scores were generated on a larger representative sample of school children between 4 and 14 years of age in 2015 and are given below.

Population Norms on Life Events Scale for Indian Children

	Mean	SD	% within ±1SD
No. of life events	5.73	2.02	20–90
Stress score	220.14	91.91	12–85

Finally, LESIC is a bilingual (Hindi and English) scale comprising 50 items, hierarchically arranged in increasing order of stressfulness score, to be administered to the parent of the child as the interview schedule or as a self-administered scale, that explores into the occurrence of events in the last one year or any time before that. All the events have been assigned weighted scores, which have to be summated for the events marked present to arrive at weighted stress scores. Two measures of stress are elicited, number of life events and stress score, and the two have a very high correlation (+0.92) value. Test-retest and inter-rater reliability of the scale is adequate ranging between +0.8 to +0.9. In addition, the scale also gives subjective stressfulness score.

Children with psychiatric disorders have greater stress score and more life events than those of normal children, which provided evidence for the validity of the scale.

BIBLIOGRAPHY

1. Coddington RD. (1972a). The significance of life events as etiologic factors in the diseases of children I. A survery of professionals. Journal of Psychosomatic Research, 16, 7–18.

2. Coddington RD. (1972b). The significant of life events as etiologic factors in the disease of children II. A study of normal population, Journal of Psychosomatic Research, 16, 205–213.

3. Coddington RD. (1984). Measuring the stressful-ness of a child's environment. In J.H. Humpherey (Ed). Stress in childhood (PP 3–18). New York: AMS Press.

4. Goodyer IM. (1990a). Family relationships, life events and childhood psychopathology. J Child Psychol Psychiat 31 (1), 161–192.

5. Goodyer IM. (1990b). Annnotation: recent Life Events and Psychiatric disorder in School age children. J. Child Psychol Psychiat 31 (6), 839–848.

6. Holmes TH. and Rahe RH. (1967). The social readjustment rating scale. Journal of Psychosomatic Research, 11, 213–218.

7. Jensen PS, Richters J, Ussery T, Blcedau L, Davis H. (1991). Child psychopathology and environmental influences: Discrete life events versus ongoing adversity. J. Am. Acad, Child Adolesc. Psychiatry 30 (2), 303–309.

8. Johnson JH. (1986). Life events as stressors in childhood and adolescence. Beverly Hills, CA: Sage.

9. Malhotra S (1993). Study of life stress in children with psychiatric disorders in India. Journal Hongkong College of Psychiatrists 3, 28–38.

10. Malhotra S, Kaur R, Mehra R (1992). Life events in psychiatrically sick children. Indian Journal of Psychiatry 34 (3), 222–23.

11. Monaghan JH, Robinson JO, Dodge JA. (1979). The Children's Life Events Inventory. Journal of Psychosomatic Research 23, 63–68.

12. Rutter M, Sandberg S. (1992). Psychosocial stresses: Concepts, causes and effects. European Child and Adolescent Psychiatry 1, (10), 3–13.

7.4 PARENTAL HANDLING QUESTIONNAIRE

A variety of factors influence the attachment and bonding between parents and children. These include the characteristics of the child (e.g. individual differences in attachment behaviour; characteristics of the parent or of the caretaking system (e.g. psychological and cultural influences); and the characteristics of the reciprocal, dynamic and evolving relation-ship between the child and the parent (Parker et al. 1979). Although a large number of adjectives are used to describe the various types of parenting but very few studies have been reported examining the most significant dimensions of this parent–child relationship. In a routine case work-up in child psychiatry, it is mandatory to enquire into the parental handling methods. However, in most instances this assessment is largely subjective without any clear guidelines into the content and method of eliciting valid information on the reported characteristics. Parker et al. (1979) have studied the constructs of significance in the parent–child bond through a factor analytic study and came out with two scales 'parental care' and 'overprotection' in their parental bonding instrument.

Roe and Sieglman (1963) studied the parental behaviour during childhood in several independent sample of children and adults. Factor analysis yielded 3 factors:

1. Affection and warmth *vs* coldness and rejection.

2. Casual *vs* demanding in relation to factors of strictness of regulation, intrusiveness and demand for high accomplishment and obedience.

3. Protective concern, not necessarily affectionate.

Shaefer (1965) in a similar study on children and adults found three factors: First relating to acceptance versus rejection, second involving psychological autonomy versus psychological control and third of firm control versus lax control.

Cameron (1977) studied the parental characteristics such as degree of parental conflicts, tensions, degree of warmth, protectiveness, permissiveness, degree and form of discipline employed. Cluster analysis yielded 8 parental clusters, described in that order of the amount of matrix variance assumed:

1. Parental disapproval, intolerance and rejection
2. Parental conflict regarding child rearing
3. Parental strictness versus permissiveness
4. Maternal concern and protectiveness
5. Depressed living standards
6. Limitations on the child's material support
7. Inconsistent parental discipline and
8. Large family orientation.

Parker et al. (1979) summarized that care has been identified theoretically and supported empirically by factor analytic studies, as the major parental dimension. The significance of an over-protection dimension has received little theoretical consideration despite findings from factor analytic studies. Starting from that basis, they empirically defined both dimensions 'care' and 'overprotection' and produced two scales of parental care and overprotection with acceptable levels of reliability and validity combined under the name of parental bonding instrument.

They suggested that parental contribution to bonding comprises two main source variables: One of care dimension and the second of psychological control over the child versus autonomy.

However, the parental bonding instrument devised by them has the limitations of making subjective judgement in a retrospective manner by the respondent. It has a low practical value because the individual is called upon to describe the behaviour and the attitude of his parents during his first 16 years of life. Such a study does not help in understanding the interactional process between parental handling and its effects on the psychological development of the child and leaves no scope for intervention in case of pathological handling.

Keeping in view these lacunae though basically accepting the theoretical model of Parker et al. (1979), it was thought to devise an instrument that would measure current parental handling. It was felt that a simple adaptation of their parental bonding Instrument would not have been sufficient because the items should be culturally relevant. It was also seen important that in our setting the items should elicit information on current handling patterns from the parent rather than the subject himself.

Development of Parental Handling Questionnaire

It was decided to devise items relating to three major areas of parental handling.

1. Care/emotional nurturance to include level of need gratification, emotional climate (whether positive or negative) and frequency of adult contact.
2. Psychological control versus autonomy to measure the strictness of disciplining, permissiveness in decision making and whether there is any inconsistency in the use of these measures.
3. Tolerance of deviance whether high or low, consistent or inconsistent.

Item Selection

Items were chosen from the multiple sources that included Parent Bonding Instrument (Parker et al. 1979); Home Stimulation Inventory (Caldwell 1975); Parental Interview Variables from New York Longitudinal Study of Thomas and Chess (1969) which define 8 parental clusters (reported by Cameron 1978); Parent Interview Schedule on Child Rearing Practices (Sears et al. 1957); and Parent Attitude Research Instrument (PARI) by Schaffer and Bell (1958). None of these scales individually was considered adequate for our use, though these formed important source of items. Detailed procedure of standardization has already been published (Malhotra 1990), which involved item analysis, pretesting and initial tryouts, testing reliability and validity and generating norms.

Initially 20 items were selected which through a process of second order factor analysis and initial try-outs were reduced to 14 items. These 14 items measured two parental handling variables namely care (10 items) and control (4 items) to be scored as 0, 1 and 2. Items were worded in a manner where higher scores depicted lower levels of care as well as lower level of control. Scoring on a three-point Likert scale '0' for yes response, '1' for sometimes and '2' for no (appendix) gave a possible range of scores as 0–20 for care and 0–8 for control. Care and control were largely independent dimensions with a very low correlation value of 0.13 to 0.23 in groups of normal and emotionally disturbed subjects, respectively. The scale is to be administered to the parent about him/her self, or it can be self-administered.

Reliability and Validity

Test-retest reliability after 2–4 weeks for care and control was +0.68 and 0.76, respectively. Inter-rater reliability for care and control was +0.82 and +0.66, respectively. Care and control had satisfactory factorial, construct and concurrent validity as reported earlier (Malhotra 1990). Care and control could discriminate between emotionally disturbed and normal groups of children significantly.

Norms

Norms that were generated and reported earlier (Malhotra 1990) were revised on a much larger sample of representative school population of children aged 4 to 14 years in the city of Chandigarh in 2015 and have been given below.

Population Norms for Parental Handling Questionnaire

	Mean	SD	% within ± 1SD
Care	13.06	2.80	18–91
Control	4.58	1.41	20–90

Thus, in the final form parental handling questionnaire (PHQ) measuring two dimensions of care and control which were found to have a sound theoretical basis in literature, has been found to be satisfactory tool (Appendix V). It was found that low care in younger age group of children contributed more to psychopathology in them. On the other hand, it was found that low socio-economic status families exercised high control. High control means low autonomy. In India, there is cultural difference in terms to degree of autonomy given to children. Most families prefer to be authoritarian and accord less autonomy to children as a cultural ideal. This was a consistent trend.

Parker et al. (1979) identified four clusters of parental bonding which have been depicted in the figure above. Children who receive high care and nurturance and low control or overprotection are the ones who are likely to stay healthy, whereas all the other combinations of low/high care with high or low control are pathological. It is apparent that patterns of parental handling and their potential to contribute to disorders are likely to vary across cultures and need to be studied in depth.

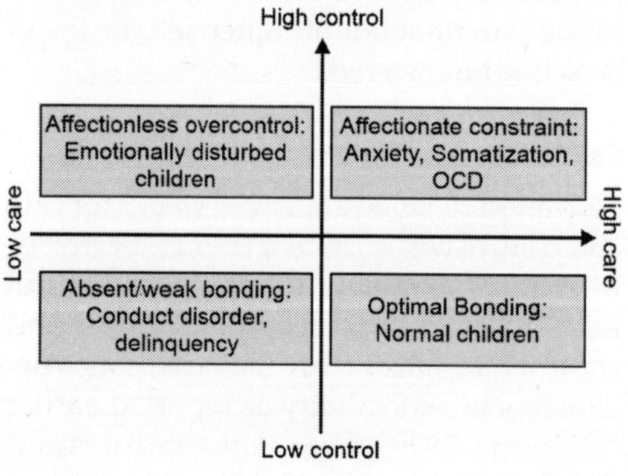

BIBLIOGRAPHY

1. Caldwell B. (1975). Home observation for measurement of environment (HOME): Instruction manual revised. (Ed.) Rittle Rock, Arkansas Centre for early development.
2. Cameron JR. (1977). Parental treatment, children's temperament and the risk of childhood behavioural problems. Amer J. Ortho, Psychiat., 47 (94): 568–576.
3. Malhotra S (1990). A Parental Handling Questionnaire. Indian Journal of Psychiatry 32 (3): 265–272.
4. Parker G, Tumpling H, Brown LB. (1979). A parental bonding instrument. Brit J. Med. Psychology, 52: 1–10.
5. Roe A. and Sieglman M (1963). A parent-child questionnaire. Child Development, 34, 355–369.
6. Schaefer ES. (1965). A configurational analysis of children's report of parent behaviour. J. Consulting Psychology, 29: 552–557.
7. Schaefer ES; Bell RQ. (1958). Development of parent attitude research instrument. Child Development, 29: 340–361.
8. Sears RR; Maccoby EE; Lewin H. (1957). Patterns of child rearing. Evanston. Illinois: Row and Paterson.

Diagnosis and Classification

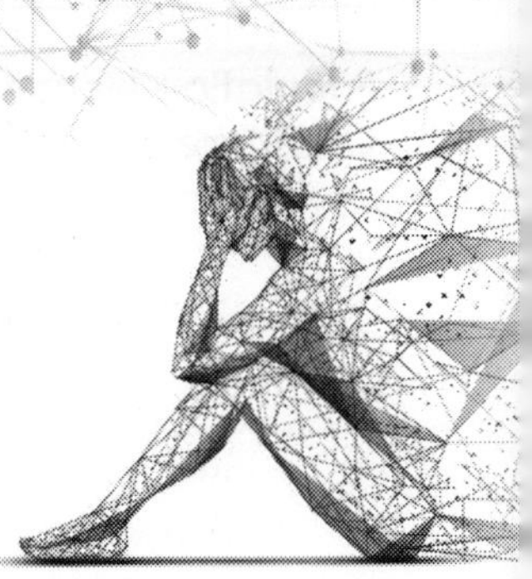

Diagnosis is a process of summarizing, labelling, organizing and categorizing information obtained through history, mental state examination and other sources of information and assessment, in a child. Diagnosis involves understanding of the case in terms of:

- Does the child have a psychiatric problem?
- What is the type or the nature of this problem?
- How does it fit in the known categories of disorders in the classification?
- What factors in the child or in the environment could have contributed to the problem?
- What are the healthy or the positive aspects of the personality, or environment of the child which are helpful in maintaining normalcy?
- Does the problem need intervention?
- What kind of intervention will be most suited?

Thus, diagnosis is not simply a process of labelling the disorder, but also involves understanding of the causes of the disorder, the probable course and outcome with or without intervention and of choosing the suitable method of intervention.

There are usually more than one, at times several diagnostic possibilities that have to be considered in a given case which is termed as the differential diagnosis. There are various reasons for possible differential diagnoses:

1. There is considerable overlap and co-occurrence of symptoms across various diagnostic categories, for example between a child can have anxiety as the main symptom but there can also be symptoms of depression, somatization, phobia, or even psychotic symptoms. In such situations one has to look at the crucial distinguishing features or take note of the predominant set of symptoms to make a diagnosis.

2. Meaning of symptoms may be different in different context. For example, school refusal could occur in a child who is scared of a harsh, punitive teacher or in whom there is significant anxiety about separation from mother. Similarly, enuresis has to be interpreted in the context of child's age. Therefore, symptoms have to be interpreted in reference to the context of the child's life and age of occurrence, and the diagnosis will differ accordingly.

3. A symptom can have several different sources of origin such as poor scholastic performance can occur due to mental sub normality or due to poor motivation in the child or due to poor attention span. One has to explore into the possibility of evidence in support of all such probable diagnoses that may be considered in any case. There is also this theoretical issue that symptoms may be non-specific manifestations of underlying pathological processes. Although our current classificatory systems such

as DSM and ICD are atheoretical, in the sense that these are based on phenomenological considerations rather than on pathological underpinnings, it cannot fully do away with issues of underlying pathology in the interpretation of symptoms. Depending upon the likely source of a symptom, its meaning and interpretation changes and so does the diagnosis.

Although traditionally it has been a standard medical teaching that one has to use the principle of parsimony in making a diagnosis in the sense, that one diagnosis that explains the entire condition of the patient should be preferred over several diagnoses to explain different aspects of illness. However, in recent years there has been a change in thinking. Depending upon meeting the required specified criteria, any number of diagnoses can be given termed as co-morbidity. These diagnoses may or may not be related to one another but would suggest presence of different clinical problems needing interventions.

Another change that occurred in approach to classification was in adopting the multi-axial system. The assumption here was that patient's condition is best described as a profile rather than by a single diagnostic label. Here, depending upon what elements are considered crucial or most relevant in evaluating the treatment needs and in guiding the treatment decisions, these are taken as separate axes or dimensions on which each case is coded. Multiaxial framework partly replaced the need for multiple category diagnoses which is found cumbersome at times. However, it did not take away entirely the system of multiple diagnoses on clinical syndrome axis. This system gave a more complete picture of the case and included such information that is important but not generally a part of diagnosis.

The process from assessment to diagnosis requires judgement and decisions at several levels. The first level of decision is to see whether there is any problem at all. Sometimes the child is referred for opinion on certain symptoms for which psychological basis may be suspected, e.g. atypical fits or seizure disorders, somatic symptoms, etc. but which on detailed evaluation may turn out to be organic or physical in nature. Occasionally, overanxious parents may bring a child to the clinic for an apparent delay in the acquisition of a milestone, e.g. absence of speech at 2 years of age, which on evaluation appears to be a normal variation in the developmental process of that child. Such a child will be considered to have no problems. Sometimes, the problems with which the child and the family have presented are minor in severity not amounting to a disorder. These fall short of the criteria for a diagnostic label and can be considered sub-threshold problems. These may be transient difficulties which get well without intervention or may represent the initial phase of a yet evolving disorder. These can be put under the diagnostic code F 99 (sub-threshold disorders). At times the index child has no problems or basic disorder but his circumstances of life or the psychosocial situation and living environment may be pathological or abnormal, e.g. child abuse, parental mental illness or alcoholism, trauma or deprivation that may constitute a serious risk or threat to the health of child and may bring the child into contact with a health facility. In such situations, the child may get positive codings on axis V, i.e. abnormal psychosocial situation which constitute the Z codes in chapter XXI of ICD-10 under the heading "Factors influencing health status and contact with health facility".

Also, there is difficulty in making distinction between normal and pathological symptoms expressions contained in diagnostic criteria. Many a times the individual's symptom itself is not inherently pathological and may be encountered in patients with mental disorder as well. Guidelines for making diagnosis and diagnostic criteria are provided in the classificatory systems like ICD or DSM.

And, there is inclusion of distress or disability to determine the diagnostic threshold as part of the diagnostic criteria. Further, assessment of severity and course of symptoms also needs to be evaluated. Multiple diagnoses whenever necessary is allowed.

If assessment provides sufficient evidence for presence of a disorder, then the second level of decision requires judgement about the prominent or the major domain(s) in which symptoms are showing manifestation and functional distress or impairment.

i. There can be predominant disturbance of emotions in which there is marked subjective distress.

ii. There can be predominant disorder of conduct and behaviour if the problems indicate disruption of family and social life.

iii. Impaired learning, memory and scholastic skills, which may be more generalized or global as in mental retardation or more specific in certain areas would suggest delays in development or specific learning disorders as the predominant diagnosis.

iv. If there is predominant problem of delay or slowness in development it can be mental retardation; and if there is deviant development or primary problems of socio-emotional communication it can be pervasive developmental disorders.

v. Sometimes, there is impaired social functioning in a selective area in a child who is basically capable of performing that function, i.e., functional capacity is preserved despite absence of function as in elective mutism.

vi. Certain symptoms may represent simply a problem of habit or behaviour such as tics, pica, etc.

Detailed analysis of all symptoms, and then delineation of the most prominent symptoms constituting a set or cluster of symptoms is done. These sets of symptoms are placed and understood in the context of psychosocial and family environment. Usually, there is overlap and often there are multiple domains of dysfunction. However, attempt is made to link their understanding as arising from one or several sources of pathology and a diagnostic label that most comprehensively describes the clinical picture is chosen. The above scheme of analysis is helpful in proceeding in a logical manner to the final diagnostic work. A form of algorithm is described in the following pages which can help the decision-making at different levels in the diagnostic process. It can be used as guide for multi-axial system of diagnosis and classification as well.

CLASSIFICATION

Classification is a way of generalizing and grouping the phenomenon into categories that share certain defined characteristics in common. It is necessary in any scientific enquiry to bring order to the vast amount of information gathered. Classification serves the purpose of reducing the complexities by organizing and arranging the information into categories according to defined criteria. As classification is a process of categorizing, classificatory categories convey basic information about the clinical features, course, outcome and treatment of the concerned disorder. It, thus, helps in understanding the basic nature of the disorder and in deciding about the management. Although each individual is unique but the disorders generally have pattern to it. By assigning a name to the disorder, i.e. "naming process", one can communicate with colleagues and with patients who feel reassured that the doctor has understood the problem. Classification is basically nosological but it may simultaneously have etiological and prognostic implications.

Classification of adult psychiatric disorders did not apply entirely to children and adolescent for several reasons. Several phenomenon and conflicts seen in childhood are a function of development which disappear with time such as separation anxiety in infancy, fears in pre-school age. Some of the concepts applicable to adults, e.g. premorbid personality did not apply to children, and many illnesses of adulthood like dementias, alcohol dependence, personality disorders, etc. did not occur in children. Moreover, there are certain disorders that typically occur or begin in childhood, for example, neurodevelopmental disorders. It has been both necessary and desirable that classification system provided categories which would suit or fulfil the needs of child patients.

Earliest classification of psychiatric disorders by Kraeplin 1896 did not cover children. Over the years, in psychiatry, two parallel systems of classification have prevailed, i.e. Diagnostic and Statistical Manual (DSM): the American System by American Psychiatric Association and the International Classification of Disease (ICD): the WHO Scheme. There have been successive revisions of DSM and ICD since early fifties from DSM-I and ICD-7 to the latest DSM-V and ICD-11 reflecting improved understanding and enhanced knowledge about disorders from time to time. Child psychiatric classification has undergone tremendous change, expansion as well as shift in these revisions.

DSM-I (1952) had only two categories specific to psychiatric disorders of childhood namely adjustment reaction and childhood schizophrenia. ICD-7 (1955) had only one diagnostic category adjustment reaction of infancy, childhood and adolescence. In DSM-II (1965) and ICD-8 (1965) there were two broad categories for children:

i. Transient situational disturbances which included, adjustment reactions of infancy, childhood, adolescence, adult and late life.

ii. Behaviour disorders of childhood several of which were defined in DSM-II and not in ICD-8, i.e. hyperkinetic reaction, withdrawing reaction, overanxious reaction, run away reaction and unsocialized aggressive reaction.

Thereafter, behaviour disorders of childhood found a separate place in classification and other categories namely childhood schizophrenia, mental retardation and special symptoms also became available. ICD-9 (1979) and DSM-III (1980) showed significant advancement in terms of inclusion of more expanded categories and definitions of various diagnostic categories. DSM-III system in general followed by DSM-III R (1987), adopted the approach of using specific diagnostic criteria which were given for childhood disorders as well. ICD-10 (1992) and DSM-IV (1994) were further elaborated to include a much larger number of diagnostic categories applicable to children and adolescents, provide a comprehensive description of the clinical concept for each category followed by differential diagnosis and diagnostic guidelines. The task here involved fitting the clinical description into the overall description of category rather than counting symptoms. Both these schemes of classification are atheoretical in approach, i.e. there are no assumptions of etiology, course or prognosis. In contrast to earlier classifications these are also non-hierarchical where symptoms do not have hierarchical value in the sense that presence of symptoms higher in hierarchical value does not preclude a diagnosis which is lower in hierarchy. Use of multiple diagnostic codes for one patient is permitted. Adult diagnostic codes have to be used wherever applicable. There have been discussions on the use of multiaxial system of classification particularly for childhood psychiatric disorders (Rutter 1969, 1975). Five axes were proposed for this purpose which are:

- *Axis I:* Clinical psychiatric syndrome
- *Axis II:* Developmental delay
- *Axis III:* IQ
- *Axis IV:* Associated medical condition
- *Axis V:* Associated adverse psychosocial situation.

It took some time to define, agree to and accept these axes and only in ICD-10, a multiaxial classification for childhood psychiatric disorders has been accepted and first published in 1996. In addition to the above five axes which are included in ICD-10 under different codes there is inclusion of a new dimension as global assessment of psycho-social disability as the sixth axis. There are some concerns about the validity of categories include in axes V and VI which are new, on which further work is needed. First four axes are same as in ICD-10 and are relatively clear.

A broad list of ICD-10 diagnostic categories applicable to children and adolescents is included here.

International Classification of Diseases—10th Revision (ICD-10): Classification of Mental and Behavioural Disorders

Chapter V of the ICD-10 relates to mental and behavioural disorder and is available in several versions for different purposes:

1. Clinical description and diagnostic guidelines for general use (CDDG).
2. Diagnostic criteria for research (ICD-10, DCR) for research
3. Version for primary health care workers
4. Multiaxial classification of child and adolescent psychiatric disorders.

ICD-10 represents a significant advancement over earlier versions of ICDs. In order to make the classification more reliable, a description of its main clinical features followed by detailed diagnostic guidelines are provided for each diagnostic category in the ICD-10 (WHO 1992).

These clinical descriptions and diagnostic guidelines are sets of signs and symptoms which can be used as a useful tool for diagnosing and classifying psychiatric disorders and for facilitating teaching and education. There is a separate version of ICD-10 to facilitate research, i.e. ICD-10 Diagnostic Criteria for Research (WHO 1993). Mental and behavioural disorders

are dealt with in section V with the alphabetical code F. There are one hundred broad diagnostic categories provided in this section (F00-99) of which a few are exclusively applicable to children (F80-89, F90-98). While the classification for adults is recommended to be tri-axial.

Six axes of classification of disorders seen in children and adolescents (WHO 1996) are described as follows. Each child should be rated on all the six axes.

Axis One: Clinical Psychiatric Syndrome

All diagnostic categories given in Chapter V of Mental and Behavioural Disorders of ICD-10 except those representing specific disorders of development (excluding PDD) and mental retardation are included in this. Since ICD-10 does not provide for a separate classification for different age groups, all the categories are in principle applicable to children as well as to adults. Thus, no separate criteria for diagnosis are given for children. There are certain diagnostic categories that are applicable specifically to children and adolescent such as Pervasive Developmental Disorders (ICD-10 code F84) and behavioural and emotional disorders with onset usually occurring in childhood and adolescence (F90-98). These are described in the list. Other diagnostic categories that apply to adults are listed for the sake of completion several of which may not apply to children.

Absence of a disorder or rating on any of the axes is coded as XX.

Axis I

Code	Category name
XX	No psychiatric disorder
	Diagnostic categories specific to children and adolescents
F84	Pervasive Developmental Disorder
F84	Childhood autism
	F84.1 Atypical autism
	F84.2 Rett's syndrome
	F84.3 Other childhood disintegrative disorder

F84.4 Overactive disorder associated with mental retardation and stereotyped movements

F84.5 Asperger's syndrome

F84.8 Other pervasive developmental disorders

F84.9 Pervasive developmental disorder, unspecified

F90–F98 Behavioural and emotional disorders with onset usually occurring in childhood or adolescence.

F90 Hyperkinetic disorders

F90.0 Disturbance of activity and attention

F90.1 Hyperkinetic conduct disorder

F90.8 Other hyperkinetic disorders

F90.9 Hyperkinetic disorder, unspecified

F91 Conduct disorders

F91.0 Conduct disorder confined to the family context

F91.1 Unsocialized conduct disorder

F91.2 Socialized conduct disorder

F91.3 Oppositional defiant disorder

F91.8 Other conduct disorders

F91.9 Conduct disorder, unspecified

F92 Mixed disorders of conduct and emotions

F92.0 Depressive conduct disorder

F92.8 Other mixed disorders of conduct and emotions

F93.9 Mixed disorder of conduct and emotions, unspecified

F93 Emotional disorders with onset specific to childhood

F93.0 Separation anxiety disorder of childhood

F93.1 Phobic anxiety disorder of childhood

F93.2 Social anxiety disorder of childhood

F93.3 Sibling rivalry disorder

F 93.8 Other childhood emotional disorders

F 93.9 Childhood emotional disorder, unspecified

F94 Disorders of social functioning with onset specific to childhood and adolescence

F94.0 Elective mutism

F94.1 Reactive attachment disorder of childhood

F94.2 Disinhibited attachment disorder of childhood

F94.8 Other childhood disorders of social functioning

F94.9 Childhood disorder of social functioning, unspecified

F95 Tic Disorders

F95.0 Transient tic disorder

F95.1 Chronic motor or vocal tic disorder

F95.2 Combined vocal and multiple motor tic disorder [de la Tourette's syndrome]

F 95.8 Other tic disorders

F 95.9 Tic disorder, unspecified

F98 Other behavioural and emotional disorders with onset usually occurring in childhood and adolescence

F98.0 Nonorganic enuresis

F98.1 Nonorganic encopresis

F98.2 Feeding disorder of infancy of childhood

F98.3 Pica of infancy and childhood

F98.4 Stereotyped movement disorders

F98.5 Stuttering (stammering)

F98.6 Cluttering

F98.8 Other specified behavioural and emotional disorders with onset usually occurring in childhood and adolescence.

F98.9 Unspecified behavioural and emotional disorders with onset usually occurring in childhood and adolescence.

Diagnostic Categories that are General and Could also be Applied to Children and Adolescents. F00–F70 and F99

F00–F09 Organic, including symptomatic, mental disorders

F00	Dementia in Alzheimer's disease
F01	Vascular dementia
F02	Dementia in other diseases classified elsewhere
F03	Dementia unspecified
F04	Organic amnesic syndrome, other than induced by alcohol or other psychoactive substance.
F05	Delirium, other than induced by alcohol and other psychoactive substances
F06	Other mental disorders due to brain damage or dysfunction or to physical disease
F07	Personality and behavioural disorders due to brain disease, damage or dysfunction
F09	Unspecified organic or symptomatic mental disorder
F10–19	Mental and behavioural disorders due to psychoactive substance use
F10	Mental and behavioural disorders due to use of alcohol
F11	Mental and behavioural disorders due to use of opioids
F12	Mental and behavioural disorders due to use of cannabinoids
F13	Mental and behavioural disorders due to use of sedatives or hypnotics
F14	Mental and behavioural disorders due to use of cocaine
F15	Mental and behavioural disorders due to use of other stimulants, including caffeine
F16	Mental and behavioural disorders due to use of hallucinogenes
F17	Mental and behavioural disorders due to use of tobacco
F18	Mental and behavioural disorders due to use of volatile solvents
F19	Mental and behavioural disorders due to multiple drug use and use of other psychoactive substances.
F20–F29	Schizophrenia, schizotypal and delusional disorders
F20	Schizophrenia
F21	Schizotypal disorder
F22	Persistent delusional disorders
F23	Acute and transient psychotic disorders
F24	Induced delusional disorder
F25	Schizoaffective disorders
F28	Other nonorganic psychotic disorders
F29	Unspecified nonorganic psychosis
F30–39	Mood (affective) disorders
F30	Manic episode
F31	Bipolar affective disorder
F32	Depressive episode
F33	Recurrent depressive disorder
F34	Persistent mood (affective) disorders
F38	Other mood (affective) disorders
F39	Unspecified mood (affective) disorder
F40–F48	Neurotic, stress-related and somatoform disorders
F40	Phobic anxiety disorders
F41	Other anxiety disorders
F42	Obsessive-compulsive disorder
F43	Reaction to severe stress, and adjustment disorders
F44	Dissociative (conversion) disorders
F45	Somatoform disorders
F48	Other neurotic disorders
F50–59	Behavioural syndromes associated with physiological disturbances and physical factors
F50	Eating disorders
F51	Nonorganic sleep disorders
F52	Sexual dysfunction, not caused by organic disorder or disease

F53	Mental and behavioural disorders associated with the puerperium, not elsewhere classified
F54	Psychological and behavioural factors associated with disorders or diseases classified elsewhere
F55	Abuse of non-dependence-producing substances
F59	Unspecified behavioural syndromes associated with physiological disturbances and physical factors
F60–69	Disorders of adult personality and behaviour
F60	Specific personality disorders
F61	Mixed and other personality disorders
F62	Enduring personality changes, not attributable to brain damage and disease
F63	Habit and impulse disorders
F64	Gender identity disorders
F65	Disorders of sexual preference
F66	Psychological and behavioural disorders associated with sexual development and orientation
F68	Other disorders of adult personality and behaviour
F69	Unspecified disorder of adult personality and behaviour
F99	Unspecified mental disorder and problems falling short of criteria for any specified mental disorder

Code	*Category name*
XX	No disorder
F80–89	Disorders of psychological development
F80	Specific developmental disorders of speech and language
F80.0	Specific speech articulation disorder
F80.1	Expressive language disorder
F80.2	Receptive language disorder
F80.3	Acquired aphasia with epilepsy (Landau-Kleffner syndrome)
F80.8	Other developmental disorders of speech and language
F80.9	Developmental disorder of speech and language, unspecified
F81	Specific developmental disorders of scholastic skills
F81.0	Specific reading disorder
F81.1	Specific spelling disorder
F81.2	Specific disorder of arithmetical skills
F81.3	Mixed disorder of scholastic skills
F81.8	Other developmental disorders of scholastic skills
F81.9	Developmental disorder of scholastic skills, unspecified
F82	Specific developmental disorder of motor function
F83	Mixed specific development disorders
F88	Other disorders of psychological development
F89	Unspecified disorder of psycho-logical development

Axis Two: Specific Disorders of Psychological Development

Conditions involving specific delay in some aspects of development such as in speech and language, motor co-ordination or learning are coded on this axis. General delay in global development as in mental retardation is not coded here. In the same manner autism is not coded on axis two, it is coded on axis one.

Axis Three: Intellectual Level

Presence of intellectual retardation whether primary or secondary and irrespective of its cause is coded on axis three. This axis basically provides description of current intellectual functioning. Subtypes are described on the basis of degree of mental sub normality into mild (IQ range 50–70), moderate (IQ 35–50), severe (IQ 20–35) and profound (IQ <20)

XX   Normal level of intelligence
F70–F79   Mental retardation.

  F70 Mild mental retardation
  F71 Moderate mental retardation
  F72 Severe mental retardation
  F73 Profound mental retardation
  F78 Other mental retardation
  F79 Unspecified mental retardation

A fourth character may be used to specify the extent of associated behavioural impairment:

F7x.0   No, or minimal, impairment of behaviour

F7x.1   Significant impairment of behaviour requiring attention or treatment

F7x.8   Other impairments of behaviour

F7x.9   Without mention of impairment of behaviour

Axis Four: Associated Medical Conditions

Non-psychiatric, medical disorders that may be present in a given case are described on this axis. Presence of a medical disease at the time of assessment (not in the past) is recorded using the same medical codes that are provided in the ICD for that disease. Concurrent presence of medical illness is recorded which does not have any implications for etiology of the associated psychiatric disorder.

Any medical disease that is associated should be coded from the general list of disorders in full ICD-10.

Code XX if there is no medical disorder associated.

Axis Five: Abnormal Psychosocial Situation

Presence of associated abnormal psychosocial situation is coded on axis five irrespective of whether these are thought to have caused psychiatric disorder or not. A wide range of possible adverse psychosocial conditions are included and are listed in the ICD-10 'Z' codes. The underlying implication is that describing the psychosocial situation would help in understandings the casual factors for psychiatric disorder and in making plan for treatment. There is no clear agreement on the time frame that should be applied to these situations which may be concurrent or in the past. The codings provided refer to life time.

Abnormal psychosocial situations listed as Z codes in Chapter XXI of the ICD-10 are included here. Separate codes are provided but original ICD-10 codes are given in parenthesis which should be referred for definitions and diagnostic guidelines.

List of Categories

00   No significant distortion or inadequacy of the psychosocial environment

1   Abnormal interfamilial relationships
  1.0 Lack of warmth in parent–child relationships (Z62.4)
  1.1 Intrafamilial discord among adults (Z63.8)
  1.2 Hostility towards or scapegoating of the child (Z62.3)
  1.3 Physical child abuse (Z61.4)
  1.4 Sexual abuse (within the family) (Z61.4)
  1.8 Other

2   Mental disorder, deviance or handicap in the child's primary support group (Z58.8)
  2.0 Parental mental disorder/deviance
  2.1 Parental handicap/disability
  2.2 Disability in sibling
  2.8 Other

3   Inadequate or distorted intra familial communication (Z63.8)

4   Abnormal qualities of upbringing
  4.0 Parental overprotection (Z62.1)
  4.1 Inadequate parental supervision/control (Z62.0)
  4.2 Experiential privation (Z62.5)
  4.3 Inappropriate parental pressure
  4.8 Other (Z62.8)

5   Abnormal immediate environment
  5.0   Institutional upbringing (Z62.2)
  5.1   Anomalous parenting situation (Z80.1)
  5.2   Isolated family (Z60.8)
  5.3   Living conditions that create a potentially hazardous psychosocial situation (Z59.1)
  5.8   Other (Z60.8)
6   Acute life events
  6.0   Loss of a love relationship (Z61.0)
  6.1   Removals from home carrying significant contextual threat (Z61.1)
  6.2   Negatively altered pattern of family relationships (Z61.2)
  6.3   Events resulting in loss of self-esteem (Z61.3)
  6.4   Sexual abuse (familial) (Z61.5)
  6.5   Personal frightening experience (Z61.7)
  6.8   Other (Z61.8)
7   Societal stressors
  7.0   Persecution or adverse discrimination (Z60.5)
  7.1   Migration or social transplantation (Z60.3)
  7.8   Other
8   Chronic interpersonal stress associated with school (Z55)/or school work (Z56)
  8.0   Discordant relationships with peers (Z55.4) (Z56.4)
  8.1   Scapegoating of child by teachers or work supervisors (Z55.4) (Z56.4)
  8.2   Unrest in the school/work situation (Z55.8) (Z56.7)
  8.8   Other
9   Stressful events/situations resulting from the child's own disorder/disability (Z72.8) (within ICD-10 these could be coded under the same categories use where these have not resulted from the child's own disorder/disability, i.e. Z62.1, Z61.1 and Z61.3, respectively).
  9.0   Institutional upbringing
  9.1   Removal from home carrying significant contextual threat
  9.2   Events resulting in loss of self-esteem
  9.3   Other

Axis Six: Global Assessment of Psychosocial Disability

This is based on the WHO Disability Assessment Schedule (WHO 1988) which has been slightly modified to make it suitable for children and adolescents. Patient's current level of functioning in the past three months in psychological social domains is recorded.

This axis refers to disability caused by psychiatric condition and not by associated medical condition. Information with regard to the child's relationships, performance in school and at home, social behaviour, coping etc. are taken into account for coding. Several categories depicting different levels of functioning are included.

Levels of Functioning

0   Superior/good social functioning
Superior/good functioning in all social domains: Good interpersonal relationships with family, peers and adults outside the family; effective coping with all social situations encountered; and good range of leisure activities and interests.

1. *Moderate social functioning:* Moderate functioning overall, but with transient or minor difficulties in one or two domains only (functioning may, or may not be superior in one or two other domains).

2. *Slight social disability:* Adequate functioning in most domains but slight difficulties in at least one or two domains (such as manifested by difficulties in friendship, constrained social activities/interests, difficulties in family relationships, less than effective social coping, or difficulties in relationships with adults outside the family).

3. *Moderate social disability:* Moderate disability in at least one or two domains.
4. *Serious social disability:* Serious disability in at least one or two domains (such as marked lack of friends, or inability to cope with new social situations, or inability to attend school).
5. *Serious and pervasive social disability:* Serious disability in most domains.
6. *Unable to function in most areas:* Needs some ongoing supervision or care from other people in order to maintain everyday functioning; unable to manage completely on own.
7. *Gross and pervasive social disability:* Sometimes unable to maintain minimal personal hygiene, or sometimes requires continued close supervision to avoid danger to self or others, or gross impairment in all means of communications.
8. *Profound and pervasive social disability:* Persistent inability to maintain personal hygiene or persistent risk of severe hurting self or others or total lack of communication.

A recent epidemiological study of adults in the United States through retrospective recall, reported that half of all lifetime cases of mental illness as per DSM-IV diagnosis start by the age of 14 and three-fourths by the age of 24 (Kessler et al. 2005). In a prospective study beginning in childhood, Jaffee et al. 2005 informed that the onset of most psychiatric disorders (apart from dementias) occurs in the first two decades of life.

DSM-IV

The fourth edition of the American psychiatric Association's Diagnostic and Statistical manual of mental Disorders on DSM-IV is meant to be a guide to clinical practice for a clinician; a system to facilitate research and communication among professionals; and an objective and reliable system of diagnosing and classifying disorders. The work groups responsible for a section of the manual on the basis of the review of empirical research data and extensive discussions and consultations with the experts and clinicians representing a wide array of perspectives and experiences recommended the diagnostic categories meeting consensus. DSM-IV is a classification of mental disorders developed for use in clinical, educational and research settings. Diagnostic criteria and categories are meant to be employed by individuals with

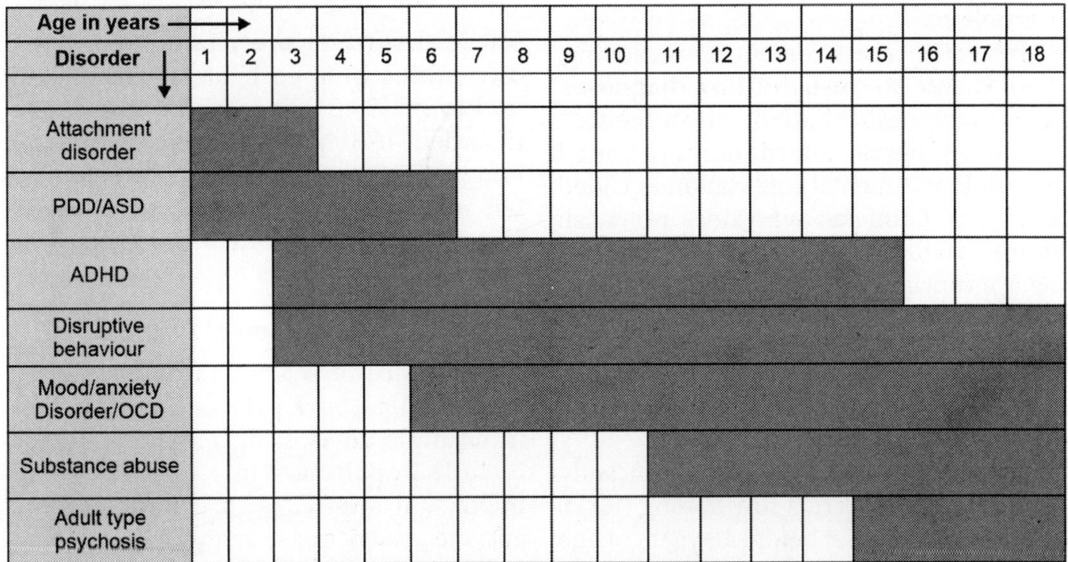

Fig. 8.1: Typical age ranges for presentation of selected disorders modified from WHO (2005)

appropriate clinical training and experience in diagnosis. DSM-IV is not meant to be applied mechanically by untrained individuals.

Although the categories describe mental disorders seen in the individuals throughout the world, it is also recognized that there may be cultural variations in symptoms and course of some disorders.

There is a broad category of disorders called "disorders" usually first diagnosed in infancy, childhood or adolescence, which covers most of the psychiatric disorders seen during these ages. There is no clear distinction between "childhood" and "adult" disorders where many so called "adult" disorders can be diagnosed in children, e.g. major depressive disorder; and many adults can have a diagnosis of disorder seen first in childhood, e.g. stuttering. DSM-IV provides a multiaxial framework for classification of disorders on five axes listed below:

- *Axis I:* Clinical disorders or other conditions that may be a focus of clinical attention.
- *Axis II:* Personality disorders and Mental retardation.
- *Axis III:* General Medical conditions
- *Axis IV:* Psychosocial and Environmental problems
- *Axis V:* Global assessment of functioning.

All disorders "usually first diagnosed in infancy, childhood or adolescence" excluding mental retardation are coded on axis I, and mental retardation is coded on axis II. Clinician who does not wish to use multiaxial format may simply list the appropriate diagnoses with principal diagnosis or reason for visit to be listed first.

The disorders included in the section are listed below:

Mental Retardation

This disorder is characterized by significantly sub average intellectual functioning (IQ 70 or below) with onset before 18 years of age with concurrent deficits or impairments in adaptive functioning.

These are coded on AXIS II and include the following categories:

Code

317   Mild mental retardation
318.0   Moderate mental retardation
318.1   Severe mental retardation
318.2   Profound mental retardation
318.9   Mental retardation, severity unspecified

Learning Disorders

These disorders are characterized by academic functioning that is substantially below that expected given the person's chronological age, measured intelligence, and age-appropriate education. The specific disorders included in this section are 315.00 Reading Disorder; 315.1 Mathematics Disorder; 315.2 Disorder of Written Expression; and 315.9 Learning Disorder Not Otherwise Specified.

Motor Skills Disorder

This includes Developmental Coordination Disorder (code 315.4) which is characterized by motor coordination that is substantially below that expected given the person's chronological age and measured intelligence.

Communication Disorders

These disorders are characterized by difficulties in speech or language and includes 315.31 Expressive Language Disorder; 315.31 Mixed Receptive Expressive Language Disorder; 315.39 Phonological Disorder; 307.0 Stuttering; and 307.9 Communication Disorder Not Otherwise Specified.

Pervasive Developmental Disorders

These disorders are characterized by severe deficits and pervasive impairment in multiple areas of development. These include impairment in reciprocal social interaction, impairment in communication, and the presence of stereotyped behaviour, interests, and activities. The specific disorders included in this section are 299.00

Autistic Disorder, 299.80 Rett's Disorder, 299.10 Childhood Disintegrative Disorder, 299.80 Asperger's Disorder, and 299.80 Pervasive developmental Disorder Not Otherwise Specified.

Attention-Deficit and Disruptive Behaviour Disorders

This section includes Attention-Deficit/Hyperactivity Disorder, which is characterized by prominent symptoms of inattention and/or hyperactivity-impulsivity. Subtypes are provided for specifying the predominant symptom presentation: 314.00: Predominantly Inattentive Type; 314.01 Predominantly Hyperactive—Impulsive Type; and 314.01 Combined Type. Also included in this section are the Disruptive Behaviour Disorders: 312.8 Conduct Disorder is characterized by a pattern of behaviour that violates the basic rights of others or major age-appropriate societal norms or rules; 313.81 Oppositional Defiant Disorder is characterized by a pattern of negativistic, hostile, and defiant behaviour. This section also includes two Not Otherwise Specified categories. 314.9 Attention-Deficit/Hyperactivity Disorder Not Otherwise Specified and 312.9 Disruptive Behaviour Disorder Not Otherwise Specified.

Feeding and Eating Disorders in Infancy or Early Childhood

These disorders are characterized by persistent disturbances in feeding and eating. The specific disorders included are 307.52 Pica; 307.53 Rumination Disorder; and 307.59 Feeding Disorder in Infancy or Early Child–hood. Anorexia Nervosa and Bulimia Nervosa are included in the "Eating Disorders" section presented later.

Tic Disorders

These disorders are characterized by vocal and/or motor tics. The specific disorders included are 307.23 Tourette's Disorder; 307.22 Chronic Motor or Vocal Tic Disorder; 307.21 Transient Tic Disorder; and 307.20 Tic Disorder Not Otherwise Specified.

Elimination Disorders

This grouping includes 307.7 Encopresis; the repeated passage of faeces into inappropriate places; and 307.6 Enuresis the repeated voiding of urine into inappropriate places.

Other Disorders of Infancy, Childhood or Adolescence

This grouping is for disorders that are not covered in the sections listed above.

- **309.21:** Separation anxiety disorder is characterized by developmentally inappropriate and excessive anxiety concerning separation from home or from those to whom the child is attached.

- **313.23:** Selective mutism is characterized by a consistent failure to speak in specific social situations despite speaking in other situations.

- **313.89:** Reactive attachment disorder of infancy or early childhood is characterized by markedly disturbed and developmentally inappropriate social relatedness that occurs in most contexts and is associated with grossly pathogenic care.

- **307.3:** Stereotypic movement disorder is characterized by repetitive, seemingly driven, and nonfunctional motor behaviour that markedly interferes with normal activities and at times may result in bodily injury.

- **313.9:** Disorder of infancy, childhood, or adolescence not otherwise specified is a residual category for coding disorders with onset in infancy, childhood, or adolescence that do not meet criteria for any specific disorder in the classification.

Children or adolescents may present with problems requiring clinical attention that are not defined as mental disorders (e.g. relational problems, problems related to abuse or neglect, bereavement, borderline intellectual functioning, academic problem, child or adolescent antisocial behaviour, identity problem). These are listed under the section "Other conditions that may be a focus of Clinical Attention".

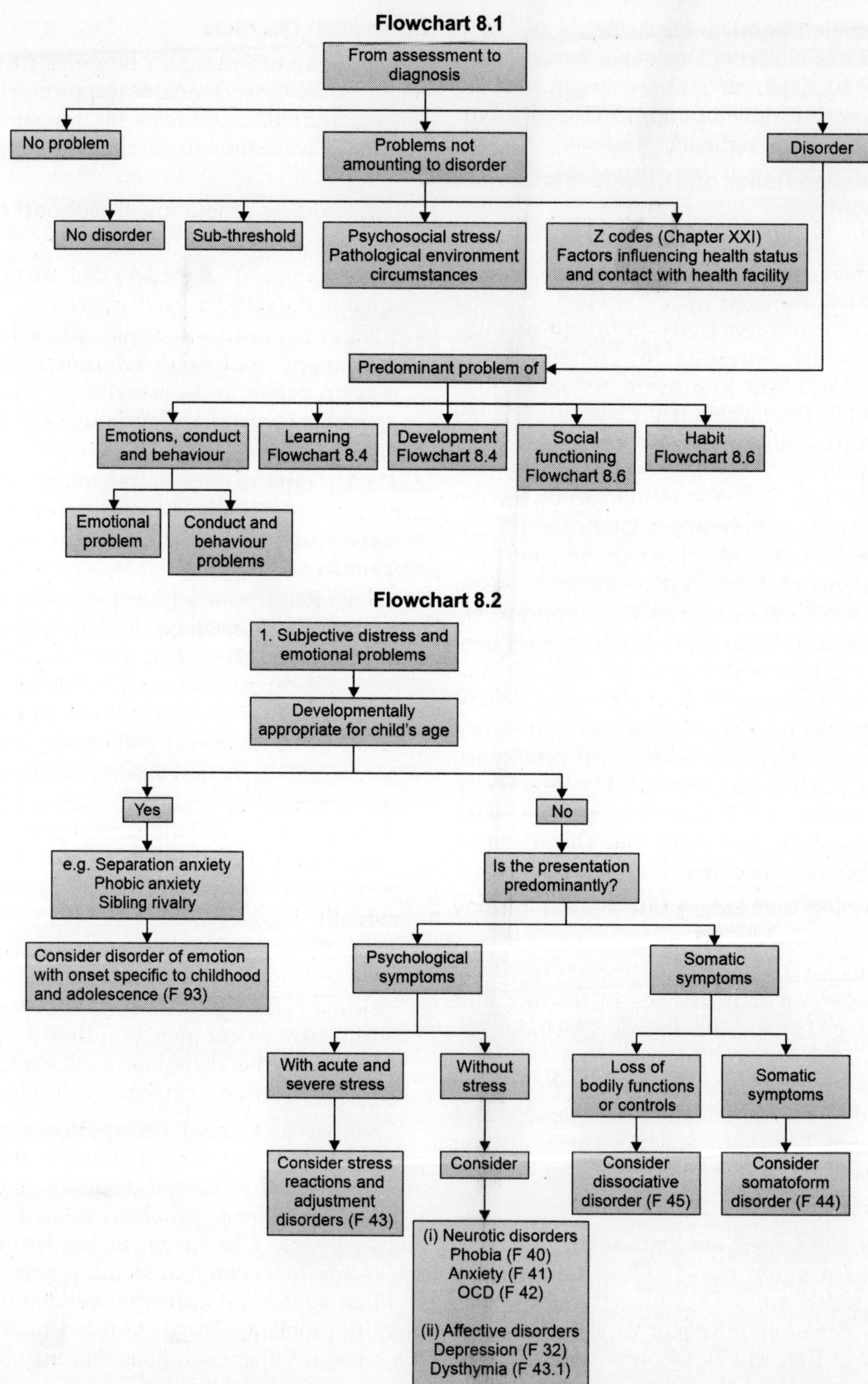
Flowchart 8.1
From assessment to diagnosis
No problem
Problems not amounting to disorder
Disorder
No disorder
Sub-threshold
Psychosocial stress/ Pathological environment circumstances
Z codes (Chapter XXI) Factors influencing health status and contact with health facility
Predominant problem of
Emotions, conduct and behaviour
Learning Flowchart 8.4
Development Flowchart 8.4
Social functioning Flowchart 8.6
Habit Flowchart 8.6
Emotional problem
Conduct and behaviour problems
Flowchart 8.2
1. Subjective distress and emotional problems
Developmentally appropriate for child's age
Yes
No
e.g. Separation anxiety Phobic anxiety Sibling rivalry
Is the presentation predominantly?
Consider disorder of emotion with onset specific to childhood and adolescence (F 93)
Psychological symptoms
Somatic symptoms
With acute and severe stress
Without stress
Loss of bodily functions or controls
Somatic symptoms
Consider stress reactions and adjustment disorders (F 43)
Consider
Consider dissociative disorder (F 45)
Consider somatoform disorder (F 44)
(i) Neurotic disorders Phobia (F 40) Anxiety (F 41) OCD (F 42)

(ii) Affective disorders Depression (F 32) Dysthymia (F 43.1)

Flowchart 8.3

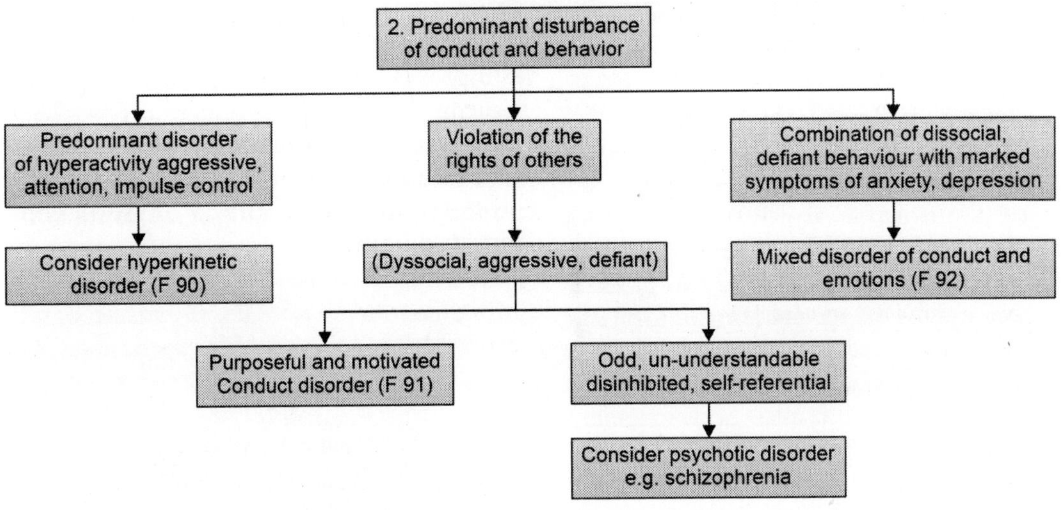

Flowchart 8.4

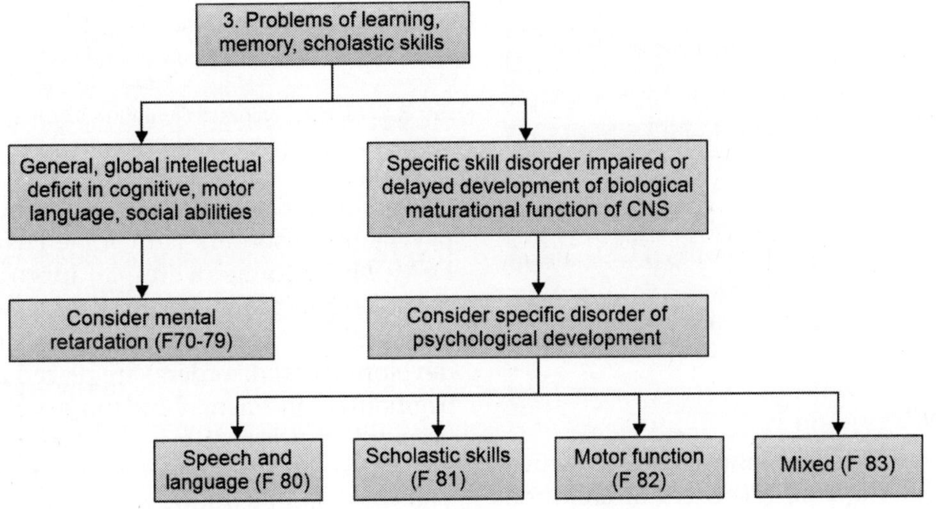

Flowchart 8.5

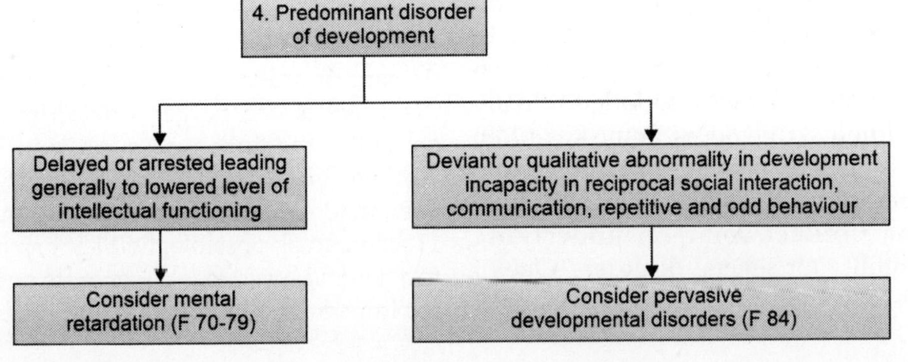

Flowchart 8.6

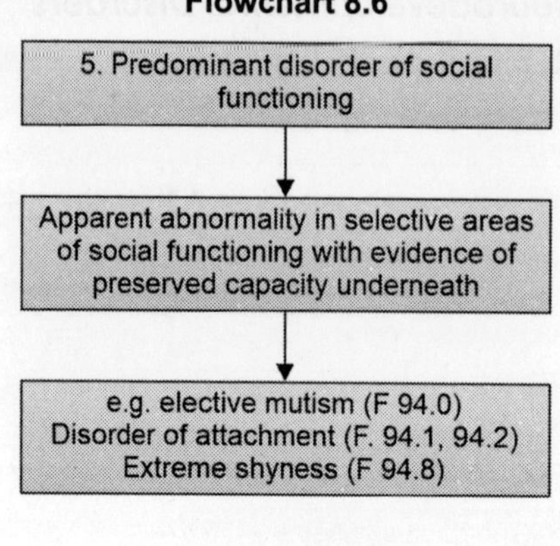

Flowchart 8.7

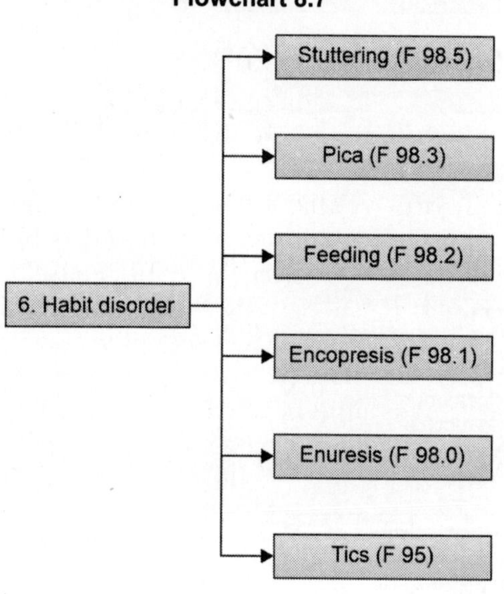

DSM-V

There has been growing acknowledgement that most mental disorders of childhood are not discreet conditions and these often do not fit completely into the diagnostic boundaries of a single disorder. These conditions are highly variable and changeable, there is considerable degree of overlap and co-occurrence of symptoms both cross-sectionally as well as longitudinally across different diagnoses. Some symptom domains such as anxiety and depression, occur across multiple diagnostic categories and may reflect common underlying vulnerability for several disorders. One of the most common psychiatric conditions of childhood is Attention Deficit Hyperactive Disorder (ADHD). In clinical practice, ADHD patients invariably also have symptoms of Conduct Disorder, Specific Learning Disorder, Intellectual Disability, Pervasive Developmental Disorder, Oppositional Defiant Disorder (See Fig. 8.2) cross-sectionally; or BPAD or Addictions longitudinally.

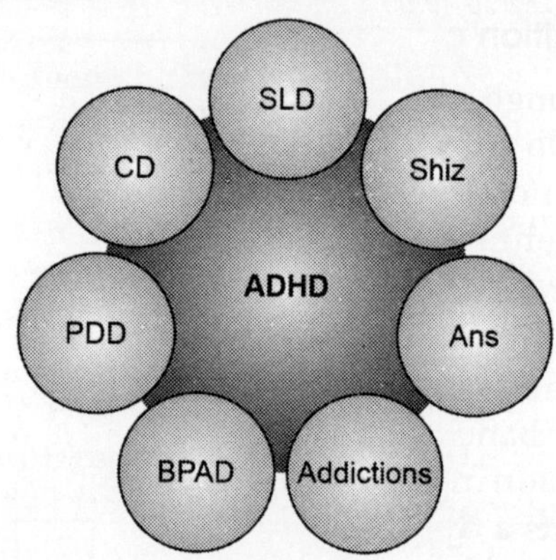

Fig. 8.2: ADHD: Hyperactivity, impulsivity, inattention

However, DSM-V (2013) continues to remain a categorical classification of psychiatric disorders with some changes. DSM-V has assumed a lifespan approach in chapter organization, where, disorders most frequently seen in childhood (e.g. neuro-developmental disorders) are placed in the beginning of the manual and those occurring later in adulthood (e.g. neurocognitive disorders) are placed later in the manual. There are subheadings on development and course providing description of how presentation may change across life span. Recent research in neuroscience and genetic linkages between psychiatric disorders has been taken into account in DSM-V. Autistic disorders, pervasive developmental disorders and asperger's disorder are all consolidated into one condition called Autism Spectrum Disorders. Efforts have been made to harmonize DSM-V with ICD 11 as much as possible. DSM-V has moved to a nonaxial system with separate notations for important psychosocial and contextual factors within the main diagnosis itself. In DSM-V, axis III is combined with axis I and II of DSM-IV, and for axis IV (for psychosocial and environmental problems), clinician should use ICD 10 Z codes. DSM IV axis V Global Assessment of Functioning (GAF) has been dropped and replaced by WHO Disability Assessment Schedule (WHODAS version 2.0).

Definition of Mental Disorder

Although no definition of mental disorders can do full justice to the entire spectrum of conditions covered under the rubric of mental disorders, DSM-V gives the following definition of mental disorder:

"A mental disorder is a syndrome characterized by clinically significant disturbance in an individual's cognition, emotion regulation, or behaviour that reflects a dysfunction in the psychological, biological or developmental processes underlying mental functioning. Mental disorders are usually associated with significant distress or disability in social, occupational or other important activities. An expectable and culturally approved response to a common stressor or loss, such as the death of a loved one, is not a mental disorder. Socially deviant behavior (e.g. political, religious or sexual) and conflicts that are primarily between the individual and society are not mental disorders unless the deviance or conflict results from a dysfunction in the individual, as described above."

DSM-V Classification (broad categories) are listed below. ICD 10 CM codes are to be used which are given preceding the category name. Disorders commonly seen in children and adolescents are only covered here to get an overview of the scheme and principle of classification and categorization of disorders. Full list of disorders can be taken from the original source (DSM-V).

A. *Neurodevelopmental Disorders*

Intellectual disability

F70	Mild
F71	Moderate
F72	Severe
F73	Profound
F88	Global developmental delay
F79	Unspecified IDD

Communication disorder

F80.9	Language disorder
F80.0	Speech sound disorder
F80.81	Childhood onset fluency disorder (stuttering)
F80.89	Social (pragmatic) communication disorder
F80.9	Unspecified communication disorder

Autism spectrum disorder

F84.0	Autism spectrum disorder

Attention deficit/hyperactivity disorder

F90.2	Combined presentation
F90.0	Predominantly inattentive type
F90.1	Predominantly hyperactive/ impulsive type
F90.8	Other specified ADHD
F90.9	Unspecified ADHD

Specific learning disorder

F81.0	With impairment in reading
F81.81	With impairment in written expression
F 81.2	With impairment in mathematics

Motor disorders

F 82	Developmental coordination disorder
F 98.4	Stereotypic movement disorder

Tic disorders

F95.2	Tourette's disorder
F95.1	Persistent (chronic) motor or vocal tic disorder
F95.0	Provisional tic disorder
F95.8	Other specified tic disorder
F95.8	Unspecified tic disorder

Other neurodevelopmental disorders

F88	Other specified neurodevelopmental disorder
F89	Unspecified neurodevelopmental disorder

B. Schizophrenia Spectrum and Other Psychotic Disorders

F21	Schizotypal disorder
F22	Delusional disorder
F23	Brief psychotic disorder
F20.81	Schizophreniform disorder
F25	Schizoaffective disorder
F06.0	and F 06.2 Psychotic disorder with other medical condition
F06.1	Catatonia
F28	Other specified schizophrenia spectrum and other psychotic conditions
F29	Unspecified schizophrenia spectrum and other psychotic conditions

C. Bipolar and Related Disorders

F31	Bipolar disorders
F34	Cyclothymic disorders
F06.33,	Bipolar and related disorders due
F06.34	to other medical condition

D. Depressive Disorders

F34.8	Disruptive mood dysregulation disorder
F32	Major depressive disorder single episode
F33	Major depressive disorder recurrent episode
F34.1	Persistent depressive disorder (dysthymia)
N94.3	Premenstrual dysphoric disorder
F06.31,	Depressive disorder due to other
F06.32	medical condition
F32.8	Other specified depressive disorder
F32.9	Unspecified depressive disorder

E. Anxiety Disorders

F93.0	Separation anxiety disorder
F94.0	Selective mutism
F40.2	Specific phobia
F40.1	Social anxiety disorder
F41.0	Panic disorder
F40.0	Agoraphobia
F41.1	Generalized anxiety disorder
F06.4	Anxiety disorder due to other medical condition
F41.8	Other specified anxiety disorder
F41.9	Unspecified anxiety disorder

F. Obsessive Compulsive and Related Disorders

F42	Obsessive compulsive disorder
F45.22	Body dysmorphic disorder
F42	Hoarding disorder
F63.3.	Trichotillomania (hair pulling disorder)
L98.1	Excoriation (skin picking) disorder
F06.8	OCD due to other medical condition

G. Trauma and Stressor-Related Disorders

F94.1	Reactive attachment disorder
F94.2	Disinhibited social engagement disorder
F43.1	Post-traumatic stress disorder
F43.0	Acute stress disorder
F43.2	Adjustment disorder
F43.8	Other specified trauma and stressor related disorder
F43.9	Unspecified trauma and stressor related disorder

H. Dissociative Disorder

F44.8	Dissociative identity disorder
F44.0	Dissociative amnesia
F44.1	Dissociative fugue
F48.1	Depersonalization/derealization Disorder
F44.8	Other specified dissociative disorder
F44.9	Unspecified dissociative disorder

I. Somatic Symptoms and Related Disorders

F45.1	Somatic symptom disorder
F45.2	Illness anxiety disorder
F44	Conversion disorder
F54	Psychological factors affecting other medical conditions
F68.10	Fictitious disorder
F45.8	Other specified somatic symptom and related disorder
F45.9	Unspecified somatic symptom and related disorder

J. Feeding and Eating Disorders

F98.3	Pica in children
F98.21	Rumination disorder
F50.8	Avoidant/restrictive food intake disorder
F50.01	Anorexia nervosa: Restrictive type
F50.02	Anorexia nervosa: Binge eating and purging type
F50.2	Bulimia nervosa
F50.8	Binge eating disorder
F50.8	Other specified
F50.9	Unspecified

K. Elimination Disorders

F 98.0	Enuresis
F 98.1	Encopresis

Other specified elimination disorder
Unspecified elimination disorder

L. Sleep–Wake Disorders

G47.000	Insomnia disorder
G47.10	Hypersomnolence disorder
G47.4	Narcolepsy
F51.3	Non-REM sleep arousal disorder: Sleep walking type
F51.4	Non-REM sleep arousal disorder: sleep terror type
F51.5	Nightmare disorder
FG47.52	Rapid eye movement sleep behaviour disorder

M. Gender Dysphoria

F64.2	Gender dysphoria in children
F64.2	Gender dysphoria in adolescents and adults
F64.8	Other specified gender dysphoria
F64.9	Unspecified gender dysphoria

N. Disruptive, Impulse-control and Conduct Disorders

F91.3	Oppositional defiant disorder
F63.81	Intermittent explosive disorder
F91	Conduct disorder
F60.2	Antisocial personality disorder
F63.1	Pyromania
F63.2	Kleptomania
F91.8	Other specified
F91.9	Unspecified

O. Substance Related and Addictive Disorders

F10	Alcohol related disorders
F15	Caffeine related disorders
F12	Cannabis related disorders
F16	Hallucinogen use disorders
F18	Inhalant use disorders
F11	Opium use disorders
F13	Sedative, hypnotic, anxiolytics use disorders
F15	Stimulant use disorders
F17	Tobacco use disorders
F19	Other or unknown substance use disorder
F63	Non-substance related disorder: Gambling disorder

In addition, there are several other conditions that may be the focus of clinical attention such as relationship problems, abuse and neglect, maltreatment, violence, occupational or educational problems, problems related to social environment, interaction with legal system etc. There are separate codes for these conditions in DSM-V.

International Classification of Diseases (ICD 11) 2022

Chapter 6 of ICD 11 refers to Mental, Behavioral and Neurodevelopmental Disorders. This chapter has 161 four-character categories. Code range starts with 0600 and is alpha numeric. Definition of mental disorder is same as in DSM-V. ICD 11 has moved towards a dimensional classification wherein most disorders are thought of as representing several interacting and underlying dimensions rather than as discreet categories. ICD 10 subtypes of schizophrenia (paranoid, hebephrenic, catatonic) are eliminated due to lack of validity. There is a major shift in understanding of personality disorders. ICD 10 had 9 specific personality disorders most of which had little validity and predictive value. In ICD 11, personality disorders are conceptualized in terms of a general dimension of severity, continuous with normal personality variation. Gender Identity disorder in ICD 10 has been reconceptualized as "gender incongruence" and is no longer considered to be a mental disorder. Gender variant behaviour and preferences alone are not sufficient for making a diagnosis. There is great degree of congruence and overlap between DSM-V and ICD 11.

ICD 11 has three versions

1. Primary care version
2. Clinical descriptions and diagnostic guidelines (CDDG)
3. Diagnostic criteria for research (DCR)

Following top level blocks are included in ICD 11:

1. Neurodevelopmental disorders (Block L1-6A0)
2. Schizophrenia or other primary psychotic disorders (BlockL1–6A2)
3. Catatonia (blockL1–6A4)
4. Mood disorders (BlockL1–6A6)
5. Anxiety or fear-related disorders (Block L1–6B0)
6. Obsessive-compulsive or related disorders (BlockL1–6B2)
7. Disorders specifically associated with stress (BlockL1–6B4)
8. Dissociative disorders (BlockL1–6B6)
9. Feeding or eating disorders (BlockL1–6B8)
10. Elimination disorders (BlockL1–6C0)
11. Disorders of bodily distress or bodily experience (BlockL1–6C2)
12. Disorders due to substance use or addictive behaviour (BlockL1–6C4)
13. Disorders due to addictive behaviours (BlockL2–6C5)
14. Impulse control disorders (BlockL1–6C7)
15. Disruptive behaviour or dissocial disorders (BlockL1–6C9)
16. Personality disorders and related traits (BlockL1–6D1)
17. Paraphilic disorders (BlockL1–6D3)
18. Factitious disorders (BlockL1–6D5)
19. Neurocognitive disorders (BlockL1–6D7)
20. Mental or behavioural disorders associated with pregnancy, childbirth and the puerperium (BlockL1–6E2)
21. Secondary mental or behavioural syndromes associated with disorders or diseases classified elsewhere (BlockL1–6E6)

There is no separation of childhood psychiatric disorders from adult psychiatric disorders in ICD 11. Disorders that occur earlier in life such as neurodevelopmental disorders, are placed first in classification; and those that occur in later life such as dementias, come later in classification. Disorders that are typically seen in children like separation anxiety disorder and selective mutism are included under the broad category of anxiety or fear related disorders. Similarly, reactive attachment disorders and disinhibited social engagement disorders typically seen in infancy are included the broad category of stress related disorders. There is no separate category of childhood onset schizophrenia. Disorders of bodily distress or bodily experience are new categories. Severity dimension is included in the diagnostic framework. Substance use disorders category is expanded with several new substances of abuse such as synthetic cannabinoids and cathinones have been added.

1. Neurodevelopmental disorders (BlockL1–6A0)
   - Disorders of intellectual development
   - Developmental speech or language disorders
   - Autism spectrum disorder
   - Developmental learning disorder
   - Developmental motor coordination disorder
   - Attention deficit hyperactivity disorder
   - Stereotyped movement disorder
   - Other specified neurodevelopmental disorders
   - Neurodevelopmental disorders, unspecified

2. Schizophrenia or other primary psychotic disorders (BlockL1–6A2)
   - Schizophrenia
   - Schizoaffective disorder
   - Schizotypal disorder
   - Acute and transient psychotic disorder
   - Delusional disorder
   - Symptomatic manifestations of primary psychotic disorders
   - Other specified schizophrenia or other primary psychotic disorders
   - Schizophrenia or other primary psychotic disorders, unspecified
3. Mood disorders (BlockL1–6A6)
   - Bipolar disorders
   - Depressive disorders
4. Anxiety or fear-related disorders (BlockL1–6B0)
   - Generalised anxiety disorder
   - Panic disorder
   - Agoraphobia
   - Specific phobia
   - Social anxiety disorder
   - Separation anxiety disorder
   - Selective mutism
   - Other specified anxiety or fear-related disorders
   - Anxiety or fear-related disorders, unspecified
5. Obsessive-compulsive or related disorders (BlockL1–6B2)
   - Obsessive-compulsive disorder
   - Body dysmorphic disorder
   - Olfactory reference disorder
   - Hypochondriasis
   - Hoarding disorder
   - Body-focused repetitive behaviour disorders: Includes trichotillomania, and excoriation disorder)
6. Disorders specifically associated with stress (BlockL1–6B4)
   - Post-traumatic stress disorder
   - Complex post-traumatic stress disorder
   - Prolonged grief disorder
   - Adjustment disorder
   - Reactive attachment disorder
   - Disinhibited social engagement disorder
   - Other specified disorders specifically associated with stress
   - Disorders specifically associated with stress, unspecified
7. Dissociative disorders (BlockL1–6B6)
   - Dissociative neurological symptom disorder
   - Dissociative amnesia
   - Trance disorder
   - Possession trance disorder
   - Dissociative identity disorder
   - Partial dissociative identity disorder
   - Depersonalization-derealization disorder
   - Other specified dissociative disorders
   - Dissociative disorders, unspecified
8. Feeding or eating disorders (BlockL1–6B8)
   - Anorexia nervosa
   - Bulimia nervosa
   - Binge eating disorder
   - Avoidant-restrictive food intake disorder
   - Pica
   - Rumination-regurgitation disorder
   - Other specified feeding or eating disorders
   - Feeding or eating disorders, unspecified
9. Elimination disorders (BlockL1–6C0)
   - Enuresis
   - Encopresis
10. Disorders of bodily distress or bodily experience (BlockL1–6C2)
    - Bodily distress disorder
    - Body integrity dysphoria
    - Other specified disorders of bodily distress or bodily experience
    - Disorders of bodily distress or bodily experience, unspecified
11. Disorders due to substance use or addictive behaviours (BlockL1–6C4)
    - Disorders due to use of alcohol
    - Disorders due to use of cannabis
    - Disorders due to use of synthetic cannabinoids

- Disorders due to use of opioids
- Disorders due to use of sedatives, hypnotics or anxiolytics
- Disorders due to use of cocaine
- Disorders due to use of stimulants including amphetamines, methamphetamine, methcathinone
- Disorders due to use of synthetic cathinones
- Disorders due to use of caffeine
- Disorders due to use of hallucinogens
- Disorders due to use of nicotine
- Disorders due to use of volatile inhalants
- Disorders due to use of MDMA or related drugs, including MDA
- Disorders due to use of dissociative drugs including ketamine and phencyclidine (PCP)
- Disorders due to use of other specified psychoactive substances, including medications
- Disorders due to use of multiple specified psychoactive substances, including medications
- Disorders due use of unknown or unspecified psychoactive substances
- Disorders due to use of non-psychoactive substances

10. Disorders due to addictive behaviours (BlockL2–6C5)
    - Gambling disorder
    - Gaming disorder
11. Impulse control disorders (BlockL1–6C7)
    - Pyromania
    - Kleptomania
    - Compulsive sexual behaviour disorder
    - Intermittent explosive disorder
    - Other specified impulse control disorders
    - Impulse control disorders, unspecified
12. Disruptive behaviour or dissocial disorders (BlockL1–6C9)
    - Oppositional defiant disorder
    - Conduct-dissocial disorder

- Other specified disruptive behaviour or dissocial disorders
- Disruptive behaviour or dissocial disorders, unspecified

13. Personality disorders and related traits (BlockL1–6D1)
    - Personality disorder
    - Prominent personality traits or patterns
14. Paraphilic disorders (BlockL1–6D3)
    - Exhibitionistic disorder
    - Voyeuristic disorder
    - Pedophilic disorder
    - Coercive sexual sadism disorder
    - Frotteuristic disorder
    - Other paraphilic disorder involving non-consenting individuals
    - Paraphilic disorder involving solitary behaviour or consenting individuals
    - Paraphilic disorders, unspecified
15. Factitious disorders (BlockL1–6D5)
    - Factitious disorder imposed on self
    - Factitious disorder imposed on another
    - Factitious disorders, unspecified
16. Neurocognitive disorders (BlockL1–6D7)
    - Delirium
    - Mild neurocognitive disorder
    - Amnestic disorder
17. Dementia (BlockL2–6D8)
    - Dementia due to alzheimer disease
    - Vascular dementia
    - Dementia due to Lewy body disease
    - Frontotemporal dementia
    - Dementia due to psychoactive substances including medications
    - Dementia due to diseases classified elsewhere
    - Behavioural or psychological disturbances in dementia
    - Other specified neurocognitive disorders
    - Neurocognitive disorders, unspecified

18. Mental or behavioural disorders associated with pregnancy, childbirth and the puerperium (BlockL1–6E2)
    - Mental or behavioural disorders associated with pregnancy, childbirth and the puerperium, without psychotic symptoms
    - Mental or behavioural disorders associated with pregnancy, childbirth or the puerperium, with psychotic symptoms
    - Mental or behavioural disorders associated with pregnancy, childbirth and the puerperium, unspecified
19. Secondary mental or behavioural syndromes associated with disorders or diseases classified elsewhere (BlockL1–6E6)
    - Secondary neurodevelopmental syndrome
    - Secondary speech or language syndrome
    - Other specified secondary neurodevelopmental syndrome
    - Secondary neurodevelopmental syndrome, unspecified
    - Secondary psychotic syndrome
    - Secondary mood syndrome
    - Secondary anxiety syndrome
    - Secondary obsessive-compulsive or related syndrome
    - Secondary dissociative syndrome
    - Secondary impulse control syndrome
    - Secondary neurocognitive syndrome
    - Secondary personality change
    - Secondary catatonia syndrome
    - Other specified secondary mental or behavioural syndrome
    - Secondary mental or behavioural syndrome, unspecified
    - Other specified mental, behavioural or neurodevelopmental disorders
    - Mental, behavioural or neurodevelopmental disorders, unspecified

With all said and done, all classificatory systems remain compromise solutions at best. Repeated modifications and alterations in underlying principles and diagnostic schemes reveals that there is no perfect method known as yet. All diagnostic categories included in DSM-V have no assumption of basis in underlying biology. At many places distinction between normal human experience and pathology is difficult to arrive or remains blurred, e.g. bereavement and depression. There is serious limitation of knowledge base in psychiatry where biological underpinnings and boundaries of various psychiatric disorders is unclear. DSM-V as well as ICD 11 still remain imperfect and far from the truth of mental disorders. Diagnostic schemes must correspond to brain mechanisms that manifest as symptoms as in Research Domain Criteria (RDoC) (Insel et al 2010). Although we are still far away from neuroscience influenced classification, ICD 11 remains a more flexible and pragmatic approach, useful in a wide variety of socio-cultural settings and global mental health.

BIBLIOGRAPHY

1. American Psychiatric Association (1994). Diagnostic and Statistical Manual of Mental Disorders. Fourth Edition. Washington DC. American Psychiatric Association.
2. American Psychiatric Association (1987). Diagnostic and Statistical manual of Mental Disorders- Third Edition - Revised. Washington DC: American Psychiatric Association.
3. American Psychiatric Association (2013). Diagnostic and Statistical Manual of Mental Disorders, Fifth Edition. Arlington, VA, American Psychiatric Association.
4. Insel T, Cuthbert B, Garvey M, Heinssen R, Pine DS, Quinn K, et al. Research domain criteria (RDoC): Toward a new classification framework for research on mental disorders. Am J Psychiatry. 2010;167:748-51.
5. Rutter M, Lebovici L, Eisenberg L, Sneznevskij AV, Sadoun R, Brooke E and Lin TY (1969). A tri-axial classification of mental disorders in childhood. Journal of Child Psychology and Psychiatry, 10, 41–61.
6. Rutter M, Shaffer D and Shepherd M (1975). An Evaluation of a Proposal for a Multiaxial Classification of Child Psychiatric Disorders.

World Health Organization Monograph. Geneva: World Health Organization.

7. World Health Organization (1988). WHO Psychiatric Disability Assessment Schedule (WHO/DAS) Geneva: World Health Organization.

8. World Health Organization (1980). Diagnostic and Statistical Manual (3rd Ed.) Washington DC American Psychiatric Association Press.

9. World Health Organization (1992). The ICD-10 Classification of Mental and Behavioural Disorders: Clinical Description and Diagnostic Guidelines. Geneva: World Health Organization.

10. World Health Organization (1993). The ICD-10 Classification of Mental and Behavioural Disorders: Diagnostic criteria for Research. Geneva: World Health Organization.

11. World Health Organization (1996). Multi-axial classification of child and adolescent psychiatric disorders: The ICD-10 classification of mental and behavioural disorders in children and adolescents with an introduction by Prof. Sir Michael Rutter. Cambridge University Press, UK.

12. World Health Organization: International Classification of Diseases 9th ed. (1977): Geneva, WHO.

13. World Health Organization: Child and Adolescent Mental Health Policies and Plans, Mental Health Policy and Service Guidance Package, 2005.

14. WHO. "International Classification of Diseases (ICD 11)". www.who.int. Archived from the original on 4 February 2022. The latest version of the ICD, ICD-11, was adopted by the 72nd World Health Assembly in 2019 and came into effect on 1 January 2022.

15. WHO Disability Assessment Schedule (2010). Measuring Health and Disability: Manual for WHO Disability Assessment Schedule (WHODAS 2.0); Eds TB Üstün, N Kostanjsek, S Chatterji, J Rehm. World Health Organization.

Management Planning

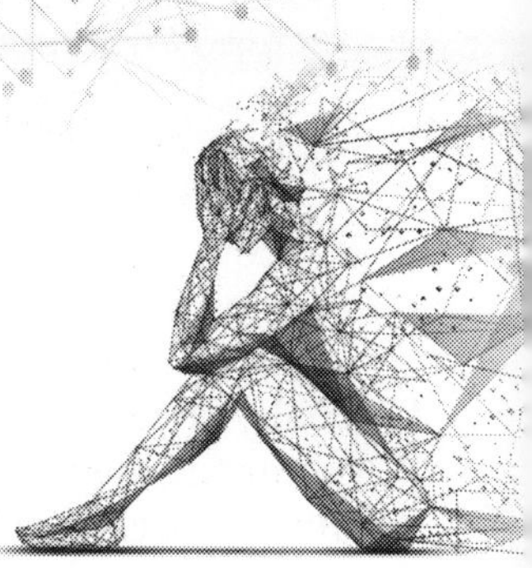

Treatment of a disorder with which the child presents to the clinic, though constitutes a large proportion of the intervention work, but that is not the whole. Management must be seen in a much broader perspective including all elements of intervention, i.e. promotive, preventive and curative, carried out at different levels and in different settings. The settings can be schools, homes, communities, and health facilities.

Prevention must address primary, secondary as well as tertiary levels of intervention, and can be instituted for the whole or a select group of population. Any treatment done for the existing disorder is called secondary prevention and it must incorporate advice for prevention of the same or other disorders in future (primary prevention) and for reduction of disability (tertiary prevention). In child psychiatry, since the treatment of current disorder in itself has preventive effects by reducing the likelihood of disorders to occur in near or distant future, there is a much greater element of primary prevention involved in the whole exercise. Universal intervention targets all children or adolescents in the given or community. Nutritional supplementation or life skills training programs for the whole school can be examples of universal intervention. The other is selective intervention where children at risk for mental health problems are targeted e.g., children with physical illness or those who live in deprivation or war zones etc. Indicated prevention targets those children who present with clinical or sub-clinical symptoms. All levels of intervention are needed from time to time. There is need for timely recognition and early management of specific vulnerabilities to reduce the burden of future morbidity.

There are a few guiding principles proposed by WHO (2005). One is integration of mental health care in general health: Mental health issues generally coexist with physical ill health and are better addressed together. It will lead to early recognition and better handling of mental health issues. It will also help to remove stigma. There should be inter sectoral coordination and access to other social, psychological, remedial, educational and occupational interventions. Child's mental health is closely linked to parental, societal, school, and community level ecosystem in which the child lives. So, the intervention plans must include the entire eco system of the child. Further, there is need to adopt a life-cycle approach where the entire life experience of the child from *in-utero* to post-natal phase should be incorporated in planning intervention. Interventions must also aim to reduce risk for mental disorder and promote resilience and effective coping.

Since treatment is linked closely with known or hypothesized aetiology of disorders, the management must address issues considered to contribute to the cause of disorders in most cases. Etiological factors contributing to the occurrence of psychiatric disorders in children generally arise from multiple sources such as biological, physical or organic, psychological and social. These should all be incorporated in the treatment plan. Thus, the treatment of necessity is multimodal and does require multidisciplinary inputs. Ideally the treatments in child psychiatry are carried out by multidisciplinary team of professionals, i.e. psychiatrist, paediatricians, psychologists, social workers, teachers. Other members of the team required are those who have specialized expertise in fields like speech therapy, art therapy, occupational therapy, remedial education, and the like.

In India, there is general dearth of psychiatrists very few of whom are involved in the care of children, and there is still lesser number of other mental health professionals to the extent that the treatment models practiced or advocated in the developed countries become inapplicable. Management approaches advocated here take into account this ground reality and represent an adaptation of the models practiced in the West. In India, we have to depend a great deal on the resource that is available in plenty, i.e. parents and families and to some extent teachers. They are, although, not trained mental health professionals, but they are, by and large, exceptionally valuable motivated, and dependable individuals who must become not only our allies in treatment but also co-therapists. Most of the treatment, therefore, depends upon the involvement of parents and other significant adults in the child's life.

In addition to lack of qualified professionals, there is also lack of sensitivity and awareness to identify psychological problems or to bring them to a service facility among population. In the absence of a psychiatric facility or due to lack of knowledge about it, most of the problems present to a general health care facility. It is often the general physician or the paediatrician who is the first point of contact and who depending upon his/her own knowledge, sensitivity and experience, also determines the need for psychiatric referral. In clinic populations, therefore, we see mostly children with neuropsychiatric or psycho-somatic problems. In schools or at the community level a wide range of emotional, behavioural and learning problems exist which may never reach a health facility. Infrequently, parents or family members directly or on advice from school teachers, bring the child over to a clinic.

In India, specialized child psychiatric services are available only in a few large metropolitan cities, varying in levels of expertise and care. An understanding of the situation about the current state of service and training in child psychiatry in India, as has been reviewed and reported (Malhotra 1998, Malhotra et al. 1992) will help in providing a perspective to the proposed treatment strategies.

Most of the treatment is and has to be done in the outpatients setting or at the community level. Inpatient treatment is available in very few places in the country.

There are no standard treatment packages. Broadly, the treatment is palliative, promotive and preventive, and not necessarily curative. General guidelines are provided to deal with most of the commonly occurring problems and disorders.

For a comprehensive treatment, one may plan intervention for diagnostic coding made on respective axes of multi-axial diagnosis. Of course, the axis I coding depicts the clinical disorder for which treatment is needed. Axes II and III point towards presence of developmental disorder or delays which may be the problem by itself or may constitute a factor of biological vulnerability that needs to be kept in mind while dealing with axis I disorders. It is essential to pay attention to the physical status of the child and deal with any associated physical disorder which is coded on axis IV. In most cases there is some disorder of psychosocial situation (Axis V) which may or may not be causally related to the clinical disorder but needs intervention.

The objectives of management of psychiatric disorders generally include:

1. Removal or minimization of symptoms
2. Enhancement of adjustment, coping and resilience
3. Reduction of impairment or handicap.
4. Promotion of optimum growth and development.

Depending upon the nature of the problems, several strategies of management can be used. Usually combinations of more than one treatment methods are used, which are targeted at the objectives of management, given above as applicable in a given case. Assessment procedure and diagnosis, particularly if done on a multiaxial framework, facilitates formulation of a management plan. Specific management in each case has to be prepared keeping in mind the nature of problems, the unique characteristics of the particular child, general background of the family and specific psychosocial and environmental factors that are relevant.

General level of functioning and psychosocial disability as coded on axis VI, measures and monitors the course and indicates rehabilitative needs.

After the diagnostic work-up, a problem-oriented analysis of the case provides the broad framework within which the case should be managed. Problems can be broadly categorized as predominantly:

- Problem of emotions causing personal distress and suffering, e.g. anxiety, depression, psychosomatic disorder, fears, dissociation, etc.
- Problems of behaviour and conduct causing disruption in family and social life, e.g. ADHD, conduct disorder, oppositional defiant disorder, delinquency or antisocial personality, etc.
- Problem of learning as in specific learning difficulties, borderline intelligence.
- Problems of development manifesting as arrested, delayed and/or deviant development as in mental retardation, pervasive or specific developmental disorders, growth retardation, etc.
- Abnormal, odd behaviour and severe disturbance of thought, affect or behaviour as in psychosis, mania stupor, aggressiveness, excitement, suicidality.
- Other problems, e.g. drug abuse.

The following description provides a method of conceptualizing, analyzing and planning treatment and gives a very broad outline of treatment approaches. A clinician must first decide on what is needed for patient and then make a specific plan on how to go about it.

Problems of Emotions

Problems of emotions are generally managed by encouraging the child to express and describe, in detail, the symptom, the emotional component associated with the symptoms, the psychosocial factors or the setting within which the problem is experienced, the events and factors that trigger or aggravate the symptoms and also those which relieve it. Although, this exercise is done for assessment, it has therapeutic value as well. This gives the child a chance not only to express and ventilate but also to focus attention on various situations and events that are closely linked to the symptoms, suggesting casual connections and thereby facilitating insight. Similar exercise undertaken with parents also serves the similar purpose and helps them to understand the symptom in the context of events. This is psycho-education and a form of supportive psychotherapy.

The next step involves making efforts to deal with specific issues in the psychosocial situation, the environment or the handling of the child, in the direction of making these suit or match the legitimate needs, desires and capabilities of the child. Here there is maximum role of parent advice, guidance and counselling and these are used extensively. In most cases the problems are often solved at this level of intervention itself.

In certain cases, where there is severe pathology in the family setting or in the social environment such as parental mental illness, alcoholism, abuse, parental discord, a systematic family therapy and treatment of parents themselves, or the environmental manipulation needs to be carried out.

Sometimes, the symptoms in the child are severe to the extent that it is difficult to engage the child in psychological therapy or the symptoms do not respond to the above measures of psychological exploration, education, parent advice, guidance and supportive psychotherapy. Medication is then used as an adjunct to psychosocial management. Depending upon the nature of symptoms and basic diagnosis, anxiolytics or antidepressants can be used. In certain instances where symptoms are deeply rooted in psychopathology or are unaffected by changes in the environment or psychosocial situation, specific symptom-oriented approach to management, i.e. behaviour therapy is instituted. Symptoms such as obsessional thoughts, rituals or behaviour repetitive behaviour, tics, habit symptoms, certain dissociative symptoms are effectively managed with behaviour therapy as the primary mode of treatment. Technique of behaviour therapy to be used is chosen after a careful behavioural analysis. It is usually a combination of therapeutic techniques that is most effective and is invariably used in the management of emotional disorders. Very young children and those who have limited repertoire of speech, play therapy is used instead of verbal psychotherapy. Details of psychotherapy, behaviour therapy or play therapy in children are given in the next chapter.

Before embarking on these formal and specific types of psychotherapies, it is important to establish therapeutic relationship. Generally, during the initial interview sessions when most of exploration into history is done, it is possible to establish a good therapeutic relationship between the child and his family and the psychiatrist. This relationship is based on faith and trust the patient has in the psychiatrist, the genuineness and concern shown by the psychiatrist; confidence in the ability of the psychiatrist to help, being non-judgmental and with an attitude of acceptance for the patient and the family despite all their difficulties and shortcomings. Sometimes there is need for an active effort on the part of the therapist to establish therapeutic relationship. In the absence of this relationship, any psychotherapy has little chance to succeed.

Parents are also dealt with using the same psychotherapeutic principles. While pointing out their shortcoming or at their contribution to problems there is need for observing great deal of sensitivity and skill in order to avoid indication of blame. Parents have be treated as partners in therapy who though are equally interested in the child's welfare but could be working at counter purposes out of ignorance, misconception, their own compulsions of personality and so on. There is need for a step-by-step correction of these attitudes imparting education, modification of their behaviour and training for a more healthy and adaptive functioning. Parent advice and counselling has both therapeutic and preventive value.

Problems of Behaviour and Conduct

Disorders that manifest with predominant symptoms (obstinacy, temper tantrum defiance, aggressiveness, impulsiveness, stealing, lying, truancy, cruelty, and the like) of behaviour and conduct require handling in multiple domains. Mild-to-moderate intensity of such symptoms can be managed with psychosocial measures alone whereas severe forms of disruptive behaviour disorders may need medication as well. Attention deficit hyperactivity disorder (ADHD) is best managed with stimulant drugs, i.e. methylphenidate, atomoxetine or pemoline. In case of non-availability or of contraindication to the use of these drugs, there are alternatives available, i.e. imipramine, buspirone, clonidine or small doses of antipsychotics (haloperidol or chlorpromazine). Medication can bring about improvement in gross symptoms so that the other psychosocial and educational inputs in therapy can take effect.

Since these symptoms indicate presence of disinhibition and dyscontrol, effort is made to structure and control the environment as well as handling methods for the child. Parents are advised to be firm, consistent, set firm limits to behaviour, and make a structured routine for the child. Use of operant conditioning principles to modify behaviour in the form of reward for good behaviour and withdrawal of reward or punishment for bad behaviour is very effective. The entire family must enter into therapy in this situation so that the whole environment can be controlled. The essential message to the child is that he cannot get away with what he does and that there are other, i.e. by behaving well, ways of achieving the desired goal. Parents are advised not to lose patience or get frustrated at the bad behaviour of the child. Child is engaged in planning of the contingency contract where the behaviour and its consequent rewards or punishments are clearly specified and agreed. The parents are advised to enforce this under supervision.

When these symptoms occur in the setting of underlying biological or organic brain disorder, as for examples, in association with birth trauma, perinatal difficulties, epilepsy, postencephlilitic sequelae, mental retardation, etc. and then medication has greater role in management. If these symptoms are seen in the setting of a pathological environment like highly restrictive or punitive parents, extreme poverty and deprivation, membership of a delinquent peer group, etc. then the predominant thrust of management is psychosocial and behavioural. Every effort is made to organize the environment in such a way that at least basic biological (food, clothes, house) and minimum psychological (care, love, education, play, security) needs of the child are met. Overall management here requires high degree of involvement and supervision by adults in whose care the child lives. These adults do well by undergoing specific training by mental health professionals.

Problems of Learning

Problems of learning and scholastic under-achievement are among the most common problems that the urban, middle class parents are concerned with. These are managed depending upon the underlying casual factors. Very often the child has low average or borderline intelligence and he/she is unable to cope with the pressure of studies. In such a situation, parent are educated and counselled to bring, down their demand and expectation to match the child's ability. Sometimes the problem is seen due to poor teaching techniques or facilities in school and poor interest and motivation in teachers. Parents are advised to either change school or arrange extra coaching to help the child. There are some children who have poor motivation to study. Many of such children come from either very rich or very poor backgrounds for whom education may have low value. There is a new trend in urban middle class who although places very high value on education but is getting increasingly attracted by the wave of consumerism and hedonism as a symbol of modernization and westernization. Children from these homes are caught in a conflict and are easily swayed by the dominant influence of adopted Western lifestyle and social media. These children lose interest in studies, and have serious problems of adjustment and relationships with parents. These problems are often seen with older children and adolescents. Management here requires family therapy in addition to individual psychotherapy for the child. Effort is made to reduce the gap between the expectations and attitudes of parents and the child. Children do well with cognitive or rational psychotherapy where they are made to see the fallacy in their own thinking and logic.

Education and learning which is the major casualty in the conflict-ridden situation, is brought back to its place of priority. Use of assertiveness training, prestige suggestion, to enhance self-esteem and self-efficacy is beneficial. For these problems, most of the therapeutic work is done with the child and the parents mainly provide support.

Another significant but ill understood and unrecognized cause of learning difficulties in the child is the group of conditions diagnosed as specific developmental disorders of scholastic skills. In these conditions there is specific difficulty in learning arithmetic, spellings, reading or writing in the child who has adequate intellectual potential to learn these skills. School-teachers as well as parents generally complain about the child as being 'careless' or 'unmotivated' rather than being incapable. Since this is a definite pathology based in biological maturational processes of the brain, these children require special or remedial education.

They require specialized methods of teaching involving, multisensory inputs, slow and systematic approach. Unfortunately, this is the area where facilities and expertise are seriously lacking in India. Even in good child psychiatry centers, not to talk of school, this facility is not available. It requires specially trained teachers who are only a handful for a vast country like India. As of now, these children remain underachievers to the great frustration and anguish of parents. The best that can be done under the prevailing circumstances is to advise parents and the child to make more effort in the direction that helps the child learn best, e.g. if he can learn better by listening or discussion rather than by silent reading then the child should

learn by reading aloud or by listening to someone. Cooperation and involvement of teachers is essential. The problem must be discussed with the teachers and strategies to help the child should be planned together. Counselling to the child and the parents help in preventing the secondary morbidity.

Problems of Development

Delayed or arrested development manifesting as mental sub normality is one of the commonest presenting problems in the clinic samples. Depending upon the degree of mental retardation and also whether it is primary or secondary, parents need to be counselled accordingly. They are given education about the nature of problems, its course and outcome, probable cause and possible intervention. They are encouraged and advised to accept the intellectual level the child has and the capabilities associated with it, and to make the best of what the child has. There is no point lamenting on what the child cannot do. Child should be helped to realize his/her full potential. Parents go through several psychological reactions themselves like guilt, anger, depression which needs to be worked through. Specific training to the child directly or through parents for teaching life and social skills is highly useful. Depending upon other associated problems like speech difficulty, behaviour problems, etc. targeted management is instituted.

Pervasive developmental disorders (PDDs) are more severe disorders involving not simple delay but also deviance in development of speech and language, social communication and certain types of behaviour problems. These are again managed by parental advice, guidance, counselling, parent training for handling of the child and for facilitating communication and language functions; specific treatment of associated problems like speech therapy for speech problems, behaviour therapy for behavioural problems; remedial education for learning difficulties. As the management of PDDs is very intensive and the progress is very slow, it is highly taxing, often frustrating for the parents as well as the therapist.

Another not so uncommon is the problem of physical growth and development, i.e., non-organic failure to thrive. As this problem is seen in families with poor education, low socioeconomic status, child neglect or abuse, the management involves family therapy and education. Parents, particularly mother needs to understand the child's nutritional needs, as well as psychological needs. Children living in abnormal situations such as in foster homes or other institutions or with foster/step parents are often victims of these problems. They need to be put in alternative care if possible. Unfortunately, in India, as we do not have many options for alternative care, we have to work with the same caretakers who are responsible for neglect. Effort is done to make them our allies in treatment.

On the whole, treatment in child psychiatry is approached not merely from the perspective of symptomatic relief, but from holistic concern aimed at managing etiological contributors in the entire eco system of the child, and fostering optimum growth and development as much as possible.

BIBLIOGRAPHY

1. Malhotra S (1992). Child Mental Health in India: Needs and Priorities. In Eds. Malhotra S, Malhotra A, Varma VK. Child Mental Health in India. Pub. Macmillan (India).

2. Malhotra S (1998). Challenges for providing mental health services for children and adolescents in India. In Designing Mental Health Services and Systems for children and adolescents: A shrewd investment. Eds. J Gerald, Young P. Ferrari. Pub. Brunner Mazel USA.

3. World Health Organization (2005). Mental Health Policy, Plans and Programme. Geneva: WHO.

Treatments

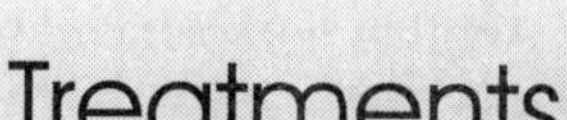

INTRODUCTION

Children and adolescents constitute about one-third of the world's population and they are particularly vulnerable to develop mental illness. Scientific studies of "normal" development carried out painstakingly for over 100 years, spanning through the late 19th and most of the 20th century, provided a firm foundation and invaluable knowledge about psychological development and notions of "normalcy" in children. Further, this knowledge has created a database to show that psychopathology is developmental in nature which in other words means that psychopathology is rooted in the course of development of the brain involving both nature and nurture.

Studies on neurobiology, gene-environment interaction; neurocircuitry and localization of brain functions; developmental neuropsychiatry; have the potential, on one hand, to unravel the mysteries of mental disorders and provide opportunities for intervention at the primary, secondary and tertiary levels for most of psychiatric disorders seen during childhood or adulthood, on the other.

According to Costello (2010), "Prevention and development are intimately intertwined: only when we understand the developmental course of a symptom or disorder can we have a solid scientific underpinning for prevention." Treatments in child psychiatry need to be developmentally appropriate and sensitive.

It is known that pediatric mental illness in children doubles to triples the likelihood to develop a substance use problem later in life. A new study from Massachusetts General Hospital (MGH) finds that treating psychiatric disorders with psychotropic medications in children and adolescents does not increase the risk of developing substance use, misuse, or substance use disorder (SUD). In fact, for at least three disorders—ADHD, major depressive disorder (MDD), and psychotic disorders—treatment with medication reduces the risk of developing a SUD, particularly when treatment is started early and for prolonged duration. So, early treatment of psychiatric disorders in children has preventive effect for later disorders of adulthood.

Treatment of childhood psychiatric disorders requires treatment of the child within and along with his/her family and the environment as much as possible. The key therapeutic principles before embarking on the specific modalities of treatment are as follows:

General principles and key points of treatment are:

1. Be positive and encouraging with the child and also the family.
2. Provide support and advice. Help the child and the parents to help understand and solve the problem.
3. Do not take over the function or role of parents.
4. Do not be authoritative or judgmental with the child.

5. Be holistic, pay due attention to biological, psychological and social issues.
6. Different children depending upon their developmental stage, temperament, IQ and social context will need different treatment approaches. So, always prepare an individualized treatment plan.
7. Different problems need different treatment approaches. There are no fixed treatment protocols.
8. Try to understand the risk and protective factors in the child, which will be the targets of intervention.
9. Apart from symptom removal, promotion of mental health, and inculcation of healthy and adaptive developmental patterns must remain the central goals of intervention.
10. Most problems are amenable to common forms of interventions.

Specific treatment methods useful in child psychiatry are briefly described below.

A. PARENT COUNSELING AND ADVICE

This is the mostly commonly used therapeutic intervention that is useful in almost all cases. Before embarking on parental counseling, it is important to understand what can go wrong in parenting. Most commonly seen family difficulties or dysfunctions contributing to the child's psychiatric problems are as follows:

1. *Lack of consonance with child's temperament or intelligence:* Each child has a unique profile of temperament and intellectual abilities. Failure to recognize the uniqueness or incongruities between this and the parental expectations and behaviour is a source of strain and conflict between the child and the parent.
2. *Overwhelmed parents and parenting inadequacies:* Many parents have their own stresses and strains in life due to which they are unable to provide necessary time, guidance or organized environment in the house for the child, leading to deficient parenting.
3. *Poor or faulty communication:* Communication can be deficient, or discordant. There may be no or minimal communication; failure to listen or to respond; loud, authoritative, snappy communication; or it may be frequently interrupting, demeaning, critical, hostile pattern; contradictory messages, or unclear, vague messages, etc. are some of the common pathological patterns of communication.
4. *Absent or unsupportive parents:* Parents could be distant or disengaged or negative so that the child feels unsupported.
5. *Emotionally out of tune:* Parents may not recognize or feel the problems of each other or of the child.
6. *Inconsistent parenting:* Parental instructions and behaviour is not consistent between each other or over time.
7. *Parental discord or disharmony:* Parents themselves have problems between them and the child is caught in the conflict.
8. *Inflexible or rigid parenting style:* This is never helpful nor conducive to achieving any goals.
9. *Pathological relationships or alliances:* Family members may have pathological alliances, e.g. child and the grand parents; or child—one parent; leading to failure of normal developmental channels.

It is important to identify the problems as a prerequisite for planning family intervention and undertaking corrective steps.

Establish Therapeutic Alliance

It is important to establish a supportive relationship with parents and other significant family members; engage them in treatment; get their cooperation and willingness; and commitment to help. Use empathy, non-judgmental attitude, attentive listening, and unconditional positive regard. Be sensitive to the emotional currents and tenor of all interactions and communications.

Provide Support

Family and the child should be supported by therapist's stance; by his/her willingness and offer to help; and by his/her ability to understand and treat the disorder. Tell the child and the family that you (the therapist) will give all the advice, guidance that will be needed to help tide over the problems, or to bring about change in their behaviour or adaptations.

Provide Advice and Guidance

This involves giving concrete advice such as changing the faulty patterns of behaviour, or communication, or to bring down the expectations or to be more consistent in approach, etc. as the case may be. This depends upon the nature of identified patterns of family dysfunctions or parenting issues in the given child.

Parental Counselling

Counselling involves explorations into the problems and issues conjointly with the parents where they themselves are able to uncover and understand the likely factors contributing to the occurrence or the precipitation of the problem behaviour. Effort is made to discuss the options for change and see which option is most feasible, useful and acceptable to them. The parents themselves find their own solution to the problem and engage in choosing the strategy where the therapist facilitates free discussion of various pros and cons of various options. The process involves analysis of difficulties, understanding the root causes of problems, and thinking of possible solutions, agreeing on the most suitable/feasible solutions; and then to implement the preferred or the desired action. Parents themselves are the agents of change. They must feel effective and confident and are likely to sustain such a change. Counseling is an active process as opposed to guidance and advice which are passive processes.

Indications

Parent counseling and advice is practically required in treatment of all psychiatric conditions. But these are especially helpful in treatment of emotional disorders, somatization, conversion and dissociation, stress and trauma related conditions. It is also useful as adjunct in treatment of psychotic disorders or other severe mental disorders.

B. FAMILY THERAPY

Family constitutes the most significant and powerful resource in India and in most cases where family is available, it should be included in the treatment. Family therapy is a more specialized treatment approach where the underlying premise holds the pathology to be within the family system rather than in the individual members. In family therapy, effort is made to change the family system instead of focusing on the individual members. There are several models of family therapy, of which parent-training model and general systems approach are most suitable and are commonly used in clinical practice.

Parent-Training Model

This model is based on the assumption that child's behaviour is primarily dependent on the reinforcements, both positive and negative, that he/she receives in everyday life and in interactions with family members. In most instances, parents are deficient in parenting skills that contributes to failure in acquisition of life skills or prosocial behaviour in children. Parent training model incorporates teaching of new skills and correction of old problematic ways in dealing with children in terms of inculcating discipline and prosocial behaviour in them. Parents are provided with direct guidance and advice on parenting skills and are supervised for practice of newer skills. Children with behaviour problems, such as disruptive behaviour or aggressive behaviour are managed with this approach.

This approach utilizes principles of behaviour modification.

Parents are given parenting skills training where they are advised to exhibit, and helped to learn, the following specific attributes:

Parenting Skills Training

Developing a positive, trusting and fulfilling relationship with the child is the key to healthy parenting. Parents should try to be good role models and inculcate the following principles in their behaviour.

1. *Know the child:* Parents must know about the intellectual potential; temperamental uniqueness; and presence of any assets/liability in the child.
2. *Listening skills:* Parents should exhibit good listening skills, i.e. that they are attentive to the child, they do not interrupt the child, be patient till the child has said what he/she wants to say. They should not ridicule or reprimand the child for what he/she has said. It is only when the child has finished, that the parents should respond.
3. Develop a positive, trusting and fulfilling relationship with the child which is the most significant factor in helping the child grow and develop in most healthy manner.
4. *Attitude:* Support an attitude of understanding, tolerance, acceptance, supportiveness, helpfulness and patience. All these help in developing a positive relationship with the child.
5. *Effective communication:* Communication between the parent and the child should be open, free, respectful and a two-way process. Parents should allow the child to speak. They should communicate their viewpoint clearly without using negative critical words for the child (parents may disagree with what the child says without ridiculing or humiliating him/her), providing logic and reasoning for their viewpoint. It is important that the child not only learns to obey parents but also learns to understand the reasoning behind their viewpoint.
6. *Control of emotions:* Parents must learn to control their own emotions and not be given into outbursts of anger, unhappiness, criticism, etc. on the child or on the other family members.
7. *Consistency:* Behaviour of parents should be consistent overtime and across situations so that the child knows clearly as to what is expected of him/her and what are the limits set by parents.
8. *Problem solving:* In situations of conflict or difficulty, parents must not leave the child in lurch or in a state of unresolvable conflict. Parents should provide/suggest solution to the problem and dissipate tension.
9. *Give reasoning to the child:* Parents are advised to give reasoning/logic for their behaviour or viewpoint to the child. This enhances the child's acceptance of parental viewpoint and also helps the child develop cognitive skills of reasoning and logic.
10. *Be a role model:* This is a very crucial strategy. Parents should understand that the child is a mirror image of their own behaviour. So, do what you would like your child to do.

A simple manual for healthy parenting is given as appendix at the end of this book.

General Systems Approach

According to this theory, the living systems are dynamically inter-dependant for homeostasis and adaptation or change. The mutual interrelatedness and reciprocity of the systems regulates the boundaries and sustenance of the components or the subsystems. In families, symptoms can occur if the boundaries of subsystems are rigid or the homeostatic mechanisms are inflexible; or if the family equilibrium is disturbed by any event; or if there is a reciprocal spiral of distortions and so on.

The central premise here is that a dysfunctional family structures and faulty communication patterns are the root cause of psychiatric symptoms. Certain pathogenic situations can universally produce a variety of symptoms. For example:

1. If the child is co-opted into alliance with one parent against the other, there is violation of the boundary of marital subsystems.
2. If the conflicts between husband and wife are played out as parental conflict regarding children.
3. If the communications between members of the family are unclear, paradoxical, distorted, critical or hostile, indirect, etc.
4. If the patterns of authority are not clearly defined or are highly lopsided.

In family therapy, effort is made to create openness, uncover and correct the family coalition patterns and alliances, correct the ways of communication, establish rules of authority and decision making, facilitate communication and discussion. Effort is made to create an atmosphere of trust, cooperation, understanding and freedom with mutual regard and respect among family members. In many instances, family therapy brings into focus, problems of another member of the family who may actually not be the patient but who may be responsible for most of the dysfunction and pathology. It is also possible that such a family member may be rigid, un-understanding and unaccommodating, making the therapy unsuccessful or impossible. In such a situation, intervention strategy must change and the focus should shift to individual therapy with the symptomatic members.

Indications

Family therapy is indicated in conduct disorders, oppositional defiant disorders, addictions, anorexia nervosa, bulimia, affective and anxiety disorders, schizophrenia and dissociative disorders.

C. Behaviour Therapy

Behaviour therapy is based on principles of learning and the types of learnings described have given the fundamental basis for the techniques of behaviour therapy so derived. Four types of learning is described below and there are corresponding techniques of behaviour therapy, that have been used in treating the various clinical problems and disorders:

1. Classical conditioning or respondent conditioning or Associative learning
2. Operant conditioning or Experiential learning
3. Conceptual or Cognitive learning
4. Social or Observational learning

Behaviour therapy approaches assume that:

1. All behaviour, adaptive or maladaptive, is learnt and therefore, can also be unlearnt and relearnt.
2. Primary focus is on external observable behaviour rather than on internal subjective experiences such as emotions or thoughts.
3. Most techniques of behaviour therapy have been derived from laboratory experiments including animal studies.
4. Focus of treatment is symptom change.
5. Environment has a role in maintaining the symptom change and should be involved in treatment.

Main aim of behaviour therapy is two folds:

1. To strengthen, develop or maintain healthy or adaptive behaviour.
2. To reduce or eliminate unhealthy or maladaptive behaviour.

Techniques to Increase, Strengthen, Develop or Maintain Behaviour

Most commonly used methods are:

1. *Reinforcement:* Giving a reward (positive reinforcement) for a positive desired behaviour increases the occurrence of such behaviour. On the other hand, aversive stimulus (negative reinforcement) decreases the likelihood of that behaviour. Reinforcement can be

tangible such as food, money, etc. or can be intangible such as praise, smile. There can be different reinforcement schedules; like every time a good behaviour is seen there is immediate reinforcement or reward given (continuous reinforcement); or the reward can be given intermittently at a fixed interval schedule (at a fixed time period), or at variable intervals. Similarly token economy is another technique, where rewards are earned systematically in the form of tokens which are later exchanged for other reinforcers that the patient likes. Reinforcement techniques are based on operant conditioning principles and are useful in inculcating skills in skill deficient children.

2. *Modeling:* Child observes a model engaged in a certain behaviour and then tries to carry out the same act or emulate the model. This technique is based on social learning theory. There can be live modeling where the child sees the actual person in real life or it can be symbolic modeling where the child sees a video film or imagines himself performing the act.

3. *Skills training:* Skills training can be for social skills or for cognitive skills. Multiple behavioural techniques are used such as positive reinforcement, modeling, instructions, role playing, behavioural rehearsal, etc. in interactive participatory sessions. Social skills training is useful in deficient social behaviour as is seen in highly withdrawn children or in mentally retarded, autistic, aggressive or antisocial children. Cognitive skills training involves techniques such as problem solving, self-control or regulation, regulation of emotions, attention, corrective self-statements, decision making, generating alternative solutions, positive self-reinforcement, etc. to be able to successfully complete the tasks. Skills training is used to deal with problems of impulsivity, aggression, fears, anxiety, low self-esteem, etc.

Techniques to Reduce or Eliminate Behaviour

1. *Negative reinforcement and punishment:* This involves withdrawal of positive privileges such as watching TV, going out to play, etc. or introducing negative or aversive stimulus like scolding, after the child exhibits an undesirable or problematic behaviour. Punishment is given immediately after the behaviour and is a useful technique in dealing with symptoms of aggressiveness, disruptive behaviour, self-injurious behaviour or for habit disorders. This technique brings down the frequency of occurrence of problem behaviour very quickly. If used very frequently, it has the risk of inducing fear of the punisher or of the therapist or of making the child withdrawn which should be avoided. Some of the punishment procedures are:

    a. *Time out:* Remove the child from the situation where the undesirable behaviour occurs and place him in a restrictive environment for brief periods where there is no reinforcement or attention to the child. In such a situation, misbehaviour comes down rapidly. Child is warned beforehand about time out and also informed about it so that he knows. Time out is a very successful technique to control disruptive or aggressive behaviour in homes or classrooms.

    b. *Response cost:* This procedure involves withdrawal of tokens or positive reinforcements for bad/ forbidden behaviour or when terms of contingency contract have been violated. For example, if the family agrees to give the child the privilege of outing for cleaning up his room, then his failure to complete the task will entail foregoing the outing. The child continues to be in a natural environment (as opposed to time out) and is encouraged to learn self-control. This technique is useful in dealing with hyperactivity, temper tantrums, aggressiveness, etc.

   c. *Overcorrection:* Child is made to correct the consequences of his 'bad' behaviour, e.g. put the room back in order after the child has created mess.

2. *Desensitization:* Child is gradually exposed in a graded fashion to the stimulus that the child is afraid of and avoids. This technique is useful in managing phobias and anxiety. Child is first trained to relax through various techniques and then exposed, step by step, to the feared stimulus which can be done either in imagination (*in vivo*) or in real life situation (*in vitro*). This technique is called systematic desensitization.

3. *Modeling:* The child can observe another child being exposed to the feared stimulus and is encouraged to do the same which is called modeling.

4. *Flooding:* In some circumstances, the child can be directly and fully placed in or exposed to the feared situation/object leading to maximum anxiety which gradually settles down in the presence of the supportive persons and environment. This method is called flooding. There have been some ethical and consent issues with this kind of technique as it can upset the child and the family.

Behavioural Assessment

Thorough behavioural assessment is essential before embarking on behaviour therapy. Behavioural assessment includes identification of the problem behaviour; specification of the target behaviour that is sought to be modified; planning and designing the treatment programme; assessing and monitoring the progress and final outcome. In depth analysis of what triggers the target behaviour, i.e. antecedents; what behaviour follows, i.e. behaviour; and what are the consequences of that behaviour on the situations of the environment, is done in a systematic manner. Choice of behavioural technique to be used depends upon the nature of target symptom or behaviour, child's intellectual and cognitive abilities, associated symptoms of anxiety, fear, depression, and the contextual factors in the occurrence of behaviour.

Behaviour therapy is useful for certain specific disorders. For many conditions, packages are available in other countries. In India, we mostly have to devise our own treatment plan.

Indications

Anxiety disorders: Generalized anxiety disorders, panic disorder, phobic disorder and obsessive compulsive disorders are amenable of behavior therapy with great success. Desensitization, relaxation training, modeling, flooding, exposure and response prevention, contingency contracting, are most useful techniques.

Depression

Children with depression have negative cognitions and the underlying assumption is that changing these negative self-attributions and negative thoughts will bring out change in the affect. Behavioural techniques useful in this situation are:

1. *Self-control training:* Child is encouraged in setting goals, using positive self-statements, refraining from negative self-defeating thoughts, attributing success to their efforts and failure to external factors.

2. *Problem-solving training:* Think of alternative methods of dealing and implementing the actions that are most suitable for a situation.

3. *Relaxation training:* Methods of relaxation are taught such as deep breathing, calming technique, meditation, graded exposure.

4. *Cognitive-behaviour therapy:* Child is made to analyze and record negative or pessimistic cognitions and related cognitive errors such as magnification, over generalization; followed by generation of alternative thoughts. Child is made to evaluate the alternative thoughts and then to change his faulty cognition

into a more plausible alternative thought. Cognitive-behaviour therapy also includes problem solving, self-control training and relaxation training; and has been found to be most effective technique in treatment of depression.

Disruptive Disorders of Behaviour

This group of conditions includes conduct disorder, oppositional defiant disorder, antisocial behaviour and ADHD. Most useful treatment techniques are contingency contracting, reinforcement, time out, response cost, over correction. Parents are required to be firm, consistent and clear in their instruction and behaviour. Child is engaged in planning the treatment and reinforcements. Initially positive and prosocial behaviour is positively reinforced; and negative (destructive, aggressive) behaviour is ignored causing extinction; child is warned once for negative consequences of non-compliance. Most of the times, it works. If not, this can be followed by punishment or negative reinforcement.

Pervasive Developmental Disorders

Techniques used to reduce/stop unwanted behaviour such as rocking, stereotypies, self-injurious behaviour include negative reinforcement, time out, over correction, punishment; and those to increase prosocial or desirable behaviour include positive reinforcement and skills training.

Mental Retardation

Mentally retarded children benefit from skills training, reinforcement techniques, and time out for undesirable behaviour.

Enuresis and Encopresis

In enuresis, conditioning technique using bell and pad method has been useful. The equipment has a pad which is sensitive to urine and there is an attached bell that gets activated by the wetness from few drops of urine. Child sleeps with a pad under his bed sheet and as soon as he/she wets the bed, the alarm bell rings, waking the child up. The child goes to toilet to urinate, makes his bed, resets alarm and sleeps again. Repeated pairing of urination and alarm, waking up the child, conditions the child to wake up before urination (when the bladder is full).

The other technique for enuresis is based on principle of token economy or positive reinforcement for dry nights. Child marks a star in calendar for dry nights and earns tokens for each successful dry night to be exchanged for rewards later on. In some instances, child puts up 'urine alarm', alarm to wake up and void at a specific time interval during sleep. He is praised for his effort and given reward for successful dry nights.

In functional encopresis, positive reinforcement, mild punishment, reinforcement for appropriate toilet training as a regular habit, periodic panty check, reinforcement for clean pants are useful.

D. COGNITIVE BEHAVIOUR THERAPY

Cognitive behaviour therapy is a combination of cognitive, behavioural, social and affective techniques aimed at changing thinking patterns as the fundamental strategy to bring about change in behaviour and emotions. Underlying assumption is that there are automatic thoughts, i.e. thoughts that occur automatically without any underlying basis and are negative and dysfunctional in nature; and that there are cognitive distortions or errors in logical thinking; and there is negative view of the world, the self and of the future. Cognitive distortions include:

- Dichotomous thinking (absolute, negative thoughts, i.e. "I will never be OK").
- Selective abstraction (responding to a part of the situation and out of context, i.e. teacher did not look at me because I am bad).
- Personalization (e.g. "I am responsible for my mother's illness.")
- Arbitrary inference (e.g. "I will never learn the subject because I have made a mistake.")

- Overgeneralization (e.g. "I cannot do anything in life if I cannot do this.")

In CBT, patients are made to engage in identification of automatic thoughts, and to analyze the cognitive errors or distortions therein through a process called as guided discovery. He/she sets or corroborates the evidence, in favour of his thoughts which is arbitrary or missing. Thereafter, the patient is made to evaluate and consciously monitor negative thoughts, generate alternative thoughts that are reality based in place of distorted ones, and then substitute these reality based interpretations instead for the situations. Change in cognitive style brings about change in affective and behavioural state. Depressive and anxiety disorders are amenable to CBT.

E. PSYCHOTHERAPY

Psychotherapy is one of the most intensive forms of psychological interventions, useful in achieving or realizing the best potential, the child is endowed with, in the realm of mental functioning. More specifically, aims of psychotherapy can include:

1. Symptom removal or reduction
2. Better coping
3. Reduce anxiety, anger or sadness
4. Improved self esteem
5. Increased frustration tolerance
6. Increased autonomy/independence
7. Improved relationships with family, peers and other adults
8. Feelings of enjoyment and pleasure
9. Improved functioning and productivity
10. Developmental optimization.

Psychotherapy entails a deliberate professional relationship between a trained therapist and a patient, using psychological means, verbal or non-verbal. Therapy is held as 30–40 minutes sessions, one to three or four times a week for periods varying from 3 months to a couple of years depending upon the aim or the technique. A thorough diagnostic assessment, assessment of the basic personality structure and a psychodynamic formulation for the

case, are the essential prerequisites to psychotherapy. The process of initial assessment for psychotherapy may take several (4–8) sessions before actual therapy can be started. In children, treatments are multimodal, done in a combination of pharmacotherapy, behaviour therapy, psychotherapy, family therapy, counseling, remediation, rehabilitation, environmental changes and so on. Usually, more than one treatment is recommended. It is only rarely that individual, intensive, psychodynamic psychotherapy alone is indicated for a child.

There are several types of psychodynamic psychotherapies based on corresponding theoretical viewpoints. However, psychoanalytic theory of Freud provides the basis for most psychodynamic psychotherapies and the underlying tenets include the uncovering of unconscious, transference, interpretation, analysis of mental mechanisms and conflicts, and working through. Several modifications in this approach have been suggested by many analysts, including involvement of cognitive, interpersonal or social perspectives. Conducting psychodynamic psychotherapy requires rigorous training of the therapist in the form of either personal psychoanalysis, or intensive individual psychotherapy supervision and systematic participation in psychotherapy case discussions/conferences, etc. Needless to say that these opportunities are rare and unavailable to most professionals in India.

Technique of Psychotherapy Involves the Following

1. *Therapeutic alliance:* Establishing a positive, trusting relationship, called as therapeutic alliance between the therapist and the child is the first and the foremost prerequisite for psychotherapy. Therapist's stance of being a non-judgmental, understanding, caring and helpful person facilitates therapeutic alliance.

2. *Setting up of contract:* Child is explained about the goals and process of psychotherapy where the child will be required to follow the rules and also engage in the process of introspection, and verbal expression of thoughts, feelings, impulses, situations or other relevant issues without inhibition, with a view to develop an understanding of his/her own psyche. Child should agree to the process and be willing to seek help to help him/herself.

3. *Uncovering of unconscious thoughts, feelings, motivations and conflicts* is the main task in psychotherapy sessions. This is achieved by using several techniques such as reflecting on the expressed statements or descriptions of situations, events, feelings or thoughts, dream analysis, free association (to speak whatever comes to the mind), or analysis of play, etc.

   During the process of uncovering of unconscious motivations and conflicts, the child re-experiences the trauma (that he/she experienced in the past and was buried in the unconscious mind) and that can rekindle the feelings the child felt then. The process can also lead to development of certain feelings towards the therapist which is called as transference.

   These thoughts and emotions are analyzed and the child reflects on them. Actually, it is these very thoughts and emotions activated by a current life circumstance/event that are the cause of current neurotic symptoms.

4. *Interpretation:* Interpretation involves interpretations of the unconscious conflicts, motivations, thoughts or feelings that manifest in the current behaviour patterns of the child in different situations or circumstances. It is a subtle process where the child is himself/herself on the verge of same interpretation as the therapist is trying to allude to. Knowing and understanding the basis of one's behaviour has tremendous therapeutic effect in itself. Interpretation is a corrective emotional experience. Moreover, with the interpretation, insight begins to develop, emotional charge is dissipated, and the thoughts/conflicts become available for conscious and rational re-evaluative mental processing; and the child begins to think differently, and is able to change his perspective.

5. *Working through:* After interpretation, there is working through process, where the child learns to practice newer ways of thinking, feeling, behaving and sees it succeed.

6. *Termination:* Once the goals of psychotherapy are achieved, termination of therapy is planned. Most often, the child's symptoms abate; he/she has acquired better understanding and control of behaviour, thoughts or emotion; has acquired better coping or handling methods and no longer feels unhappy or distressed.

Improvement in psychotherapy is often a clinical judgment and can never be perfect or absolutely complete. The most important step in psychotherapy is to embark on a journey of self- awareness, self-improvement and self-correction which can go on for life.

Psychotherapy is highly effective and beneficial in enhancing levels of happiness, satisfaction and calm. Most recent research on psychotherapy supports the evidence for its definite efficacy and also for its neuro-biological underpinnings making it a robust, scientifically proven form of therapy.

F. PLAY THERAPY

Play therapy is a form of psychodynamic psychotherapy where play is used as a medium of exploration, communication and change. Play serves several normal developmental functions in children. Normally all children play and through play they learn to master the environment, develop motor control and coordination, expand then cognitive processes, learn symbolism, enact relationships, express emotions, indulge in role play, develop object relations, reality testing and other ego functions. Play stimulates and facilitates cognitive, affective and motoric development in children. Children have a natural tendency and a biological need for engaging in age appropriate play.

Use of play in therapeutic situation was first described by Hug-Hellmuth (1921), and was further expanded by Melanie Klein (1932); Anna Freud (1946) and Virginia Axiline (1947). Goals of play therapy are more restricted than those of psychotherapy. Play provides an interface between the inner world of the child and the external experience.

Setting of a play room: Physical environment for play needs to be safe, bright, open and quiet. There should be basic furniture such as child chairs, table, a rug, some shelves, etc. Toy material should include drawing and colouring material, a doll house and doll family; stuffed human figures of both genders, and of adults and children; toy vehicles; toy animals; a rocking horse; some jig-saw puzzles; blocks and beads, etc. If possible a sandpit is also useful. Toys should be simple and safe to handle but not very fancy or alluring. Toys are used as a means for communication and not for their seductive appeal.

Therapy session: During the therapy sessions, it is important to establish therapeutic alliance and to assess the child's level of development, psychological organization, his style of stress response, defenses and adaptations.

Child is called to the playroom and parents normally wait outside. Child is encouraged to become active without specifically offering any toy to him/her. Child scans the environment and chooses the activity or toy that interests him.

A child can then get absorbed in play. Children can play by themselves irrespective of the therapist; or they can play alone but expect or desire therapist's attention.

Children may engage the therapist in play in a structured or in an unstructured manner. The therapist pays attention to the choice of play, manner of choosing the play, body language and communication during the play and the content of play. It is for the play therapist to see what the child is doing (content), 'how' is he doing it (style or manner), and with what 'intent' (motivation). The therapist tries to assess the child's body language or affective response, cognitive ability and skills and the behaviour. The therapist also tries to see the creativity, or imaginativeness, abstraction and symbolism involved in the child's play. The therapist can engage the child in conversation regarding his/her play acts and gradually try to mould the thoughts, feelings or behaviour of the child through alternatives in the form of suggestions, prompting or rephrasing. Non-threatening, non-coercive environment facilitates free expression of child's inner feelings/traumata. Feelings of safety, security and anxiety free and soothing environment further helps the child to open up psychologically. Play provides an opportunity for catharsis or ventilation. The therapist gradually and softly guides the child's emotions or thoughts into conscious awareness and then into alternative expansions or interpretations. Gradually, having dissipated the emotional charge, the child learns to accept the reality and begins to control or modulate behavioural and emotional reactions as also to acquire autonomy and ego strength.

Play therapy is used in children who are cognitively less mature such as those below 7–8 years of mental age; or in those who have problems of communication and speech such as in pervasive developmental disorder or specific delay in speech development; or who have severe problems in social, interpersonal relationships; or in those who have severe psychopathology where motivation for change is minimal such as in anorexia nervosa, dissociative disorders, etc.

Play therapy is very useful and effective technique for young and cognitively less mature children.

G. PHARMACOTHERAPY

With the advent and expansion of psycho-pharmacology in adult psychiatry, there has been increasing use of psychotropic drugs in treatment of psychiatric disorders in children and adolescents. Although, there has been extrapolation from adult psychopharmacology for use in children with similar indications, more and more research studies and clinical trials have been conducted on children in recent years. As the biological etiology of many psychiatric disorders of childhood is still not fully understood, most of the drug treatment indications and targets remain empirical. There are ethical and moral concerns in the families and society on the use of psychotropic medication in children, who by virtue of their immaturity are unable to give informed consent for themselves. Most of the times, children and adolescents are kept, out of clinical drug trials leading them to be either deprived of the benefits of potential treatment or to be subjected to off label use of drugs in them. Moreover, most efficacy studies are done on a limited time scale basis, not addressing the effects of such drugs on neurological and psychological development. Moreover, effect size of therapeutic benefit, except for ADHD, is moderate at best. Further, medicines can have considerable side effects. Therefore, extreme caution must be observed while using psychotropic drugs in children and adolescents.

There are, however, many disorders or situations where psychotropic drugs have vital role and need be used in children with considerable benefit. Further, drugs alone by itself are never complete or sufficient treatment for childhood psychiatric disorders. Non-pharmacological treatments must always be used in addition to medication.

General principles for using psychotropics in children are:

1. It is advisable to start on a low dose and slowly increase it.
2. Use monotherapy as much as possible.
3. Assess the need and indication carefully; identify the target symptoms for drug therapy.
4. Do not use drugs with contradictory neurotransmitter profile simultaneously, e.g. not to use agonist and antagonist of same neurotransmitter together.
5. Combining two agonists can compound major side effects, e.g amitriptyline and thioridazine can accentuate anti-cholinergic side effects.
6. Individualize treatment protocol for each case.
7. Use the principle of parsimony, i.e. as few drugs and as low dosages as possible, for as short a duration as possible.

Psychotropic drugs act by correcting the underlying dysfunction that lead to disorder, or by acting on complex pathways in neurochemical or neuroendocrine functions at the cellular and molecular level in the brain that produce psychiatric symptoms and psychopathology. Therefore, one drug may be beneficial in many even dissimilar disorders, e.g. imipramine can help in depression, in enuresis and even in ADHD.

One must obtain consent of parents or legal guardian and assent of the child for prescribing psychotropics to them.

Baseline assessment of height, weight, vital functions (pulse, BP, respiration and temperature) as well as general physical and systemic examination should be done before starting drugs. It is advisable to do hemogram, routine urinalysis, serum biochemistry and liver function tests. ECG, EEG, renal function tests and thyroid function tests are indicated if there is plan to use lithium.

Given in Table 10.1 is a brief account of the drug(s), disorder wise, and its indication for use. Indications are derived from the available research evidence on its efficacy and usefulness in a particular condition.

	Drug	**Dosage**	**Side effects**	**Caution**
Table 10.1: Drugs, dosages and side effects				
Antipsychotics				
Typical	Haloperidol	0.5–5 mg/day for child or 0.05–0.2 mg/kg/day 0.5–15 mg/day for adolescents	Sedation, extrapyradmidal symptoms, neuroleptic malignant syndrome	Monitor liver function tests
Atypical	Risperidone	0.5–3 mg/day or 0.015–0.05 mg/kg/day	Weight gain, metabolic syndrome,	Monitor total leukocyte count with clozapine
	Olanzapine	2.5–10 mg/day or 0.1–0.20 mg/kg/day	EPS, NMS	
	Quetiapine	25–400 mg/day	Low seizure threshold (more so with clozapine), hepatotoxicity	
	Aripiprazole	2.5–15 mg/day		
	Ziprasidone	5–40 mg/day		
	Clozapine	50–400 mg/day or 3–5 mg/kg/day		
Antidepressants				
SSRIs	Sertraline	12.5 mg–150 mg/day or 0.5–2.5 mg/kg/day	Headache, insomnia, drowsiness, dry mouth, agitation, mania, suicidal behaviour, nose bleed	Monitor ECG
	Fluoxetine	5 mg–40 mg/day or 0.15–0.5 mg/kg/day		
	Citalopram	2.5 mg–15 mg/day 0.3–0.6 mg/kg/day		
	Escitalopram	2.5 mg–10 mg/day		
	Paroxetine	5 mg–30 mg/day or 0.2–0.5 mg/kg/day		
	Fluvoxamine	50 mg–300 mg/day or 1–3 mg /kg/day		
SNRIs	Venlafaxine	1–4 mg/kg/day		
Trycyclics				
	Imipramine	1.0–3 mg/kg/day	Dry mouth, constipation, tachycardia, decreased seizure threshold, cardiac arrhythmias	
	Amitriptyline	0.5–1.5 mg/kg/day		
	Clomipramine	1–3 mg/kg/day		
Psychostimulants				
	Methyl-phenidate	10–40 mg/day or Up to 1 mg/kg/day max	Insomnia, anorexia, weight loss, headache, tachycardia, palpitation, precipitation of tics	
	Atomoxetine	10–80 mg/day	Dry mouth, constipation, tachycardia, cardiac arrhythmias, decreased seizure threshold	

Contd.

	Drug	Dosage	Side effects	Caution
Mood stabilizers				
	Lithium	200–1000 mg/day Serum levels to be 0.4–1.2 meq/L	Nausea, vomiting, polyuria tremors, hypothyroidism, ataxia, dysarthria, delirium in toxicity	Monitor serum levels, renal function tests, thyroid function tests.
	Sod. valproate	200–800 mg/day or 10–20 mg/kg/day Blood levels to be 50–100 mg/ml	Hepatoxicity, blood dyscrasias, nausea, vomiting, sedation, hair loss, weight gain, polycystic ovaries	Monitor complete blood counts and LFTs and blood levels
	Carbama-zepine	Start with 10 mg/day, build up to 20 mg/day Blood levels 4–12 mg/ml	Drowsiness, nausea, rash, ataxia, tremors, irritability, vertigo	Monitor blood counts, LFTs and blood levels
Anxiolytics				
Benzo-diazepines	Clonazepam	0.1–2 mg/day or 0.01–0.02 mg/kg/day	Drowsiness, disinhibition, addiction, confusion, decreased memory	Use extremely sparingly and for very short time. Abuse and addiction potential is very high
	Lorazepam	0.25–1.5 mg/day		
	Diazepam	0.5–2 mg/day or 0.1–0.9 mg/kg/day		
	Alprazolam	0.6–25 meq/kg/day		
L-adrenergic receptor agonists				
	Clonidine	0.25–0.4 mg/day or 0.2–0.5 cg/kg/day	Sedation, bradycardia, hypotension, stomach ache, withdrawal hyper-tension	Avoid sudden stoppage
B-adrenergic receptor antagonists				
	Propranolol	10–120 mg/day or 0.5–2 mg/kg/day	Sedation, dizziness, bronchoconstriction, bradycardia, hypotension abdominal pain	Contraindicated in asthma, diabetes, hypoglycemia
	Buspirone	0.5 mg/kg/day		

Table 10.1: Drugs, dosages and side effects

Autistic Spectrum Disorders

Basically there are no drugs for treatment of autism and autistic spectrum disorders. Medication can be used for control of troublesome symptoms which are often present and can be quite varied. Choice of medication depends upon the type of symptom targeted. Associated comorbidity may require medication separately. For example:

Aggression: Aggression is managed with antipsychotics (risperidone, haloperidol, olanzapine) or with antidepressants such as SSRIs or amitriptyline; or with lithium. Clonidine or clonazepam can be given for acute/severe aggression.

For anxiety symptoms, SSRI's, Buspirone, tricyclic antidepressants (amitriptyline) or benzodiazepines can be used.

For depression, use SSRIs or venlafaxine. Carbamazepine helps in stereotypies.

For comorbid hyperactivity and inatten-tion, methylphenidate or clonidine can be given.

Lithium is useful in self-injurious behaviour.

Obsessive symptoms can be treated with SSRIs.

ADHD

Psychostimulants such as methylphenidate or dexamphetamine (no more available in India) are the first line drugs in ADHD. Methylphenidate acts by blocking reuptake of dopamine and increasing noradrenaline levels in pre frontal cortex. The non-stimulant atomoxetine, a selective noradrenaline reuptake inhibitor (SNRI), is an alternative when tics, Tourette syndrome, anxiety disorder, stimulant misuse or risk of diversion are present, or where methylphenidate is ineffective or not tolerated. Atomoxetine is also useful in ADHD with social skills deficits. In an open clinical trial of use of Buspirone in ADHD for 6 weeks, there was significant improvement in all subjects, in all symptoms of ADHD, i.e. hyperactivity, inattention, impulsivity and disruptive behaviour and a favorable side effect profile (Malhotra and Santosh 1998). In cases with marked impulsiveness, aggression or tics, clonidine can be used. Guanfacine is an alpha-adrenergic receptor agonist pharmacologically similar to clonidine. Side-effects can include somnolence, hypotension, bradycardia and weight gain. Consequently, careful monitoring of weight, pulse and blood pressure is necessary. Amitriptyline or venlafaxine can be used as second and third line drugs. Rarely risperidone can be used in extreme cases.

Anxiety Disorders

SSRIs and 5HT2A antagonists, i.e. sertraline, citalopram, fluoxetine, paroxetine, fluvoxamine are recommended as first line drugs to manage anxiety disorders including social anxiety, separation anxiety, generalized anxiety in children and adolescents. Venlafaxine or amitriptyline can be used as second line drugs. As a general rule,

benzodiazepines (alprazolam, clonazepam) should not be used (except to tide over acute crisis situation), and if at all these have to be prescribed, it is for very short period of time. Occasionally, in brain damaged or intellectually impaired children, small doses of risperidone or olanzapine may be used. Clonidine can be given in PTSD or in acute stress reactions. Buspirone can also be used as a safe option in treating anxiety.

Depressive Disorders

SSRIs (sertraline, fluoxetine, citalopram) are the main drugs. Fluoxetine is most studied and preferred medication. Citalopram and sertraline can be used if there is no response to fluoxetine. Venlafaxine and paroxetine are avoided due to possible suicidal risk. In psychotic depression or marked agitation, use risperidone or olanzapine in addition. Vortioxetine, vilazodone and ketamine are only in trial stage.

OCD

Use or SSRI's (fluvoxamine, clomipramine, sertraline, fluoxetine or paroxetine) as first line drugs is recommended. Most drugs are approved for ages 6 and above, fluvoxamine from age 8 years and above. Best results are seen with combination of SSRI and clomipramine. Again, olanzapine or haloperidol can be combined in severe cases. In case OCD occurs in the background of ADHD or PDD, clonidine can be used. Many patients require more than one anti obsessional drug. In some patients with impulsivity and/or compulsivity, addition of naltrexone or memantine is useful.

Tourette's Disorder

Antipsychotics are the drugs of first choice. Haloperidol is preferred if there is concomitant OCD or OCD symptoms are made worse by atypical antipsychotics. Risperidone or Olanzapine are the drugs of first choice except when there are prominent symptoms of OCD. Clomipramine can be tried if there is comorbid, resistant OCD. In case of comorbid ADHD, clonidine (α-2, agonist) is helpful.

Aggression

Aggression can be present in a wide variety of diagnoses, i.e. psychotic disorders, schizophrenia, bipolar affective disorders, brain damage or mental retardation, PDDs, ADHD, conduct disorders. Aggression can be treated by effective management of the basic disorder but at times symptoms of aggressiveness can be targeted by a careful choice of the drugs for the primary disorders. In case of psychotic disorders including schizophrenia or brain damage; risperidone or olanzapine can be given. Give haloperidol or IV diazepam for acute sedation, clonazepam can be given for acute psychotic excitement. Carbamazepine can be given if there is brain damage or intellectual impairment or head injury. In ADHD with aggressiveness, methylphenidate, or clonidine can be given. Lithium can be given in cases where there is primary aggression as in personality disorder or in impulse control disorder or when bipolar affective disorder is present.

Psychotic Disorders Including Schizophrenia

Atypical antipsychotics, clozapine and aripiprazole have been recommended for use in children and adolescents and are the drugs of first choice. In a study on use of clozapine in five cases of childhood onset schizophrenia (CoS), it was found that there was substantial global clinical improvement and no side effects (Malhotra et al (2000). It was highlighted that clozapine can be recommended as the first-choice antipsychotic for treatment of CoS. However, risperidone, olanzapine, and quetiapine are equally effective and also are used. Amisulpiride and haloperidol are second line drugs. In case, there is major affective component which is recurrent, then lithium or anticonvulsants can be used.

Bipolar Disorders

Lithium and anticonvulsants (carbamazepine, sodium valproate, lamotrigine) are the first-line drugs in most cases. Aripiprazole is used in acute mania. Risperidone, olanzapine, quetiapine has also been used particularly if there are associated psychotic symptoms. Since young age bipolar disorder patients are often rapid cyclers, use of SSRIs and tricyclic antidepressants has to be very careful. In rapid cyclers, sodium valproate or carbamazepine is preferred for short term as well as for long-term prophylaxis. Lithium is preferred in all BPAD for prophylaxis. In bipolar depression, combination of fluoxetine and olanzapine is beneficial, whereas quetiapine has not shown much promise.

Substance Use Disorders

Treatment of substance use disorders in children and adolescents is highly challenging. Most common substances of abuse in India are tobacco, alcohol and opiates. Cannabis use is now becoming more popular due to liberalization. Most difficult problem is to identify the problem and then to get them into treatment. Outpatient treatment involves detoxification, managing withdrawal symptoms, and managing associated medical problems. Initial contact may be with pediatrician or general physician for medical issues. Motivation to quit the substance is generally low. Children are usually brought by parents, whereas, adolescents sometimes are brought by friends without the knowledge of their parents. We must respect the adolescent's wish for confidentiality and privacy and work with them to make them agree to bring parents in treatment. In the initial stage, there is need to build trust and cooperation to engage in treatment. Use empathic approach exhibiting genuine concern rather than an authoritative or challenging approach. Motivational interviewing, motivation enhancement therapy and building insight are necessary steps for all cases. Inpatient treatment may be necessary if the problem is severe, or when outpatient treatment has failed, or when there is dysfunctional family, or danger to self. Psychosocial and behavioural interventions remain the first line of treatment. Medications are used to relieve withdrawal symptoms, manage craving, treat comorbid psychiatric conditions (such as ADHD, depression, impulse dyscontrol, aggression, insomnia), or to make drug use aversive. There is no evidence to suggest that adolescents have to be treated differently than adults for treatment of addictions. Same practice guidelines are followed as in adults. Buprenorphine-naloxone combination (2 mg buprenorphine and 0.5 mg naloxone to be uptitrated as per need) and N-acetlycysteine (1200 mg twice a day) have been shown to be relatively safe and effective for reducing craving and use of opioids and cannabis, respectively. Fluoxetine (20 mg daily) for co-occurring major depressive disorder, methylphenidate (standard dose 18 mg per day, maximum 72 mg) and atomoxetine (25 mg 100 mg per day) for co-occurring ADHD have been shown to be relatively safe, well-tolerated, and efficacious. Family therapy and CBT are very helpful. Adolescent substance use is often associated with polysubstance use, high risk sexual behaviour, educational failure and illegal activities. Treatment must address multiple risk behaviours. Overall treatment results are generally poor.

Following table provides the list of drugs, recommended dosages, common side effects and cautions (if any) to be observed. General recommendation is to start on a low dose and then gradually build. All dosages are lower than those used in adults.

Caution

Dosage ranges are given for children up to adolescent age. Dosages for children are very low and should be calculated at mg/kg body weight. All medications must be started at half or one-third of the recommended therapeutic dose and built gradually up to therapeutic dose level. Dosages given here are adjusted for Indian population. In general, and in clinical experience, dosage requirement is lower in Indian population than those recommended for western subjects.

Side Effects

For the sake of convenience and understanding, side effects of drugs (Table 10.1) can be categorized into syndromes comprising of several clusters of symptoms as listed below (Lask, Taylor and Nunn 2003):

1. The sedation syndrome
2. The cerebellar syndrome
3. The anticholinergic syndrome
4. The extrapyramidal syndrome
5. The serotonergic syndrome
6. The lithium toxicity syndrome
7. The hemopoietic depletion syndrome
8. The weight escalation/metabolic syndrome
9. Syndrome of inappropriate antidiuretic hormone (ADH) secretion
10. Drug interactions

These syndromes can occur across different groups of drugs and are briefly described below:

The Sedation Syndrome

It is characterized by tiredness, sleepiness, yawning, hypersomnia, difficulty in staying awake, fatigue, respiratory depression, unduly deep sleep, even sleep apnoea. Phenothiazines, tricyclic antidepressants, benzodiazepine, and anticonvulsants can cause sedation syndrome. It is managed by either reduction of dosage or change of medication to a less sedating one or by completely stopping the offending medicine.

The Cerebellar Syndrome

- Feeling of unsteadiness and drunkenness
- Wide-based gait, slurred speech
- Clumsiness in motor movements, decreased muscle tone (a slouching slumped posture), are indications of cerebellar involvement due to drugs.

Cerebellar syndrome occurs most commonly with lithium, carbamazepine and other anticonvulsants and benzodiazepines. The condition is managed by reduction or complete stoppage of medicine and then restarting at a low dose, building up very gradually to a minimum effective level.

The Anticholinergic Syndrome

It is characterized by dry mouth, blurred vision, tachycardia, hypotension, constipation, difficulty in passing urine, even urinary retention, fine tremors, prolonged QT interval on ECG, seizures, confusion, delirium, stupor, or coma vigil.

Tricyclic antidepressants and phenothiazine group of antipsychotics can cause this. Complete stoppage of medicine and supportive management is warranted. Bromocriptine or physostigmine can be given to treat anti-cholinergic syndrome.

The Extrapyramidal Syndrome

Several symptoms involving muscle tone and involuntary movements are included as extrapyramidal syndromes. These are:

- *Dystonia:* There is acute increase in muscle tone involving tongue, jaw, neck limbs or eyes, leading to torsion movement. It occurs within first few days of starting antipsychotic medication particularly with typical antipsychotics or can occur even with atypical antipsychotics (if given in high doses) and occasionally with SSRIs. The condition is managed with anti-cholinergic drugs and benzodiazepines.
- *Akathisia:* It is motoric and psychological restlessness causing discomfort and occurs in the early part of treatment with antipsychotics given in high dosages. The symptom is managed with dose reduction of the incriminating drug and use of propranolol or benzodiazepine or anticholinergic agents.
- *Parkinsonism:* Typical features of parkinsonism like bradykinesia, rigidity, mask like face, short shuffling gait, sialorrhoea, low pitch speech can occur with antipsychotics. Though it is more common with typical antipsychotics but can also occur with atypical ones if given in high doses. Symptoms are treated with dose reduction, or change of drug to one with low EPS potential and with use of anti-Parkinsonian drugs.
- *Tardive dyskinesia and dystonia:* These are a late development occurring after several months to years of antipsychotic use. Tardive dyskinesia symptoms involve involuntary repetitive movements of tongue or mouth, limbs or trunk leading to slow or jerky movements of twisting or writhing quality. Tardive dystonia involves symptoms such as torticollis, retrocollis or blepharospasm. The condition responds poorly to treatment, therefore, prevention of tardive dyskinesia (TD) remains the main focus of treatment. TD can increase with anticholinergics and may not respond adequately to tetrabenazine which is advocated as the treatment.

It is important to be aware of this potentially treatment refractory side effect and monitor the dose and duration of antipsychotic drugs to a minimum essential level. Once it occurs, the strategies involve substantial reduction in the dose or change of the antipsychotic drug to a lesser EPS producing type; if possible, stoppage of drug and institution of propranolol, or benzodiazepine can be done. Clozapine or olanzapine are safer alternatives. Tardive symptoms take time to improve.

Neuroleptic Malignant Syndrome (NMS)

NMS occurs rarely in children or adolescents. The condition has classical presentation of confusion, altered sensorium, fever, fluctuating BP and pulse, increased sweating, muscle rigidity, occurring in the background of recent antipsychotic use particularly typical antipsychotics. There is elevated creatinine phosphokinase. The condition is serious, potentially fatal and has to be managed in emergency or ICU type of set up. Treatment involves stoppage of incriminating medicine, conservative management and care of vital functions, and use of bromocriptine.

The Serotonergic Syndrome

This is a rare or uncommon side effect occurring with use of SSRIs in high doses over a prolonged period of time. There is restlessness, agitation, tachycardia, increased sweating, headache, confusion, tremors and shaking, hyper reflexia, diarrhoea, abdominal cramps, nausea, ataxia, incoordination and seizures.

This condition can mimic NMS except that rigidity, sialorrhoea, autonomic instability is not seen in the serotonergic syndrome. Patient has to be hospitalized and managed with supportive, conservative regimen.

Lithium Toxicity Syndrome

Acute lithium toxicity presents as nausea, vomiting, diarrhoea, tremors, delirium, seizures, hypertonia, ataxia, incoordination, slurred speech, and cardiac instability. It occurs when the serum lithium levels exceed the therapeutic range limits, i.e. >1–2 mEq/L but at times can also occur in patients with lower serum lithium levels. It is, therefore, essential that therapeutic monitoring should include clinical monitoring in addition to monitoring of serum lithium levels. Treatment involves complete stoppage of lithium, increase in salt intake, IV fluids to flush out lithium from the body and general conservative management of vital bodily functions done in an inpatient setting.

Chronic toxicity with lithium can lead to hypothyroidism, diabetes insipidus and leucocytosis. These are managed by adding thyroid supplements and reassessing the need for lithium and considering the alternative mood stabilizer.

The Syndrome of Inappropriate Antidiuretic Hormone Secretion

This syndrome can occur with use of carbamazepine or phenothiazines, tricyclic antidepressants and even with SSRIs. The condition presents as fluid overload and cerebral oedema leading to symptoms of nausea, headache, malaise, confusion, low urine output, weight gain, coma, seizures. The condition requires inpatient management with fluid restriction, and correction and maintenance of electrolyte balance.

Neuroadaptation Syndromes

Sometimes there is loss of treatment response after few weeks of clear response to medication. Dose escalation is required to get the response again. This is not an addiction phenomenon as there are no withdrawal symptoms. Here, the nervous system gets adapted to the drug. This condition requires change of drug or drug rotation.

Drug Interactions

There is need to be aware of the drug interactions within the commonly used psychotropic drugs in children and adolescents. Most drug detoxification in the body is mediated through the cytochrome P450 (CYP 450) enzyme.

There is research evidence that people and populations differ in their metabolic systems. Asians and Afro-Americans are slow metabolizer, than the Caucasians, thus, supporting the clinical evidence of lower dosage requirements in Asian and African subjects as compared to the Caucasians.

Management of Learning Disabilities and Developmental Disorders

Learning disabilities or specific developmental disorders of learning are lifelong conditions for which there is no cure and the deficits persist through adulthood. In many instances there is associated neurological disorder such as epilepsy, neurofibromatosis or Tourette's disorder; or other neurodevelopmental psychiatric disorder such as ADHD; or there may be secondary emotional, social or behavioural disorder. Treatment of primary condition of learning disabilities involves special education and remediation.

Special Education

Special education focuses on alteration in the teaching approaches depending upon the nature of disability. Teaching approaches include simplification of learning task, involving multisensory inputs, building associations, giving practice sessions, etc. Special education incorporates highly technical approaches in education and is carried out by qualified special educators. Unfortunately, there are very few special educators available in India. Thus, the main burden of educating learning disabled children falls on parents and school teachers. It is recommended that teachers in regular school should be sensitized to the problems of learning among children and should also be well-versed in general principles of special education. It is now recommended as per the CBSE (Central Board of Secondary Education) guidelines that every school should have a counselor and a special educator. Parents should inform themselves of this special need of their child and try to access services from the schools as much as possible. Many mothers themselves undertake short courses in remediation or special education to help their child.

Remediation

Remediation means to compensate for the disability through alternative channels of sensory input and learning. Parents and teachers should understand the child's difficulties and help him rather than criticize him for not learning. Positive understanding approach helps to build child's selfesteem and also helps prevent secondary, emotional, behavioural or social difficulties. Parents and teachers must work together to reset goals and provide remediation. Associated comorbidity needs to be managed accordingly.

Remediation involves strengthening of the process weaknesses or of the deficient underlying functioning such as impaired visual discrimination, impaired auditory processing, eye movements, deficit in fine motor skills, etc. In learning disabilities there is difficulty or absence of ability to perceive, integrate and remember information in the auditory and visual domains during the listening, speaking, reading or writing tasks. Assessment for SLDs involves identifying specific strengths and weaknesses in auditory and visual processing related to academic functioning. Treatment approaches include:

i. Psycho-educational approaches
ii. Neuropsychological approaches
iii. Cognitive psychological approaches
iv. Linguistic approach
v. Behavioural approach

Psycho-educational approaches: It involves modification in teaching methods by taking into account the child's area of strength or preferences such as auditory, visual or kinesthetic; and where the deficit lies, i.e. whether it is verbal or nonverbal; oral or written. Effort is made to use and exploit the child's areas of strength as much as possible.

Neuropsychological model: This approach requires understanding of efficacy of underlying brain regions or systems that sub serve the various academic tasks. The effort is made to design instructions in a way that will engage the intact neural systems bypassing the areas of dysfunction.

Cognitive psychological model: This is based on the assumption that SLD children are unable to engage efficient and appropriate cognitive strategies for learning. They are made to understand the demands of the task and to recruit cognitive principles such as simplification, fragmentation, building associations, over practice, etc. for efficient learning.

Linguistic model: Several SLD children have underlying deficiency in language functions in the form of phonological coding or memory for linguistic material, leading to difficulties in reading, writing and spellings. Effective speech therapy is useful for such children.

Behavioural approaches: Here, academic tasks are considered as skills to be acquired and SLD is viewed as a skill deficit situation. Efforts are made to use principles of learning theory for acquisition of academic skills.

In most cases, a comprehensive approach involving an admixture of all or several of the above-mentioned approaches are used. There are programmes for SLD children, viz. Otto and Smith (1980) for remedial math's teaching; Gillingham and Stillman (1973) phonetic method for reading and writing; Fernald's Multisensory approach (1943) for reading and writing; Rosario (1991) for scholastic backwardness.

Most children with learning disability are intellectually bright and many a times they can learn to overcome or compensate for their learning disabilities. If approached in a positive and supportive way, most children with learning disabilities can grow up to become successful adults. Parents must be conveyed this information so that they do not harbour a pessimistic view of the situation, and stop engaging in their own efforts for remedial teaching.

Parents should be helped to access special concessions for children by the CBSE for their board exams for such children.

Autistic Spectrum Disorders (ASD)

Treatment of ASD includes early detection, and multimodal intervention. After diagnosis is disclosed, parent guidance and support is most essential as it can devastate parents and families. There should be systematic teaching of skills and education for the child depending upon his/her needs and deficits. It is advisable to make a structured routine and timetable for the child. Learning environment should be supportive and child friendly. Parental attitude should be moulded towards acceptance of the child's problem, understanding of the

child's deficits or difficulties, accessing help and guidance, engaging in the treatment program as a co-therapist or a facilitator or a teacher. Many parents undertake to learn the treatment approaches by attending parent training workshops or courses for autism. Child has to be taught basic skills of verbal or preverbal (as the case may be) communication; engage in play and social interaction; pay attention to stimuli and respond; and then learn the routine self-care and social skills in a step-by-step fashion. Many techniques of behaviour therapy are useful in acquisition of skills or in unlearning of undesirable behaviour such as rocking or stereotypic movements, etc. Treatment is multimodal where elements of pharmacotherapy, behavior therapy, family therapy, skills training are used. It is also multidisciplinary in that the psychiatrist, pediatrician, psychologist, play therapist, speech therapist, occupational therapist, physiotherapist and parent and families work together. In a study on treatment of autistic children using modified TEACCH technique using behavioural principles, structured environment, visual cues, supportive intervention along with medication was used and was found to be effective (Malhotra, Chakrabarti and Nehra 2002).

Individualized treatment plan is made for each child. Every professional undertakes to provide the necessary and appropriate therapeutic inputs, for example, speech therapy for speech and language deficits; physiotherapy for motor coordination and motor skills, occupational therapy for sensory processing, integration and occupational skills, and so on. Medication can be given for associated psychiatric symptoms if present. For example, antipsychotics can be given for aggression, agitation, irritability and self-injurious behaviour; SSRIs can be given for obsessional symptoms, anxiety, depression or social isolation; methylphenidate for hyperactivity or inattention; clonidine for hyperactivity, aggressiveness or sleep dysregulation; buspirone for autonomic dysregulation and anxiety; melatonin for sleep problems and so on. Intranasal oxytocin has been tried to improve social behaviour and bonding in ASD children with some benefit.

ASD and learning disabilities are covered under the National Trust for welfare of persons with Autism, Cerebral Palsy, Mental Retardation and Multiple Disabilities Act 1999, where several concessions and services are admissible to them. Parents and families should be encouraged and helped to access these services.

Mental Retardation

Aim of treatment in mental retardation is to make the child function at the level of intelligence that the child possesses or in other words to optimize his functioning to his/her best potential. Treatment involves learning of personal/selfcare skills, social skills and education up to the level that the child has the potential to reach. Parents and families should be educated to know, understand and accept the condition that mental retardation is. A change in their attitude towards becoming positive, accepting, supportive and helpful to the child should be inculcated. Parents and families need help to overcome their own anger, sorrow, denial or frustration. They should become partners in treatment and help the child learn the skills necessary for life and independent living. They should set realistic goals and ambition for the child, be protective and supportive to the child. Depending upon the intellectual level, the child can be sent to a regular school (as much as possible) or a special school.

In addition, speech therapy, occupational therapy or physiotherapy can be undertaken as per need. Efforts are made to build on the strengths of the child and to make him as much self-reliant as possible. Medication can be used for associated/comorbid psychiatric symptoms as the case may be and as per the guidelines already given.

Parents should be helped to access services and benefits or concessions given by the state or central governments for the care of disabled children under the purview of the National Trust for welfare of persons with Autism, Cerebral Palsy, Mental Retardation and Multiple Disabilities Act 1999 or the Persons with Disabilities (equal opportunities, protection of rights and full participation) and Act 1995.

H. ELECTROCONVULSIVE THERAPY (ECT)

Use of ECT for treatment of several psychiatric disorders is well established in adults, but is an uncommon treatment for children and adolescents. Use of ECT in children and adolescents is less well-described, mainly because many ethical/moral and safety concerns have precluded its use. It has been argued that ECT may interfere with brain development and maturation. But it is also known that untreated mental illness itself is detrimental to neuronal function causing progressive damage. There are mostly case reports or small sample series describing use of ECT in children and adolescents, but with positive results. ECT has been described to be an effective treatment for severe mood disorders when other treatments have been unsuccessful. ECT can be considered usually as a last resort after two or more trials of pharmacotherapy have failed or when the condition of the patient is incapacitating or life-threatening in cases of depression, bipolar disorders, catatonia, psychosis, or self-injurious behaviour or suicidality. Response rates for ECT in depression and catatonia in children and adolescents is much higher as compared to that in psychotic disorders. ECT is usually not recommended under the age of 11 years. In a review article on ECT in children and adolescents (Malhotra and Singh, 2000), it has been found that ECT is sparingly used in this age group, whenever used it is the treatment of last resort, for indications like major depression, bipolar disorder and schizophrenia, and often effective with low levels of side effects. Consent of parents and assent of the child is essential for instituting ECT. In India, ECT for minors is a prohibited treatment as per the new Mental Health Care Act 2017. It has to be approved by the Mental Health Review Board. So, the legal guidelines have to be followed.

G. NEWER TRENDS

Newer trends are seen in compliance with supporting, protecting, augmenting neuronal function and neuroplasticity. Several compounds and approaches are currently under examination that look beyond psychotropics or repurpose psychotropics cutting across diagnostic boundaries. This is the new arena or revolution deriving interventional approaches based on dysfunctions at neuronal, synaptic, cellular or molecular mechanisms occurring due to multiple etiological factors operating at different stages of brain development.

These treatment approaches, as listed below, are holistic and applicable to both child and adult psychiatric disorders.

- Strategies for neuro-protection, neuro-modulation, neural-integration
- Stimulation of neuronal plasticity and neurogenesis
- Manage environment and stresses such as trauma, toxins, inflammation
- Provide enriched environment

Following intervention strategies are derived from the above approaches:

- Cognitive training
- Neuro-modulation
- Neuro-protection
- Pro-cognitive agents
- Cellular function modulation
- Astrocyte function modulation
- Hippocampal modulation
- Stem cell therapies
- Enriched environment
- Diet
- Physical exercise
- Yoga/meditation
- Spiritual practices

Neuroprotective agents: Some of the neuro-protective agents are listed below and are potentially useful.

- Antioxidants like ascorbic acid, toco-pherol;
- Anti-inflammatory drugs i.e., methy-lprednisolone, carbamylated erythro-poietin;
- Nutraceutical (L carnosine, phosphatidyl choline, proteins and peptides, omega 3 fatty acids, N-Acetyl cysteine)
- Neuronal membrane stabilizers, e.g. citicholine
- Opioid antagonists, e.g. naloxone
- Mitochondrial fortifier co-enzyme Q10

Pro-cognitive agents: There are studies to show benefits of these agents.

- Glycine agonist D-serine
- GlyT1 inhibitor sarcosine
- Piracetam
- Modafinil
- Donepezil

Cellular Function Modulation

- Phospholipids, essential fatty acids, sphingolipids have a role in cell function and neural plasticity.
- Use of nutritional and other strategies to modulate the function and regulation of PUFA, phospholipids, sphingolipids can be used as strategies to improve functioning, symptom control and outcome in psychiatric disorders, as well as use it for preventive strategies.

Astrocyte Function Modulators

- Astrocytes are involved in neurogenesis, synapse formation and synaptic transmission during development and in later adult life.
- Drugs modulating astrocyte functions can have a role in treatment of mental disorders.
- Drugs targeting astrocytes include clozapine, desipramine, fluoxetine, paroxetine, amitriptyline, riluzole.

Hippocampal Modulation

- Hippocampus is involved in learning, memory and mood regulation.
- Active neurogenesis takes place in hippocampus.
- Environmental factors such as exercise, enriched environment, calorie restriction increase adult hippocampal neurogenesis.
- Stress, low grade inflammation, oxidative stress, ageing decrease neurogenesis in hippocampus.

Non-invasive Neuromodulation

Neuromodulation has been an area of interest in recent years. From the growing evidence of safety and efficacy of non-invasive neuromodulation techniques such as transcranial magnetic stimulation, deep brain stimulation, transcranial direct current stimulation, vagal nerve stimulation in treatment of adult psychiatric disorders, interest has evinced for applying these methods on children and adolescents. However, application of these treatments and research is still in nascent stage. Neuromodulation techniques have been considered in children with depression, autism spectrum disorder, attention-deficit hyperactivity disorder, and other neuropsychiatric disorders (Doruk Camsari et al 2018). But more research is needed to establish the efficacy and safety.

Stem Cell Therapies

- Progenitor cells lining the walls of the cerebral ventricles, and stem cells, can give rise to new neurons in hippocampus, an area consistently implicated in memory processing.
- Neural stem cells can repopulate the injured nervous system with tissues that has the capacity to develop into a variety of different organs including brain cells.
- Stem cell therapies have theoretical promise but are yet to be found useful in clinical setting for treatment of psychiatric disorders in children.

Enriched Environment

- Human brain grows in response to multi-sensory stimulation, challenges, new learning, novelty, laughter, human love, exercise.
- Animals raised in enriched environment have more neurons, more synaptic connections, greater number of blood capillaries and more mitochondrial activity.
- Enriched environment promotes development of cognitive, emotional and behavioural abilities and integration of neural networks in humans as well.
- Several studies have shown that children exposed to enriched environment make significant gains in intelligence and emotional functioning.

Diet

- Diet affects hippocampal neurogenesis and function, and inflammatory processes.
- Foods rich in omega 3 FA, flavinoids, antioxidant rich berries, resveratrol stimulate neurogenesis, reduce oxidative activity and down regulate proinflammatory processes, thus reducing neuro degeneration.
- Poor diet (saturated fats and refined carbs) is associated with smaller hippocampus, increased risk of depression and cognitive decline.
- Biological pathways through which diet operates are inflammation, oxidative stress and gut microbiome.
- Nutritional compounds like fish, olive oil, legumes, dairy products, nuts, fruits, vegetables have been found to have inverse relationship with depression and can be considered to be helpful in alleviating symptoms. On the other hand, western diet comprising of sweetened beverages, processed meats, baked products have been shown to be associated with an increased risk of depression in longitudinal studies (Khanna et al 2019). Diet and nutrition

can be a crucial component of treatment and prevention of mental disorders. Saffron, the dried stigmas of *Crocus sativus L.* plant, has been found to have antianxiety and antidepressant properties in several preclinical and clinical studies. A number of clinical trials have demonstrated that saffron possess antidepressant properties similar to those of current antidepressant medications such as fluoxetine, imipramine and citalopram, but with fewer reported side effects (Shafiee M et al 2018). Similarly, Curcumin, active compound in turmeric, has been found to have antidepressant properties in some studies.

- *L-Carnosine:* L-Carnosine is an amino acid containing β-alanine and L-histidine. It is an over-the-counter food supplement, which has been proposed to have neuroprotective, antioxidant and anti-convulsive properties that may benefit children affected with neurodevelopmental disorders. Studies are limited and results are equivocal, with indication of some benefit in children with ASD and ADHD. A pioneering study by Chez et al. (2002) in 31 children with ASD showed that eight weeks of carnosine supplementation (800 mg daily) decreased autism severity scores compared with placebo, especially behaviour, socialization, and communication sub-scores. Improvements in receptive language and impression of change (as reported by parents) were also observed. In the experience of the author, there is evidence of benefit in improving communication and eye contact in children with autism. One RCT has examined L-carnosine supplementation (800 mg/day for eight weeks) as adjunctive therapy in previously drugnaïve children with ADHD. Results showed modest but significant improvements in clinical symptoms of the disease (especially in

the inattention subscale) as assessed by parents (Ghajar et al 2018). Although, it is limited data, but there is evidence from at least three RCTs in children with ASD, that suggest that carnosine may be effective in improving core as well as secondary symptoms of ASD either alone or in addition to antipsychotic treatment (Schoen et al 2019).

- N-acetylcysteine (NAC) is another compound of interest in psychiatric disorders based on its role as a precursor to the antioxidant glutathione, and its action as a modulating agent of glutamatergic, dopaminergic, neurotropic and inflammatory pathways. In a systematic review it has been reported that in trials testing the use of NAC, mainly as an add-on treatment, in cannabis use disorder in young people, depression in bipolar disorder, negative symptoms in schizophrenia, and excoriation (skin-picking) disorder, there are promising results (Minarini et al 2017).

Physical Exercise

- Physical exercise increases neurogenesis, angiogenesis, BDNF
- Physical exercise is associated with increased hippocampal volume and increased hippocampal N-acetyl aspartate, a marker for neural integrity.

Yoga and Meditation

- Yoga and meditation stimulate neurogenesis and synaptogenesis.
- There is evidence of increased regional cerebral blood flow (rCBF) in pre-frontal cortex in people who meditate.
- It increases levels of serotonin, dopamine.
- Hath yoga is shown to be associated with increased energy levels and increased cognitive functioning amongst its practitioners.
- Yoga practitioners exhibit larger hippocampal size and dorsolateral prefrontal cortex.

Other Approaches

- Spiritual practices
- Alternative systems of medicine

Benefits of spiritual practices and alternative systems of medicine have not been well studied although empirical evidence or personal accounts may point towards that. These cannot be or rather should not be discarded, and there is definite merit in studying these as methods of treatment or of promoting mental wellbeing.

BIBLIOGRAPHY

1. Axiline V. Play therapy. Boston, Houghton Mifflin, 1947.

2. Chez M.G., Buchanan C.P., Aimonovitch M.C., Becker M., Schaefer K., Black C., Komen J. (2002). Double-Blind, Placebo-Controlled Study of L-Carnosine Supplementation in Children With Autistic Spectrum Disorders. J. Child. Neurol.17:833–837. doi: 10.1177/08830738020170111501.

3. Costello E. Jane (2010). Grand Challenges in child and neurodevelopmental psychiatry, Frontiers in Psychiatry, vol. 1, Article 14, pp 1–2. www. frontiersin.org. doi.10.3389/fpsyt.2010.00014.

4. Doruk Camsari D, Kirkovski M, Croarkin PE. 2018) Therapeutic applications of noninvasive neuromodulation in children and adolescents. Psychiatr Clin North Am. 41:465–77.

5. Fernald G M (1943). Remedial Techniques in basic School subjects. Mc Graw Hill, New York.

6. Freud A: The psycho-analytical Treatment of Children. London, Imago, 1946.

7. Ghajar A, Aghajan-Nashtaei F, Afarideh M, Mohammadi M.R., Akhondzadeh S. L-carnosine as Adjunctive Therapy in Children and Adolescents with Attention-Deficit/Hyperactivity Disorder. J. Clin. Child. Adoles. Psychol. 2018;28:331–338. doi: 10.1089/cap.2017.0157.

8. Gillingham A. and Stillman BW. (1973). Remedial training for children with specific disability in reading, spelling and penmanship. Cambridge, Mass. Educators Publishing Service. Inc.

9. Hug-Hellmuth H von: On the Technique of Child Analysis. Int J Psychoanal 2:287–305, 1921.

10. Jaffee S, Harrington H, Cohen P and Moffitt TE (2005). Cumulative prevalence of psychiatric disorder in youth. J. Am. Acad. Child Adolesc. Psychiatry 44, 406–407.

11. Khanna P, Chattu VK, Aeri BT. Nutritional aspects of depression in adolescents—a systematic review. Int J Prev Med. 2019;10:42.

12. Kessler RC, Berglund P, Demler O, Jin R and Walters EE (2005). Lifetime prevalence and Age of onset distributions of DSM IV disorders in the National Co-morbidity survey replication. Arch. Gen. Psychiatry 62, 593–602.

13. Klein M. The Psychoanalysis of Children. London, Hogarth Press, 1932.

14. Lask B, Taylor, Nunn K (2003). Practical Child Psychiatry: The Clinician's guide. Pub: BMJ Books London pp 298.

15. Malhotra S, Singh G ((2000). Efficacy of electroconvulsive therapy in children and adolescents. Archives of Indian Psychiatry. 6(1) 115–118.

16. Malhotra S, Santosh PJ (1998). An open clinical trial of Buspirone in children with Attention Deficit Hyperactivity Disorder. J Amer Acad Child Adolesc Psychiatry, 37 (4) 364–371.

17. Malhotra S, Chakrabarti, Nehra A (2002). Psychological intervention with parents of autistic children. Indian J Psychiatry, 44 (2), 108–117.

18. Martin Schön, Aya Mousa, Michael Berk, Wern L. Chia, Jozef Ukropec, Arshad Majid, Barbara Ukropcová, and Barbora de Courten (2019) The Potential of Carnosine in Brain-Related Disorders: A Comprehensive Review of Current Evidence. Nutrients. Jun; 11(6): 1196. doi: 10.3390/nu11061196.

19. Minarini A, Ferrari S, Galletti M, Giambalvo N, Perrone D, Rioli G, Galeazzi GM. (2017). N-acetylcysteine in the treatment of psychiatric disorders: current status and future prospects. Expert Opin Drug Metab Toxicol. 2017 Mar;13(3):279–292. doi: 10.1080/17425255.2017.1251580. Epub 2016 Nov 2.PMID: 27766914.

20. Otto W and Smith RJ (1980). Corrective and remedial teaching (3rd ed.) Boston; Houghton Miffin.

21. Persons with Disabilities (equal opportunities, protection of rights and full participation) Act 1995, Ministry of Social Justice and Empowerment Govt. of India, New Delhi

22. Rosario J (1991). Intervention strategies for scholastic backwardness, Doctoral thesis, Bangalore University, Bangalore.

23. Shafiee M, Arekhi S, Omranzadeh A, Sahebkar A (2018). Saffron in the treatment of depression, anxiety and other mental disorders: Current evidence and potential mechanisms of action. J Affect Disord.;227:330–7.

24. The National Trust for Welfare of Persons with Autism, Cerebral Palsy, Mental Retardation and Multiple Disabilities Act 1999, Ministry of Social Justice and Empowerment Govt. of India, New Delhi.

Special Issues in Adolescence

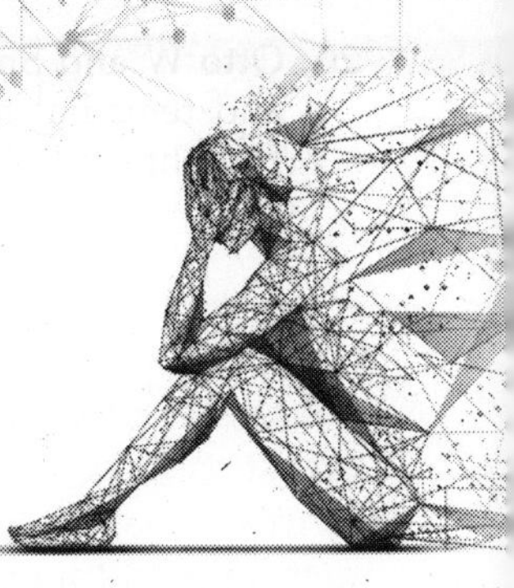

Adolescence is a phase of transition between childhood to adulthood. It is a transition from state of dependence to full independence. Onset of puberty marks the beginning of adolescence. Conventionally, adolescence has been taken as 11–18 years of age. Adolescence in many ways represents a form of discontinuity in development in biological, psychological and social domains setting it apart from childhood on one hand and adulthood on the other. Adolescents are physically, cognitively, and socio-emotionally more advanced than children but are prone to behave in manners that are inconsistent with adult values and norms. In earlier times, in many communities there were rituals marking the termination of childhood and entry into adulthood, and adolescents were seen as no different from adults. Now adolescence is seen as a distinct phase in the developmental course. Puberty symbolizes as one important milestone heralding adolescence. Further, adolescence requires adaptation to biological and psychological changes occurring within the body and the mind of the person, and incorporation of sociological expectations and demands. In recent years, with the advancement in age of puberty and prolongation of the period of preparation involving advanced study and training before entering the adult roles and occupations, period of adolescence constitutes a rather prolonged period of partial responsibility extending from age 10 through early twenties. In Indian philosophy, first 25 years of life have been considered to constitute what has been called as 'brahamcharya' which is supposed to be a period of learning under strict observance of austerity and celibacy.

Considerable importance has been accorded to the adolescent phase of life. It is a phase of transition where considerable changes take place in physical built and physiology; intellectual ability and verbal and social skills; emotional and sexual development; family and society's expectations and so on. Historically, and still in some cultures, adolescence is a brief ritualized transition from childhood to adulthood where children are expected to follow in parent's footsteps. However, in technologically advanced societies, it is an extended period of education, learning and training. Conflict between the biologically determined propensities and socially dictated expectations is the core of what is called as 'adolescent crisis'. Developmental changes occurring in adolescence are summarized below.

PHYSICAL DEVELOPMENT

Physiological Changes

Puberty refers to sexual maturity to procreate and is marked by growth and development of secondary sexual characters, genital organs and apparatus where the ovum and the sperm become viable. Puberty which means acquisition of capacity to reproduce, marks the onset of adolescence. There is marked increase in the tempo of growth which is different for boys and girls; increase in hormone secretion particularly androgens with its multiple effects like increase in libido, increase in skin thickness and oily secretion from sebaceous glands leading to acne. There are marked physical or bodily changes in the form of development of breast, public and axillary hair, and onset of menstruation in females. In addition to getting public and axillary hair, moustache and beard, and enlargement of penis and scrotum, boys begin to get spontaneous erections and night emissions. Usual age of menarche now is seen to be 11–13 years in females and growth spurt is also seen at the same time. Height spurt among boys starts around 12 years and peaks at 14 years.

There is activation of hypothalamic functions which stimulates gonadotrophic hormones of pituitary. In the brain, dendritic connections attain their adult level and alpha rhythm of adult mature pattern gets established in EEG.

Overall, there is a trend these days from many communities in Europe and America toward earlier puberty among girls as compared to earlier times. This change has been attributed to better diet. Puberty occurs in girls about 2 years earlier than in boys and the process is complete in 3–4 years.

Early maturers have, on an average, a slightly higher level of intelligence than do the late maturing children. Exact reasons are not fully understood. Some American studies have shown that early maturing boys have a slight advantage in personality. They were found to be more popular, more relaxed, more good natured and generally more poised. In contrast, late maturers were found to feel less adequate, less self-confident, and more anxious. In girls, personality adjustment is most satisfactory in those who mature around the average time, whereas early and late maturers show worse outcome. These differences are explained to be more social-psychological rather than biological. In boys, it is a matter of pride with added social benefit

to be physically sturdy and good at sports, whereas girls in whom development may appear deviant in its pace, are more sensitive to other's opinion about their physique. Clear cut relationships between age at puberty and psychiatric disorders have not been demonstrated.

Increase in the secretions of androgens by adrenals at puberty in both the boys and the girls, is mainly responsible for marked increase in eroticism and sex drive at this time. However, individual difference in libido after puberty is not related to differences in hormone levels. Animal studies indicate that androgens influence assertiveness and dominance as well as sex drive in both sexes. These effects are two-way: Sex hormones influence social behaviour and social experiences influence testosterone levels. Emotional and behavioural consequences of changes in oestrogen and progesterone levels during adolescence are less well understood. However, there is indirect evidence of such a relationship does exist, when we look at other settings, e.g. premenstrual depression and irritability, post-partum psychiatric disorder, oral contraceptives induced depression.

COGNITIVE DEVELOPMENT

There is an accelerated development of cognitive functions during adolescence. Cognitive functions include a large array of functions such as memory, attention and concentration, knowledge, perception, language, reading and mathematical skills, intelligence and thinking. The striking advance in mental ability that takes place in puberty and adolescence has been attributed not to any simple spurt in intellectual level but to a qualitative development in thinking and reasoning (Coleman 1980). According to Piaget, adolescence is the period of formal operations in which there is development of abstract thinking, ability to construct hypothesis and propose alternatives, and distinguish from each other the beliefs, fantasies, possibilities and probabilities.

Moral and Political Thinking

Studies have shown that there is increase in altruistic behaviour during adolescence. The adolescent can think in terms of freedom versus anarchy; compromise versus radical change; patriotism versus internationalism; idealism versus expediency; and matters which continue to tax the wisdom of his or her elders (Steinberg 1983). Their political thinking becomes more abstract, complex, and humanitarian, which when coupled with high altruism and strong conviction about right and wrong makes them very capable of influencing the world they live in, and support what is morally right and politically desirable.

Education

Most important change is increased emphasis on education and performance; concern about examination and career is foremost in the mind of the adolescent. Those who continue into education show greater increase in intellectual ability. Development of abstract thinking and intelligence is not uniform among all children, i.e. the rate of maturation and development varies. Some studies suggest that only 10% of 14 years hold and 35% of 16–17 years olds achieve the Piagetian stage of formal operations. Further, 60% of those categorized as gifted adolescents achieve formal operations which is in contrast to the average adult population, in which only 25–33% attained formal operations (Dulit 1972). These developmental changes contribute to several social and psychological issues that are the hallmark of adolescence. More prolonged period of dependence on parents may cause strain. Adolescents earning their own livelihood are likely to feel more independent financially. Those who remain unemployed experience marked discouragement and demoralization.

EMOTIONAL DEVELOPMENT

Adolescence is characterized by emotional turmoil, mood swings, intense emotional outbursts, strife, and consequent behavioural disruption. They often come in conflict with parents and society. Most of it is due to the surge of sexual drives stimulated by sexual maturity and hormones of puberty. More recent studies however (Oldhum 1978) have suggested that long exposure to parental values has significant effects on long-term adaptation in adolescents indicating that late teenage remains to be a highly impressionable phase of life. Emotional functioning is inseparable from physiological, behavioural and social aspects of functioning and needs to be understood in that context.

A large body of knowledge and theories exists to explain the emotional development in childhood and adolescence, i.e. temperamental model, behavioural model, psychodynamic model, psychosocial model.

PERSONALITY DEVELOPMENT

Apart from cognitive and emotional development, personality tends to crystallize during the period of adolescence and young adulthood. Characteristic and enduring patterns of behaviour, relationships, sexuality, identity and self-concept, and social relationships become manifest.

Sexuality

There is marked upsurge in sexuality at puberty. In most societies masturbation is an almost universal occurrence in adolescent boys and it is less common in girls. There is intense attachment to members of the same sex initially, which may occasionally turn into transient homosexuality. Although there is marked increase in heterosexual interest but sexual behaviour is determined by a large number of social and cultural factors, values, norms and opportunities. Adolescents experience intense sexual drive, untamed because of poor inhibitory control due to immature pre-frontal cortex, can indulge in sexual experimentation, transient promiscuity, impulsiveness in decision making and high-risk behaviour. The adolescent generally gets his knowledge of sexual behaviour and reproduction from friends rather than parents or teachers. Their sexual knowledge can be inaccurate or fraught with misconceptions which further adds to problems. Teenage pregnancies though were common in the West, are now seen much more often in India than before, and have its own added psychological and social problems.

Friendships

Friendships become more durable and more intense during adolescence. Initially it is with same sex peers later on it becomes mixed sex groups. Friendships among girls are generally more exclusive than in boys. Gradually adolescents spend less and less time with their family members and more and more time is spent with friends. Heterosexual attractions and friendships are very common to the extent that most adolescents are seen grappling with their emotional turmoil on account of relationship issues.

Emotions

The capacity to experience and express emotions depends on the developmental level and it surges during preadolescence and adolescence, as part of overall maturation. There has been a prevailing belief that adolescence is characterized by psychological upheaval and disturbance which often appears similar to mental illness. However, this is an exaggerated view. General population surveys have shown that most adolescents do not show emotional disorder. On the other hand, an adolescent feels things more deeply, is prone to marked mood swings and often feels self-conscious. They are sensitive about other's opinion about them, are concerned about their appearance and social behaviour, that can lead to them feeling awkward or socially withdrawn at times. In the famous Isle of Wight study by Rutter, et al. (1976),

over 2/5th of adolescents reported feelings of misery and sadness; 1/4th reported feelings of self-reference. Such feelings are more commonly experienced in adolescence rather than in middle childhood or later adult life. Due to intensity of their emotional reactions, their experience of bereavement is longer and more intense. The reason for this increase in depth and intensity of emotional experience is attributed to biological factors.

Identity and Self-Concept

Erickson has suggested that main psychosocial task of adolescence is the achievement of a stable identity of self-concept. According to him, this stage of 'identity crisis' is both necessary and desirable. Identity and self-concept include important components of self-esteem; commitment to a particular occupation, religion or political belief; view of one's own personality, physical attractiveness; sex role identity; and so on. There is an effort to develop autonomy, a sense of self, a view of their own capabilities, opinions, values, a sense of belonging. Identity formation is extremely important to build the foundation for adulthood. During adolescence, they experiment with and try out, a variety of looks, hair styles, attitudes, activities, friends and hobbies; and then begin to slowly grasp and understand what appearance or styles, interests or friends work for them. Then there is consolidation and acceptance of the concept of self and feeling of inner comfort at the individual level. This individual self-concept gets integrated with social-cultural-religious values that one lives in leading to development of strong commitments and ideologies. Formation of identity and self-concept are important building blocks that shape personality. Problems in identity formation and self-concept can lead to major challenges in mental health including mental illness.

One of the common issues with impaired identity formation is absence of identity formation or what is called as "identity diffusion". Such adolescents have not explored or experimented with options or made commitment to identity. Such adolescence become drifters in later life and remain aimless with little purpose in life. On the other hand, some parents may make decisions for their children and do not grant them the opportunity to participate or experiment with these choices. Sometimes, teenagers may strongly identify with their parents or elders and may follow in their footsteps. In such situations, without active and intentional participation in multiple alternatives, their commitments may not be as strong or durable.

Relationship with Parents

Adolescents strive for autonomy and individuation from their parents as a developmental task and as a step towards maturity. This requires redefining their relationship from the standpoint of authoritarian control to a mature egalitarian relationship. This transition is difficult for both sides, the parents and the adolescent. Cognitive and brain development pushes the teen to question parents on their jurisdiction in personal choices and facilitates reorganization of parent–adolescent relationship from it being vertical where parents have more knowledge and power, to it being horizontal, where parent and adolescent have equal and reciprocal relationship. This situation invariably leads to conflict where parents continue to negotiate for authority and adolescent continues to seek autonomy. This constant renegotiation eventually leads to mutually settling down of expectations, reduction of conflict and re-establishing closeness in relationship.

It has been popularly believed that adolescents usually become increasingly estranged from their families, become cut off from the rest of the society and develop a subculture of their own. However, systematic studies do not support this view. Many studies reviewed from America and Britain have shown that although adolescents would like their parents to be less restrictive and less old fashioned, and although there may be frequent arguments about clothing, length of hair, pop music, etc. but the great majority of teenagers showed core values as common with their parents, retain harmonious family relationships and respect the need for discipline.

The process of negotiating emotional conflict and its resolution towards a more egalitarian relationship happening within the safe environment of the family provides an opportunity for learning skills of emotional regulation in the adolescent. These are adaptive processes.

Adolescence, therefore, is not just puberty. It includes biological, social and psychological development and adaptations that are critical for this stage of life. It was described that 23% have smooth and continuous growth; 35% show surgent growth and 21% have tumultuous growth; and remaining 21% could not be classified (Offer and Offer 1975).

Adolescence is also a time for exploration and risk-taking; intense idealism and rejection of many of social norms and standards. This idealism may include an element of rebellion against home.

Exploration and risk taking increases during this period. They indulge in adventurous activities, that give them excitement as well as thrill. In addition this is the period of intense idealism rejection of social norms and standards, and radical thinking.

Psychiatric disorders in adolescence

These can be divided into three categories:
1. Disorders of adulthood which make their first appearance around adolescence, e.g. schizophrenia, depression, anorexia nervosa, substance abuse, anxiety, phobia and OCD, etc.
2. Disorders of childhood which continue into adolescence, e.g. conduct disorder, hyperkinetic syndrome, autism, specific learning disabilities, etc.

3. Disorders peculiar to adolescence which present in a variety of symptoms related to mood, behaviour and conduct. These are relatively less well-defined disorders.

Epidemiological data differs for each of these categories of disorders described.

PSYCHIATRIC DISORDERS IN ADOLESCENCE

There is increase in the risk for serious psychiatric disorders in adolescence. There is a sharp rise in the occurrence rates for depression, schizophrenia, bipolar affective disorder, anorexia and bulimia, substance abuse, antisocial behaviour and obsessive-compulsive disorders. Globally, it is estimated that 1 in 7 (14%) 10–19 year-olds experience mental health conditions (GHDx).

Emotional disorders are common among adolescents. It is estimated that 3.6% of 10–14-year-olds and 4.6% of 15–19-year-olds experience an anxiety disorder. Depression is estimated to occur among 1.1% of adolescents aged 10–14 years, and 2.8% of 15–19-year-olds (WHO 2019). Depression and anxiety share some of the same symptoms, including rapid and unexpected changes in mood. Depression can lead to suicide.

Behavioural disorders are more common among younger adolescents than older adolescents. Attention deficit hyperactivity disorder (ADHD), characterized by difficulty paying attention, excessive activity and acting without regard to consequences, occurs among 3.1% of 10–14-year-olds and 2.4% of 15–19-year-olds (GHDx). Behavioural disorders can affect adolescents' education and conduct disorder may result in criminal behaviour.

In two studies conducted on adolescents, the Isle of Wight study (Rutter et al. 1976) and Blackburn study (Leslie 1974), individual psychiatric diagnoses were made for adolescents. About 40% of those with psychiatric disorder showed emotional disorder of some kind like anxiety, depression, or affective disorder. OCD, hysteria, phobia, and tics were seen in few. Conduct disorder was diagnosed in another 40%. Enuresis, encopresis and hyperkinetic disorder was seen in few. Psychoses were rare. However, clinic based figures show a different trend. There is a larger number of psychotics and depressives in clinic samples.

Eating disorders, such as anorexia nervosa and bulimia nervosa, commonly emerge during adolescence and young adulthood. Anorexia nervosa can lead to premature death, often due to medical complications or suicide. Symptoms of psychosis most commonly emerge in late adolescence or early adulthood. Suicide is the fourth leading cause of death in older adolescents (15–19 years) (WHO 2019). Many risk-taking behaviours for health, such as substance use or sexual risk-taking, start during adolescence. Cannabis is the most widely used drug among young people with about 4.7% of 15–16-years-olds using it at least once in 2018 (World Drug Report 2020).

Internalizing mental disorders are more common in girls; these include depression, social anxiety, and eating disorders (prevalence ranges from 12% to 23%), whereas disruptive disorders, e.g., disorders of social behavior, are more common in boys, with a worldwide prevalence of approximately 5% to 10%.

Most of these disorders may be viewed as exaggerations or distortions of normal behaviors and emotions. Exploration into the etiology of psychiatric disorders among adolescence, indicates that there is a significant contribution from biological vulnerability factors as well as from family and social adversity factors including affiliation with "bad company or peer circle".

Protective factors that contribute to resilience include easy and conducive temperamental or personality disposition, a healthy and supportive family environment, good physical health, high IQ, economic advantage, and absence of any neuro developmental problems.

LESS WELL-DEFINED PSYCHIATRIC DISORDERS

There are certain emotional, conduct and behaviour problems encountered in adolescence which may bring the child to professional attention, but are difficult to be clearly defined as psychiatric disorders. A large proportion of adolescent population manifest such non-specific emotional or behavioural problems, many of which may improve by themselves through the processes of development and maturation, and may never come to psychiatrist's attention. Sometimes parents bring such problems to mental health professional, and these respond to certain general measures like changes in social conditions or methods of upbringing, general support and guidance, family intervention, changes in educational or recreational systems and so on without actual treatment being instituted for the patient. Thus, it becomes difficult to even label these disturbances as psychiatric disorders. However, on the other hand, this may be an area for preventive psychiatry where a timely and appropriate intervention may stall the future occurrence of psychiatric disorder. Therefore, it is necessary as well as important to recognize and understand these problems.

These generally present as emotional problems, relationship issues with parents, educational problems or sexual problems.

Emotional Problems

Emotional problems in the form of feelings of misery unhappiness, self-depreciating ideas and ideas of reference are very common (20–40%) which have been often described as the "inner turmoil" of adolescence. Feelings of sadness, apathy, emptiness, loneliness, boredom and isolation from peer groups may occur in normally adjusted young people. Dysphoric mood and non-specific sadness are common but not a reliable indicator of psychiatric disorder. Atypical depressive forms may be common, e.g. aggression, drug abuse, somatic complaints, sexual promiscuity etc. Self-poisoning is usually seen in females, which is more of an impulsive act, precipitated by some stress. Accident proneness is common and may be a manifestation of impulsiveness or depression.

Parent–Adolescent Estrangement and Social Alienation

It is common for adolescents to have hostility and conflict with parents. Issues involved are adolescent's demand for independence, parental disapproval and disappointment with their behaviour and developing personality, overreaction to adolescent's life style. They generally adopt a particular cult or a lifestyle which is a product of social, political and economic trends in contemporary time frame. Parent–adolescent alienation does not necessarily lead to psychiatric disorder. They often exhibit anti-authority and challenging behaviour which to some extent represents the normal developmental process of growing up.

Sexual Problems

One of the important tasks of adolescence is to accept the adult sex roles. Anxiety and guilt about sexual thoughts and activities, homosexuality of a transient nature in boys, worry over masturbation are common and may have all pervasive effects over his activities. Problems involving incest, rape and other forms of sexual abuse are coming more frequently to psychiatrist's attention. It is likely that increased sexual permissiveness in the last few decades in the society has complicated the sexual adjustment of adolescents causing sexual experimentation at a much younger age.

Problems in School

Disenchantment with conventional education leading to truancy and other conduct disorders, academic problems including examination anxiety, under achievement, etc. are common.

CHANGES IN PATTERN OF PSYCHIATRIC DISORDERS AT ADOLESCENCE

Disorders with strong developmental component, e.g. enuresis, encopresis become much less frequent in adolescence.

Emotional disorders get more differentiated in their symptomatology during adolescence with closer resemblance to adult neurotic conditions.

Sex ratio changes from equal proportion before puberty to female preponderance after puberty, particularly for depression and dissociative disorders.

Conduct disturbances and delinquency rises to its peak in teens particularly in boys. There is marked increase in truanting, absconding. Violent crimes, drunkenness and drug offences become commoner in later adolescence and early adulthood.

Results of the follow-up studies have shown that:

1. Most psychiatric disorders during adolescence run true to type and marked fluctuations in symptoms are not seen.
2. Prognosis varies markedly according to diagnosis.
3. Prognosis for adolescent psychiatric disorders is not much different from that for similar disorders in early childhood or adult life.

Some of these psychiatric disorders start in infancy and childhood, and continue into adolescence, others are adult disorders with onset in adolescence and some disorders are first manifest only in adolescence.

Adolescent disorders are classified as in general classification of psychiatric disorders. Generally the same diagnostic scheme and approach as for other disorders is applied. It has been found that adolescent adjustment reaction is generally a non-specific over diagnosed label. Many of these patients could fit in with the criteria for other specific disorders. Personality disorder, if presenting with characteristic picture can be diagnosed in adolescence though theoretically personality is not fully formed at that age.

Etiology of adolescent psychiatric disorders is not very different from that for most other psychiatric disorders. It is generally multifactorial with significant contribution coming from developmental and psychosocial factors.

THERAPEUTIC APPROACHES

General approach to treatment requires the therapist to be non-judgmental, using participatory/collaborative approach rather than an authoritarian approach. Bringing the adolescent to treatment net can be a challenge. Many a times they want to be seen alone without knowledge of their parents which should be honoured. Confidentiality is a big issue for them. However, if there is a situation where there can be harm to self or others, then the adolescent has to be told to inform parents or the psychiatrist informs them. Adolescents often set limits or conditions what treatment they will accept, which the therapist may have to work through and negotiate. Use of patience, openness, discussion and reasoning often help to break any impasse.

Multidisciplinary team work approach involving treatment, training, education, care and control are the significant elements suggested for treatment of adolescents. Thorough and realistic appraisal of objectives should be made. Full range of psychiatric treatments used with adults or children can be used with adolescents. Most disorders seen in adolescence are managed with a combination of psychotropics and psychological methods or with psychological methods alone without medication.

Drugs have an important place in a range of adolescent psychiatry disorders. Psychotropics are used as in adults for respective indications. They are preferably used for relatively specific therapeutic effects, and it is legitimate to use them in the following situations:

a. Symptomatic management to relieve distress, e.g. in anxiety, depression, OCD, PTSD etc.

b. To manage destructive or self-destructive behaviour such as violence, aggression, self-harm, refusal to eat, high risk situation in patients when nothing else works.

c. To treat specific psychiatric disorders like ADHD, psychosis, BPAD, schizophrenia etc.

Psychostimulants such as methylphenidate, pemoline, or non-stimulant medication like atomoxetine are indicated for hyperkinetic syndromes as primary treatment and also as an adjunct to other therapies. These are particularly indicated when there is poor attention span, overactivity and disorganized behaviour and psychological, physiological or EEG evidence of brain dysfunction. Seventy-five per cent adolescents show improvement on short-term use, and also give long term help in social, academic and psychological adjustment.

Neuroleptics are indicated in schizophrenia, mania and other psychotic-disorders, in aggression, anxiety, excitement, severe conduct disorder, in Tourette's syndrome and tic disorder.

Antidepressant drugs have much larger ranger range of effects and are used in many conditions like depression, phobic disorder, OCD, enuresis, PTSD, and anxiety.

As a general principle, anxiolytics, sedative and hypnotic are not used except in unusual circumstances, e.g. severe anxiety, severe psychotic or manic excitement or catatonia.

Lithium is indicated in BPAD, and some episodic behaviour disorders, impulse control disorders and anorexia nervosa. Similarly, anticonvulsants can be used for treatment and prevention of BPAD, and some episodic behaviour disorders, impulse control disorders.

ECT can be used for severe, retarded, delusional depression or suicidality particularly if drugs have failed. ECT is also indicated in Catatonia.

Buprenorphine with or without naloxone combination can be used for opiate dependence.

Psychotherapy: Individual psychotherapy is very useful.

Behaviour therapy, relaxation, cognitive restructuring, group therapy is especially beneficial when applied to adolescents.

Parental and family therapy: Greater reliance is placed on family therapy rather than psychoanalytic individual psychotherapy while treating adolescents. Engagement of family and parents is often crucial in treatment.

Establishing school liaison is extremely important specially in problems related to academic functioning such as learning disorders, ADHD, intellectual disability, or those related to peers like bullying.

Residential or in-patient treatment is mostly indicated for patients with severe symptoms as in schizophrenia, mania, depression, dissociation or anorexia nervosa; or when the patient does not respond to outpatient treatment. In-patient treatment is also indicated in those with severe family pathology.

Preventive and Promotive Interventions

These include adopting healthy sleep patterns; exercising regularly; developing coping, problem-solving, and interpersonal skills; and learning to manage emotions. Protective and supportive environments in the family, at school and in the wider community are important.

In a scoping review from India, it was reported that school-based programs using a life skills curriculum and coping skills and resilience curricula showed improvement in depressive symptoms, cognitive abilities, academic stress, problem-solving, and overall mental well-being in adolescents (Mehra et al 2022).

In conclusion, adolescent age has been often described as age of follies, misadventures, misdirectedness and has attracted criticism of elders. It, however, should be recognized as a phase of genuine transition, where biological factors and developmental changes are at its peak, effects of which get worse or more complicated by misdirected approach in handling of the adolescent. An adolescent requires understanding, tolerance, flexibility in the attitude of adults; a non-authoritarian and rational approach to deal with their turmoil and rebellion. They can be more usefully involved in the social and constructive tasks provided their energy and motivation is properly harnessed.

BIBLIOGRAPHY

1. Coleman JC. (1980). The Nature of Adolescence. London: Methuen.
2. Dulit E. Adolescent thinking a la Piaget: the formal stage. Journal of Youth and Adolescence 4: 281–301, 1972.
3. Institute of health Metrics and Evaluation. Global Health Data Exchange (GHDx).
4. Leslie SA. (1974). Psychiatric disorder in the young adolescents of an industrial town. British Journal of Psychiatry, 125, 113–124.
5. Mehra D, Lakiang T, Kathuria N, Kumar M, Mehra S, and Sharma S, (2022). Mental Health Interventions among Adolescents in India: A Scoping Review. Healthcare (Basel). Feb; 10(2): 337.
6. Offer B, Offer JB. From Teenage to Young Manhood: A Psychological Study. New York, Basic Books, 1975.
7. Oldham DG. Adolescent turmoil: a myth revisited, in Adolescent Psychiatry: Developmental and Clinical Studies, Vol. 6. Edited by Feinstein SC, Giovacchini PL. Chicago, IL, University of Chicago Press, 1978, pp 267–279.
8. Rutter M, Graham P, Chadwick O, Yule W. (1976). Adolescent turmoil: fact or fiction. J. Child Psychol Psychiat 17, 35–56.
9. Rutter M. (1979). Changing youth in a changing society. Patterns of adolescent development and disorder. London: Nuffield Provincial Hospitals Trust.
10. Steinberg D (1983). The Clinical Psychiatry of Adolescence. Pub. John Wiley and Sons.
11. WHO Global Health Estimates 2000–2019.
12. World Drug Report 2020.

Infant Mental Health

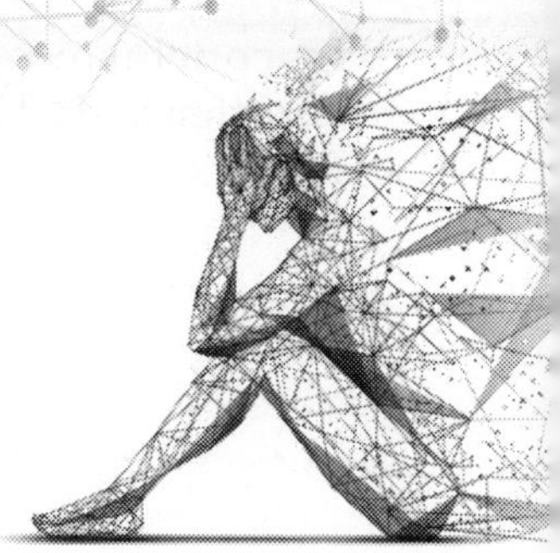

Infant mental health refers to how well a child develops socially and emotionally from birth to three years of age. Infant mental health is the study of mental health of infants, toddlers and their families. Mental health of infants is as important as their physical health and essential for the growth and maturity of their brain and body as well as for their social and emotional development now and for the whole lifetime. Research in neuroscience, biological, genetic and social science in the last 2 decades has shown unequivocally that infancy (up to first 3 years) are foundational in terms of brain development. Origins of mental disorders are found in the biological and developmental disruptions occurring during early years of life. This happens by cumulative damage or by biological embedding of adversities during sensitive developmental periods.

'Infant mental health' or 'infant brain health' has been defined as *"The developing capacity of the child from birth to five years of age to: Form close and secure adult and peer relationships, experience, manage and express a full range of emotions, and explore the environment and learn all in the context of family, community and culture"* (Zero to three 2012).

Infant mental health (IMH) is a rapidly evolving new discipline with sufficient knowledge and scientific foundation focusing on the first three years of life. Infants have mental life in the context of their early relationships with mother or mother figure, that has been amply explored and described by Anna Freud, John Bowlby and Donald Winnicot. Development of the field of IMH has paralleled research on the consequences of child abuse and neglect and infant development (Steele 1986, Zeanah et al 1989). There is international consensus that the first 1,000 days of life i.e., the period of development from conception to age two, represent a crucial period of rapid physical, psychological and neurological growth (Moore et al, 2017). Infant mental health is 'the young child's capacity to experience, regulate and express emotions, form close and secure relationships, explore the environment and learn (Zero to Three, 2001). There are several important developmental skills or tasks (listed below) for babies to learn. We have already discussed this in earlier chapter on neurodevelopment (Chapter 1). They have to learn to:

- Manage and express emotions
- Manage impulses and regulate their behavior
- Establish close, secure relationships with people
- Learn to identify and begin to understand own feelings
- Learn to recognize feelings and emotions in others
- Develop empathy
- Make friends
- Develop confidence, cooperativeness and the capacity to communicate

- Learn to explore and gain knowledge about their environment, including their family community and culture.

Babies are dependent on adults for experiencing the environment in an optimal and positive manner. While both physical and mental development relies on nutrition, a child's physical growth requires exercise and the opportunity to explore and interact with the physical world. A child's social, emotional, and intellectual development depends on a loving environment that promotes self-awareness, social awareness, problem-solving, intellectual curiosity, and the ability to focus attention.

The brain grows most rapidly in the first years of life, that is both qualitatively and quantitatively different than at any other time of life. At birth the baby has 25% of adult brain weight and 75% of our brain structure is added after birth. By age 2 years, brain is 80% of adult size. Brain development is driven by unfolding of the evolutionarily conserved genetic programming. Environmental influences or experiences comprising of molecular, cellular, hormonal, microbial, interpersonal, social environment, during in-utero and postnatal periods, influence brain development. Further, the dyadic relationship between the infant and the caregiver in the first years of life has direct and enduring effect on the child's brain development and behaviour. In the first few months of life, just as parents are learning to read the baby's cues, the baby is also learning to read the parent's emotional cues. Infant's sensory systems are more advanced than motor systems. Young infants experience sadness, fear, and a whole range of human emotions. We are just beginning to understand the depth of feelings, emotions, stress responses that infants can experience. During first year of life, a close relationship with mother helps in development of those neural networks that underly attachment and bonding, safety and danger, and core sense of self identity. Neonatal reflexes get translated into more advanced skills like gazing, smiling, imitating, which are the building blocks of emotional bonding and communication. Prolonged sharing of emotional gaze stimulates growth of networks of attachment in brain. Building of social brain is driven between 18–24 moths in the form of unconsciously organized neural networks that constitute the core. These experiences are visceral, pre-verbal and hence more resistant to change. As the mother and child touch and separate and touch again, endorphin levels rise and fall leading to alternate feelings of well-being and distress that helps in development of emotional awareness and cognition in the baby. Emotional/social development starts immediately after birth, even before birth when the mother looks at or relates and talks to the baby. Exposure of the fetus to stress hormones of the mother primes and sensitizes its nervous system, which on repeated exposures, can become dysregulated and hypersensitive.

Infants are endowed with very high ability of sense perception and discrimination. Infants very early learn to sense and respond to their mother's moods and emotions. Infant's language lacks words, but it is rich in terms of expressions. They communicate without words, through facial expression, gaze aversion, crying, cooing, gurgling or withdrawal behaviour in states of distress. Young infants can experience and exhibit evidence of sadness, fear and a whole range of human emotions (Gopnik et al 2000). When their needs are successfully met by a responsive caregiver, infants learn that they can rely on that person, and the social bond builds. Babies smile when mother or caregivers smile. Young children cry when another child cries. Toddlers will want to cuddle or give hugs when their mother or caregiver is sad.

Environment influences the genes by altering gene expression and through the process of epigenesis. No other stage of life depends more on external environment for growth and development as infancy. Early experience gets embedded in the brain that shapes the brain to an extent that it has lifelong consequences for health, learning and socio-emotional relationships. Ultimately every individual brain is a built uniquely through life experience and customization.

We have already discussed the attachment theory of development in earlier chapter. It is abundantly clear that the attachment relationship or emotional bonding between infant and mother or caregiver(s) is extremely crucial to development. A secure, warm, responsive and predictable relationship with at least one caregiver in early infancy influences the formation of neural structures in the brain that lead to positive infant well-being. Secure attachment also positively affects the development of the hypothalamic pituitary axis, which regulates stress. Secure attachment provides a safe haven and secure base for learning and social, emotional and cognitive development. Secure attachment also protects the brain from harm. Infants are unable to regulate their physical and emotional states independently on their own. Secure parent–child relationships provides the infants, toddlers and young children strong (or weak) foundations for all emotional, cognitive, and social development, positive physical health and resilience for all times to come. Development of a sound social and emotional base in infancy goes a long way in assuring positive learning experience and establishing positive relationships in adult life.

Risk Factors for Developmental Pathologies

If there is lack of positive, protective, secure and consistent relationship between the infant and the mother or caregiver due to any reason, such as maternal absence, poverty, unpredictability or violence, it can lead to insecure attachment or bonding and that has several deleterious effects on the child like social difficulties, reduced stress tolerance, anxiety, relationship difficulties. Exposure to traumatic or abusive events in childhood are associated with depression, cardiovascular disease, cancer, alcoholism and drug abuse in adult life, personality disorders, dissociation, somatization disorders, and risk-taking behaviours later in adolescence and adulthood. Infants exposed to abuse, neglect, substance abuse, domestic violence, mental illness, and an incarcerated primary caregiver, have a lifelong impact, and are linked to obesity, smoking, heart disease, diabetes and other illness and risky behaviors in adults. Infants who receive a poor-quality care due to depression or mental illness in the mother or care giver become less responsive to environment. Infants who are not spoken to sufficiently lag in language skills and social relationships.

Lack of sensitive and responsive care-giving can occur under several conditions, when there is:

- Mental illnesses such as depression or psychosis in the caregiver
- Caregiver's own history of neglect and abuse
- Single parenthood without social support
- Temperament adversity/mismatches between infant and caregiver
- Financial stress
- Alcohol or drug abuse in the caregiver
- Marital discord or dysfunction between parents

Mother's mental and physical and mental health status during pregnancy is extremely crucial for IMH. Her use of alcohol or other intoxicants during pregnancy, and her exposure to toxins such as lead, mercury or organophosphates, or exposure to intimate partner violence during pregnancy are other significant risk factors for mental ill health of infants.

Risk factors for poor mental health in infants, involve the interaction between the individual child's genetics, temperament and environment (McLuckie et al., 2019).

Family based risk factors include parenting interactions that are insensitive, lack of warmth, controlling parents, or over involvement or over protection. Other factors include overly harsh or punitive disciplining, parental mental health problems or stress, parental substance abuse, family violence, limited parental education, and parental conflict or separation/divorce. The experience of trauma during infancy, including maltreatment, exposure to domestic violence, and disruption of attachment relationships are significant developmental risk factors that lead to vulnerabilities and mental health problems later on. Epigenetic studies have found that early childhood maltreatment is linked to higher methylation of key genes related to the stress response. These methylation changes place children at risk of cancers, cardiovascular disease, autoimmune disorders, and psychiatric disorders. Environmental stressors such as war, natural disasters and family dislocation also place infants and young children at risk of mental health difficulties.

High and prolonged stress leads to activation of HPA Axis and prolonged increase of glucocorticoids which disrupt neural function. Glucocorticoid receptors in brain regions associated with emotional learning, self-regulation, reward processing, executive control such as amygdala, hippocampus, prefrontal cortex are most susceptible to stress and impair the development of these functions. Reduction in volumes of amygdala, hippocampus and pre-frontal cortex is seen in children who are Reduction in volumes of these areas is seen in children who are maltreated, or institutionalized early in life or faced toxic stress in childhood. Toxic stress such as poverty, abuse and trauma, hinders the brain's development and child's capacity to regulate behaviour, emotions and attention; and impacts a child's other body systems, which in turn impacts the physical health as well. It also impairs the child's ability to learn. Early nutritional deficits have negative impact on cognitive development. Persistent poverty is a primary cause of toxic stress in children. Other causes include abuse, chronic neglect, domestic violence and parental mental illness.

Early childhood temperament is a recognised risk factor for depression in both preschool and at older ages. Research has also shown that infants with temperament characteristics of social withdrawal, high intensity of responsiveness, low threshold, negative mood and high persistence have greater likelihood of developing anxiety, depression, somatization disorders. On the other hand infants exhibiting high activity, high intensity of responsiveness, low attention span, high distractibility, low threshold of responsiveness have greater likelihood of developing externalizing disorders like conduct disorder, ADHD, substance use disorder later on.

Many disorders of childhood and adolescence have onset as early as preschool age. The first signs of mental health difficulties can be manifest in infancy, emphasizing the importance of understanding and identifying both protective and risk factors particularly in pregnancy and the early postnatal period. Research has shown that preschool-onset internalizing disorders are well defined, well-described, and validated conditions that are linked to behavioral issues and brain functioning later in life. Developmental psychopathology manifesting in the form of emotional dysregulation, inability to change or adapt, inability to form relationships, get soothed, sleep problems, feeding problems, and developmental delays. Other issues are lack of resilience, poor social competence, or aggression and temper tantrums can even be enduring.

Common mental health concerns seen in infancy are:

- Poor sleep patterns
- Difficulties with feeding
- Persistent or unremitting crying

- Restlessness
- Gastric disturbance
- Anxiety and tension
- Distress and fear
- Lack of weight gain or failure to thrive
- Failure to meet expected developmental milestones

Red flag signs for mental health problems are:

Infant (birth through 1 year)

- Excessive fussiness-very difficult to soothe/console
- Limited or no interest in things or people
- Failure to gain weight
- Consistent strong reactions to touch, sounds or movement
- Sleep problems
- Feeding problems

Toddler (1–3 years)
(Includes the above issues in addition to the following)

- Displays very little emotion
- Unable to calm self
- Does not turn to adults for comfort or help
- Excessive fearfulness or excessive sadness
- Withdrawal or excessive clinging
- Aggression toward self or others
- Impulsiveness and hyperactivity
- Excessive tantrums or defiance
- Language delays
- Interference with typical developmental tasks

Preschool (3–5 years)
(Includes the above issues in addition to the following)

- Consistently prefers not to play with others or with toys
- Destructiveness
- Hurts animals
- Limited use of words to express feelings

Most often mental health difficulties begin in the preschool years. Children exhibit signs of anxiety disorders, phobias, attention-deficit hyperactivity disorder (ADHD), depression, post-traumatic stress disorder (PTSD) and other mental conditions at a very early age. Pre-school anxiety, a very common condition at that age, has to be differentiated from normative situational fears. Fear response includes physiological responses such as increased heart rate, fearful expressions or crying, these responses serve important adaptive functions to provide cues to caregivers to promote protective behaviors. Many of these are normative fears which follow a well-defined developmental trajectory and disappear as the child grows. For example, stranger anxiety emerges at around age nine months, while separation anxiety occurs in the first year or two of life. Anxiety in infants and pre-schoolers manifests as crying, anger, avoidance, freezing, school refusal, clinging, or tantrums. Most studies estimate the prevalence of preschool anxiety disorders in the range of 10–20% (Franz et al 2015, Paulus et al 2015). Anxiety disorders are widely acknowledged as the most prevalent class of psychiatric illness during the preschool period and across the lifespan; and retrospective studies report the median age of onset for anxiety disorders around 6 years of age (Petresco et al 2004, Kessler et al 2005). Eggar and Angold (2006) in a review article on the presentation, nosology and epidemiology of behavioral and emotional psychiatric disorders in preschool children (children ages 2 through 5 years old), focused on the five most common groups of childhood psychiatric disorders: attention deficit hyperactivity disorders, oppositional defiant and conduct disorders, anxiety disorders, and depressive disorders. Rates of preschool psychopathology were compared with the rates of psychiatric disorders in older children. There was convincing evidence that the rates of the common child psychiatric disorders and the patterns of comorbidity among pre-schoolers are similar to those seen in later childhood. It has been reported that children <6 years of age have a similar rate of mental illness as older children and youth (14% to 20%). Research has also established that infants and toddlers can suffer from mental health disorders that require treatment in their own right (Warner and Pottick 2006, Zero to Three, 2012).

Egger and Angold (2006) found rates of preschool depression ranging from 0–2.1% depending on the sample and assessment measure used. Most other studies have reported prevalence rate of depression in pre-schoolers to be about 2% (Levigne et al 2009, Buffered et al 2011). Symptoms of depression include withdrawal, refusal to eat, crying, reduced social responsiveness, irritability, sleep problems. Low frustration tolerance, anger and temper outbursts predict later onset of oppositional defiant disorder. In a study by Whalen and colleagues (2015) suicidality was studied in a sample of 306 children between the ages 3 and 7, and it was found that preschool suicidal ideation was concurrently associated with several child psychopathologies, including depression, anxiety disorders, ADHD, ODD, and CD. It has also been seen that prenatal maternal depression may lead to an intrauterine environment that is not conducive to healthy fetal development, thereby increasing risk for mental health issues in childhood. Common presentations are dysregulated emotional or behavioral patterns including anger, aggression, or anxiety that interfere with a child's ability to interact with family and the environment. These problems rarely resolve spontaneously without intervention but often respond to therapy and family support.

Management

Raising children is complex, needs hard work and a time intensive responsibility where parents, grandparents, extended family, other caregivers and the whole community plays significant roles. Indicators of mental health issues become apparent very early in life i.e. infancy and preschool years. Thus, infancy and preschool years provide a major opportunity for preventive and promotive interventions. Early interventions are effective in improving outcomes in health and cognition. Interventions started early in infancy have a more powerful and lasting impact than interventions at later ages. Prevention of mental health difficulties before they arise, particularly during the earliest stages of life when intervention has the greatest capacity to bring about change is the most crucial strategy. Prevention and treatment are intricately inter related in this age group. Every or any intervention will have preventive effect as well.

Management of infant's mental health issues focuses on treatment of three parties: the Infant; the Parent/Caregiver; and Infant-parent relationship.

Assessment includes assessment of the:
Infant: the developmental level of the infant, temperament of the infant, physical status
Mother/caregiver: Mother's or caregiver's personality, mental state, attitude towards child care and expectations.
Infant-parent relationship: Assess the mother-infant dyad in terms of warmth, physical and emotional contact, response to baby's needs, sensitivity to cues, communication both quantitatively and qualitatively and so on.

Parents and child health professionals should be aware of an infant's developmental benchmarks so they can accurately monitor their mental development in various domains like motor skills, social milestones, linguistic skills and adaptive skills. Knowledge about temperamental characteristics and assessment is essential for IMH. Temperamental variations and mismatches with parenting styles can majorly contribute to emotional and behavioural problems arising during infancy. Babies who are temperamentally unhappy, hyper responsive, with intense reactions and high persistence are hard to soothe, are frustrating for the care giver who may feel incompetent and develop negative reactions towards the baby. This negative reaction may lead to reduced or compromised care which further aggravates the problem.

Mental health and emotional development in babies and very young children is enhanced through relationships which are warm and help them feel loved and protected. The more young children are able to safely explore and experience the world around them, the better they feel about themselves. There is need for a good structure and reliability around them. So, for the warmth part, you should advise parents to enjoy your baby, enjoy your child, play with them, talk to them, cuddle them. Doing those things will make the child feel good, and you feel good. This interaction releases natural hormones that help bonding with the baby.

General guidelines for healthy parenting are:

- Promoting safe, and effective parenting practices;
- Promoting healthy parent and family communication styles;
- Promoting effective communication with babies;
- Sensitive and responsive care giving;
- Ensure safety of the child;
- Tune in to your child's cues and interests;
- Talk more—describe the world around them;
- No exposure to TV, mobile phone or screens;

To nurture healthy social and emotional development in infants:

- Surround children with positive, nurturing relationships
- Create a trusting, secure environment through stable, predictable routines
- Provide stable/consistent caregiving at home, in child care and in school
- Have realistic expectations
- Respond to infant and young children's cues
- Spend quality, unhurried time together without distractions such as television, phone or computer

- Comfort and reassure infants and young children when they appear scared, upset, angry or hurt
- Be consistent in behaviour
- Use judicious punishment or disapproval
- Be a good role model in terms of healthy relationships and healthy ways to manage conflict in the family
- Think how your behaviour and emotions may be affecting your infant or young child
- Identify early signs of potential mental health problems

Treatment of preschool mental disorders include both parenting interventions and psychotherapeutic interventions. Healthy parenting guidance is extremely important for both prevention as well as treatment. Parenting is a hard task. Most people do it intuitively or how they have experienced it in their childhood. However, parenting is something that everybody should learn how to do.

Play therapy is widely used with very young children in a host of problems presenting in early childhood. Parent–child relationship therapy using behavioral and play therapy techniques to enhance relationship quality and parent's ability to set nurturing and effective goals with the child are helpful.

Psychotropic drugs have not been tested nor tried in this age group.

If the mother/caregiver is feeling overwhelmed or suffer from anxiety, depression or stress, they should definitely manage their own stress and mental health condition including seeking support or professional help. Effective treatment of the mother's or caregiver's mental illness should be carried out. There are several successful programs for parents imparting psychoeducation, practical skills training, working on the co-parenting relationship, developing secure attachment, and enhancing parental reflective functioning. Many perinatal and infancy prevention/early intervention programs have been developed and evaluated, with some designed for universal implementation and others designed for population at increased risk of poor social and emotional development. Since early developmental years of a child's life have the capacity to influence themselves into adulthood, there is reason and scope for early interventions during this period so that their future life trajectory can be set up on a positive and healthy path.

Advanced interventions: Technology for development of induced pluripotent stem cells (iPSCs) to derive neurons using tissue obtained from a living person, maintaining person's genetic constitution and diversity, shall allow the study of human neural development for individual genome *in vitro*. Technology for stem cell therapy for treatment of some psychiatric and neurological disorders is available. However, application of this iPSCs though promising, for neurodevelopmental disorders (ASD, ADHD, Tourette's, SLD) remains to be proven for efficacy.

Infant Mental Health has not been in the forefront of global attention or advocacy. Allocation of resources is related to disease burden, and not to preventive or promotive strategies. Survival took priority over quality of survival or thriving. There is need for focusing attention on IMH as a strategy for preventive and promotive intervention in psychiatry as a whole. There is a strong case for starting early parenting and parenthood programs; as well as genetic and molecular biological research and stem cell research in India.

BIBLIOGRAPHY

1. Bufferd SJ, Dougherty LR, Carlson GA, Klein DN. Parent-reported mental health in preschoolers: findings using a diagnostic interview. Compr Psychiatry. 2011;52(4):359–369. doi: 10.1016/j.comppsych.2010.08.006.

2. Egger HL, Angold A. Common emotional and behavioral disorders in preschool children: presentation, nosology, and epidemiology. J Child Psychol Psychiatry. 2006;47(3–4):313–337. doi: 10.1111/j.1469-7610.2006.01618.x.

3. Franz L, Angold A, Copeland W, Costello EJ, Towe-Goodman N, Egger H. Preschool Anxiety Disorders in Pediatric Primary Care: Prevalence and Comorbidity. J Am Acad Child Adolesc Psychiatry. 2013;52(12):1294–1303.e1. doi: 10.1016/j.jaac.2013.09.008.

4. Gopnik A, Meltzoff AN, Kuhl PK. In: The Scientist in the Crib: What Early Learning Tells Us About the Mind.New York: William Morrow–Harper Collins; 2000.

5. Kessler RC, Berglund P, Demler O, Jin R, Merikangas KR, Walters EE. Lifetime prevalence and age-of-onset distributions of DSM-IV disorders in the National Comorbidity Survey Replication. Arch GenPsychiatry. 2005;62(6):593–602. doi: 10.1001/archpsyc.62.6.593.

6. Lavigne JV, LeBailly SA, Hopkins J, Gouze KR, Binns HJ. The Prevalence of ADHD, ODD, Depression, and Anxiety in a Community Sample of 4-Year-Olds. J Clin Child Adolesc Psychol. 2009;38(3):315–328. doi: 10.1080/15374410902851382.

7. McLuckie A, Landers AL, Curran JA, Cann R, Carrese DH, Nolan A, et al. (2019). A scoping review of mental health prevention and intervention initiatives for infants and preschoolers at risk for socio-emotional difficulties. Syst. Rev. 8:183. 10.1186/s13643-019-1043-3.

8. Moore T, Arefadib N, Deery A, West S (2017). The First Thousand Days: An Evidence Paper.Parkeville, VIC: Centre for Community Child Health.

9. Paulus FW, Backes A, Sander CS, Weber M, von Gontard A. Anxiety disorders and behavioral inhibition in preschool children: a population-based study. Child Psychiatry Hum Dev. 2015;46(1):150–157. doi: 10.1007/s10578-014-0460-8.

10. Petresco S, Anselmi L, Santos IS, et al. Prevalence and comorbidity of psychiatric disorders among 6-year-old children: 2004 Pelotas Birth Cohort. Soc Psychiatry Psychiatr Epidemiol. 2014;49(6):975–983. doi: 10.1007/s00127-014-0826-z.

11. Steele BF (1986). Notes on the lasting effects of early child abuse throughout the life cycle. Child Abuse Negl. 10(3):283–91.

12. Warner LA, Pottick K.J. (2006). Functional impairment among preschoolers using

mental health services. Children Youth Serv. Rev. 28473–486. 10.1016/j.childyouth. 2005.11.008

13. Whalen DJ, Dixon-Gordon K, Belden AC, Barch D, Luby JL. Correlates and Consequences of Suicidal Cognitions and Behaviors in Children Ages 3 to 7 Years. J Am Acad Child Adolesc Psychiatry. 2015; 54(11):926–937.e2. doi: 10.1016/j.jaac. 2015. 08.009.

14. Zeanah CH, Anders TF, Seifer R, Stern DN (1989). Implications of research on infant development for psychodynamic theory and practice. J Am Acad Child Adolesc Psychiatry. 28(5):657–68.

15. Zero to Three (2012). Making It Happen: Overcoming Barriers to Providing Infant-Early Childhood Mental Health. Washington, DC: Zero to Three.

Psychiatric and Behavioural Emergencies

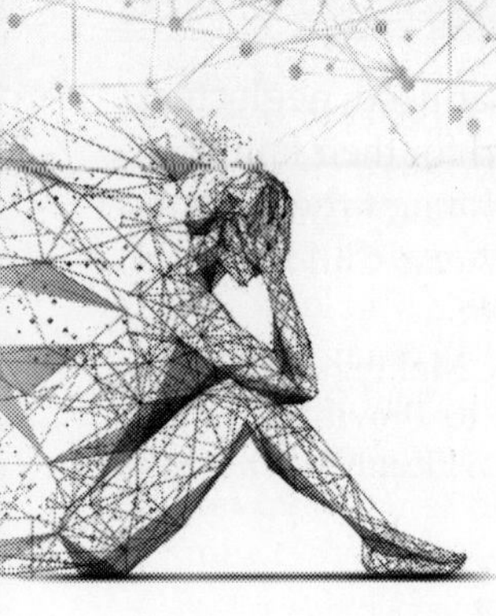

Psychiatric emergencies in children are those clinical situations where there is direct and immediate threat to the health or life of the child, or of the family or society, with or without physical harm, arising from such distressing or disruptive psychiatric or behavioural symptoms that need emergency attention. Emergency situations can arise in the background of a psychiatric disorder or of any crisis. Immediate concern in emergency situation is safety of the child/ adolescent and/or of the family and society.

Sometimes, healthy children when faced with adverse and sudden life situations, such as crisis, disaster, bereavement, breakdown of family, or child abuse, may develop serious disturbances in emotions, behaviour or adjustment. On the other hand, a child may develop acute symptoms of clear psychiatric disorders, e.g. acute psychotic breakdown, anorexia nervosa, severe depression, conduct disorder, etc. which are so disruptive or distressing to the child or the family or the society that immediate control is necessary. All such situations are broadly considered as emergencies.

Since most children and adolescents are basically dependent on their parents, it is they and not the children themselves who perceive the situation as an emergency and seek help. This issue is important because if the parents feel too anxious or overwhelmed or inadequate to help or control the child, they may declare the situation as emergency seeking immediate help. Of course, certain situations are emergencies in its own right, e.g. acute psychosis, severe depression, etc. However, certain situations present as emergencies particularly when parents or teachers are unable to handle it, or are overwhelmed by it.

Occasionally older children or adolescents, or school-age children may directly report for help. It is more likely to happen particularly when they come from non-supportive environment or homes where they have non-supportive or abusive parents or where parents are absent. Apart from parents, it may sometimes be teachers, pediatricians and rarely police or other social agencies who may refer children for emergency help. Most of the psychiatric and behavioural emergencies present to the hospitals in general medical emergency rooms, or in paediatrics or psychiatry departments depending upon the availability of service. Nevertheless, a large number of these clinical problems, remain unrecognized and unattended in the community with the concomitant toll of distress, disease and even death, unknown to people and professionals alike. Those that come to attention need to be recognized, evaluated and treated.

Most emergencies occur within the family or the school setting and often give warning signals before becoming emergent. Many a times, it is a chronic lingering maladjustment or disturbance that assumes such proportions so as to be considered an emergency. For example, parental discord, culminating into divorce that puts the child's interest into jeopardy; anxiety, maladjustment in school leading to school refusal and somatoform disorders, etc.

The institution of family has a strong and powerful influence on the development of children. Apart from providing nurturance, protection and safety, the family performs the vital functions of acculturation, i.e. imparting the cultural and social values to the child, of laying the foundation of social relationships in adult life, of providing channels and methods of communications, and so on. The adequacy or the success in achieving these goals varies a great deal from family to family and that shows the strength or weakness of a family unit. Dysfunctional families are characterized by disorganization and chaos, absence of emotional bonds. There may be absence of supportive, responsible and competent adults. Such families are unable to contain the disturbance, mitigate the effects of the emotional trauma and are more likely to end up in acute emergency or crisis.

The symptoms in the child reflect only the tip of the iceberg where longstanding problems of disturbed and chaotic family communications, impaired parent–child relationship may have existed. Frequently such families focus only on the symptoms in the child and deny underlying family pathology and to recognize that the problems in the child are a result of their behaviour. Problems like suicide, drug abuse, aggression and conduct disorder occur commonly in dysfunctional families. Parent–child communication may breakdown and the problems are not solved within the family system. It is the perceived absence of alternatives in such a situation that may culminate into a crisis.

The child may have some basic problems in himself/herself like low intelligence, specific learning disability, attention deficit hyperactivity disorder, autism, or psychosis, etc. which the parents may have failed to recognize or cope with.

Such children may be abused, neglected, punished and condemned for their failure to come up to the expectations of the parents or teachers may develop major emotional and behavioural difficulties. A supportive and understanding approach of parents towards children with such handicaps or disabilities is likely to facilitate adjustment and mitigate breakdown.

In certain situations, the child has no problems basically; he is simply a victim of the circumstances or events happening in his/her life, as for example, death of a parent, disaster, poverty and deprivation, etc. These are the conditions where the family structure may be broken or there is extreme adversity which leads to high degree of stress for the victims including the child. Severe stress can lead to breakdown of coping even in normal and healthy individuals.

Families that are well integrated and cohesive in their functioning, that have access to resources (financial, social, legal, medical) have good social support, cope better with adversity. Parental mental illness may in itself lead to an unbearable situation at home for the child. Children of parents suffering from schizophrenias, particularly paranoid subtype or affective disorder may be so overwhelmed by their unpredictable psychotic behaviour that they may develop acute anxiety, panic reactions. At times, the child may be physically or emotionally abused by his/her parents. In such situations the child may have a serious risk to life and would require protection.

Therefore, while evaluating a case with psychiatric and behavioural emergencies full assessment of the psychological, social and family factors must be done.

Problems that are Likely to Present as Emergencies

Some of the conditions, commonly seen in children, listed below are likely to culminate into emergency at some stage and present itself to emergency rooms of paediatric medical or psychiatric hospitals. Emergencies can be understood as primarily psychiatric (that arise basically from some psychiatric disorder in the child), or psychosocial (that arise from circumstances outside in the environment).

Psychiatric emergencies	Psychosocial emergencies
Severe depression and suicide	Parental discord, divorce
Dissociative disorders	Maltreatment, abuse, neglect
Anxiety and panic disorder	Sexual trauma
Psychotic disorders	Parental mental illness, alcoholism, criminality
Conduct disorders	Victim of terrorism, war, natural disasters
Post-traumatic stress disorder	Death of close family member or friend
Drug abuse	Poverty, hunger, abandonment, homelessness
Anorexia nervosa	Relationship issues, bullying, threat, extortion

It has been reported that three fourths of patients presenting with psychiatric/behavioural emergencies have a primary psychiatric diagnosis. There is sharp rise in recent years in suicide attempts and self-harm behaviour presenting in emergencies.

The clinical manifestations of various disorders may take several forms irrespective of the diagnosis, and may present as any of the following emergent clinical problems:

1. Non-epileptic fits or impaired consciousness
2. Abnormal behaviour
3. Suicidal behaviour such as bodily harm, poisoning, drug overdose
4. Aggression and violence
5. Paralysis, paresis, loss of bodily sensations
6. Refusal to eat and severe weight loss
7. Hyperventilation syndrome
8. Acute anxiety and panic
9. Acute non-organic pain
10. Non-accidental injuries and neglect.

These presenting symptoms do not necessarily correspond to a specific psychiatric diagnosis. These are symptoms of child's distress or disease or loss of control on the situation. Usually, the child or the adolescent is brought to the emergency service of the hospital accompanied by a parent or a close relative.

General Guidelines for Emergency Management

For managing emergencies in the Emergency Room, there should be quiet or seclusion rooms, with continuous observation, medication for agitation, and physical restraint (if necessary to contain patients from risk to themselves or others), available. Other precautions are decreasing ambient stimulation (e.g. lights, noise, other people, etc.), removing dangerous objects (including sharps and hard/heavy objects) from the vicinity.

Physical safety of the patient is to be ensured. Medical issues if any such as in cases of poisoning, self-harm, injuries etc. have to be addressed and managed. Standard medical work up with investigations as required should be performed. Psychiatric interview with patient and family should be done in a private, quiet space, where patients and families feel more at ease and comfortable, which facilitates disclosure of psychiatric symptoms, stresses or precipitating conflicts. Psychiatric assessment of children and adolescents must also include an understanding of cognitive, emotional, and physical development.

Sometimes these emergencies arise for admitted children receiving inpatient treatment for a medico-surgical illness where psychiatric help is sought. Immediate task upon receiving a patient with any of the above complaints is to assess the seriousness of the risk to life that warrants medical treatment. Most of the symptoms listed above that are commonly associated with psychiatric and behavioural emergencies can also occur in physical illnesses. The physician must, therefore, conduct a thorough physical examination and necessary investigations to rule out the underlying organic causes. Psychiatric causes are considered only after excluding the organic causes. At times this clinical judgement is difficult to make, in which case a cautious approach is suggested. Clinical evaluation must focus not merely on diagnosis in the child but also on the parents, and the concomitant psychosocial situation. For effective intervention, management of psychopathology in the parents and the general/specific life situation of the child must also be attempted.

Non-Epileptic Fits or Impaired Consciousness

This is one of the common and most dramatic presentations in emergency where a child or an adolescent is brought with the complaints of "fits" characterized by varying symptoms, i.e. impaired consciousness, abnormal movements or behaviour. These are usually episodic disturbances lasting for variable periods of time (varying from few minutes to few hours) interspersed with periods of recovery. The nature of the abnormal movements or abnormal behaviour does not conform to any known pattern of epilepsy or related disorders. Consciousness is usually impaired but not totally lost and the patient might show evidence of response to deep painful stimuli or preservation of memory partial or full. Presence of typical tonic-clonic seizures, complete amnesia for the episode and presence of marked perceptual disturbances particularly depresonalization and derealisation, visual distortions, etc. point towards an epileptic disorder. Sometimes children present as trance like states and do not remember chunks of their behaviour and might even exhibit psychotic like phenomenon such as

visual and auditory hallucinations, feeling of being controlled by external forces. These non-organic clinical disorders are called as dissociative disorders. These occur in children who have experienced acute or chronic stress of abuse of a severe degree. Children when overwhelmed by stress or when they feel caught in an inescapable traumatic situation spontaneously drift into dissociative states. Overtime this behaviour may generalize to other situations leading to an unpredictable pattern.

Since dissociative disorder occurs in the setting of hostile, threatening and abusive environment; the clinician must determine whether the child is still under danger or threat, and he/she needs to be protected from the environment. If the symptoms are severe and disruptive, hospitalization is necessary. Apart from environmental intervention, such a child is treated with a variety of psycho-therapeutic methods including play therapy and behaviour therapy.

Immediate relief from symptoms can be obtained by providing a reassuring non-threatening and protective environment, isolation, establishing communication with the child and encouraging him/her to express feelings which generally are of anxiety, fear, anger or unhappiness. Development of therapeutic relationship or rapport at the initial stage sets the tone for subsequent psychotherapeutic intervention. Drugs have a limited role. SSRIs are helpful in anxiety reduction as well as in improving stress tolerance and coping. Reassurance and explanation to the family members is crucial who may be equally distressed. Parents need to be informed about the psychological nature of illness in such a manner that they understand the problem in the right perspective. The risk is that it may lead them to think that the child is feigning or that they are to blame for the child's problems. Both these reactions are countertherapeutic and must be avoided.

Suicidal Behaviour

Suicidal behaviour is one of the common reasons for emergency evaluation in adolescents. Most children under the age of 12 who threaten or attempt suicide may not kill themselves. Suicidal behaviour may take any of the forms i.e., bodily harm (wrist slashing), poisoning, drug overdose, and rarely more violent methods like hanging, drowning or gun shooting. Lethality of the method indicates the severity of the intent. While more lethal means for suicide planning or attempt are to be taken very seriously, in many instances suicidal ideation or threats are transparent attempts to achieve some goal, or to coerce the friends or relatives to give reprieve to the patient from intolerable stressors. However, some children and adolescents do kill themselves. Therefore, all suicidal children must be assessed for their psychiatric status and for family's ability to supervise and monitor the behaviour, and for the potential risk of suicide. The assessment must refer to the totality of the events and circumstances surrounding the act. Severe and persistent suicidal ideation or intent, lethality of the act, presence of underlying depression or conduct disorder, drug abuse, prior suicidal attempts, family history of suicide, access to weapons, indicate a high risk for suicide. All suicidal gestures indicate presence of decreased impulse control, low self-esteem, or manipulativeness, as for example conduct disordered and anti-social boys who abuse alcohol and drugs. Nevertheless, suicidal behaviour points towards existence of severe psychopathology and pervasive maladjustment, and can be viewed as an extreme though misguided and maladaptive step to attract the attention of a dysfunctional family or circumstance.

A detailed psychiatric history, mental status examination and an assessment of family functioning must be carried out with a view to establish the general risk and need for hospitalization.

High-risk factors are listed below and point towards the need for hospitalization:
- History of multiple suicide attempts
- Persistent suicidal ideation
- Presence of depression
- Presence of alcohol or drug use
- Impulsive or aggressive behaviors
- Physical or sexual abuse.

Suicide attempt with drug overdose or physical harm requires immediate medical management, hospitalization in a paediatric emergency unit, and treatment of injury or medical consequences of poisoning. After the medical complications are adequately managed, need for psychiatric hospitalization must be assessed.

Psychiatric admission is necessary for patients who have:
1. High risk of suicide,
2. Who show evidence of psychosis or depression,
3. Who show persistent suicidal ideation or ambivalence,
4. Who have made prior suicidal attempt, or
5. Who come from chaotic and dysfunctional families.

If the family members are sensitive, responsible and supportive; the child shows no evidence of severe depression or psychosis and no further suicidal ideation, the patient can be taken in outpatient treatment. However, psychiatric consultation and follow-up appointment must be fixed before discharge from emergency. High surveillance for repeated attempt must be maintained for a few days after the current attempt irrespective of the child being in hospital or home. Medication for primary psychiatric disorder if present in the child must be started, e.g. antidepressants if there is severe depression, antipsychotics if the child has psychotic disorder, etc. Further treatment of these and other functioning that may be present is carried out by psychiatrist.

Apart from suicidality, self-inflicted injury is a common problem seen as a result of stereotypic behaviour such as cutting, head banging, biting, burning, or scratching in developmentally disabled children. This may be method for them to express distress, or self soothe themselves or to manipulate the environment. Behavioural management is often useful in such conditions.

Common syndromes of drug overdose are described below (Fader and Mroczkowski 2020).

Substance	Toxic syndrome
Salicylate	• Dizziness, nausea, vomiting, tinnitus, tachypnea, tachycardia, fever, lethargy, coma, seizures, cardiopulmonary failure, death
Acetaminophen/ Paracetamol	• Within 24 hours after ingestion: May initially be asymptomatic; nausea, vomiting, diaphoresis
	• Between 24–72 hours after ingestion: right upper quadrant pain, transaminitis, elevated INR, renal damage
	• Longer than 72 hours after ingestion: fulminant liver failure, hepatic encephalopathy, coagulopathy, hypoglycemia, renal failure, death
Diphenhydramine	• Less than 0.3 grams: somnolence, tachycardia, nausea, vomiting, dizziness, blurry vision, urinary retention, constipation, xerostomia • Between 0.3–1 gram: agitation, confusion, hallucinations, QTC prolongation • Greater than 1 gram: delirium, psychosis, seizure, cardiac arrhythmia, coma, death
SSRIs	*Serotonin syndrome:* • Altered mental status (anxiety, agitation, disorientation) • Neuromuscular dysfunction (tremor, hyperreflexia, myoclonus, rigidity) • Autonomic instability (hypertension, tachycardia, tachypnea, hyperthermia, diaphoresis, xerostomia, mydriasis, gastrointestinal distress, flushing, arrhythmia)
Lithium	• Dizziness, vomiting, diarrhea, nystagmus, tremor, ataxia, tachycardia, confusion, muscle weakness, arrhythmia, seizures, hypotension, death

In drug intoxication/overdose, take care of vital functions, manage metabolic and electrolyte dysfunction, manage intoxication or withdrawal, manage agitation or distress.

Aggressive and Violent Behaviour

Aggressive and violent behaviour in children can occur due to a multitude of etiological factors. It may be a manifestation of underlying psychotic disorder like schizophrenia or bipolar affective disorder; attention deficit hyperactivity disorder, delirium or seizures. It may be a reaction of the child to interpersonal difficulties with parents, peers or teachers. Children or adolescents who have low frustration tolerance, poor impulse control, underlying personality difficulties of borderline or antisocial type or those with conduct disorder, oppositional defiant disorder or drug abuse, etc. might show aggression and violence. The aggression and violence, even if due to underlying biological factors, is often modified by psychosocial environment.

The first task in such an emergency is to assess the risk and safety of the child and of those around him (parents, staff). Usually if the child is approached in calm, non-threatening, and non-judgmental manner where he is encouraged to speak, minimizing his anxiety and fear, the child becomes calm. During this process, assessment is made of the underlying mental state specially looking for signs of major psychiatric illness. The patient who also exhibits abnormal speech, irrelevant talk, delusions and hallucinations is obviously psychotic, whereas a child who has gross disorientation to time, place, memory impairment, gross incoherence of speech, confused ill organized acts of violence, and sphincter in continence, is likely to have organic brain pathology or delirium. Under these circumstances, the child must be given medication for calming him/her down and measures like physical restraint and isolation should be employed to protect him and the surroundings from causing harm. Oral or may be parenteral (if patient is uncooperative) medication in the form of I/M or I/V injections of haloperidol, chlorpromazine or lorazepam is recommended for quick relief. Hospitalization may be needed to tide over the crisis. Management of delirium is to be done keeping in mind the symptom presentation, underlying medical causes, and risk and benefits of medications. Melatonin and Clonidine are useful for agitation and insomnia. Antipsychotics can be used and second-generation antipsychotics like risperidone, olanzapine, quetiapine are useful for controlling agitation. Benzodiazepines can relieve anxiety but are not preferred due to respiratory depressant effects and dependence potential.

Table below summarizes the management guidelines for aggressiveness and agitation modified from Fader and Mroczkowski (2020) to suit the Indian conditions:

Clinical diagnosis	Supportive intervention	Medication
Delirium	• Keep staff consistent • Family by bedside to help orientation • Clocks, calendars to orient • Adequate light, • Minimum noise or clutter • Comfortable ambient temperature • Cluster care to minimize sleep disturbance	• PO: Quetiapine, Risperidone, or Clonidine • IM: Olanzapine or Chlorpromazine or Haloperidol • IV: Haloperidol or Lorazepam
Substance intoxication or withdrawal	• Safe and reassuring environment • Offer food and/or beverages • Ask parent/family to stay • Search and remove any possible substance from possession. • Maintain hydration, intake/output • Monitor vitals • Comfortable ambient temperature	• Unknown substance: Lorazepam +/− Haloperidol • Urine toxicology negative (suspect synthetic cannabinoids or cathinones): Lorazepam +/− Haloperidol or Chlorpromazine • PCP intoxication: Lorazepam • Alcohol/benzodiazepine withdrawal or stimulant intoxication: Lorazepam +/− Haloperidol • Opiate withdrawal: Clonidine or Opiate replacement (Buprenorphine or Methadone) • Add symptomatic treatment

Contd.

Clinical diagnosis	Supportive intervention	Medication
Developmental disability or autism spectrum disorder	• Thorough medical screening • Provide fidget and sensory tools • Toys or games • Keep family/parent • Computer Tablet/TV	• Extra dose of current medication • PO: Clonidine • PO/IM: Diphenhydramine • PO/IM: Antipsychotic (Risperidone, Chlorpromazine, Olanzapine)
Clear underlying psychiatric diagnosis	• Offer food and/or beverages. • Ask parent/family to stay	Specific treatment of the psychiatric condition
Unknown etiology	• Offer food and/or beverages. • Ask parent/family to stay • Behavioral and environmental strategies to de-escalate	• Moderate: Diphenhydramine or Lorazepam or Olanzapine • Severe: Chlorpromazine or Haloperidol + Lorazepam or Olanzapine

Patients with neurodevelopmental disabilities like ASD or ID may present with agitation and aggressiveness. Such patients may not be able to describe their distress verbally. Invariably in such conditions, underlying cause of agitation/ aggression is medical. The child may have pain abdomen, severe constipation, seizures, ear infection, dental infection, problem in ear, nose, throat, head or any part of the body, urinary tract infection, sleep problems and so on. It is important to look for physical pathology in all such cases. They may present as delirium or catatonia and should be managed with small dose of risperidone or aripiprazole or olanzapine.

In certain situations where aggression and violence has occurred due to conflict between the parents and the child, gentle and calm approach, allowing the child to talk out his difficulties brings down the aggression and medication may not be needed.

Assessment is also made of the degree to which the child appears or feels in control of his emotions and behaviour. Many children can say that they are feeling alright and can control themselves. They then have to be handled psychologically where a communication is established with a therapist, and an understanding is reached to resolve the issues during therapy sessions. Emergency management of aggression and violence must be followed by longer term treatment with a psychiatrist.

Table below gives symptoms of intoxication, withdrawal and recommended

Substance	Intoxication	Withdrawal	Treatment
Alcohol Sedatives Hypnotics	Sedation, dizziness, ataxia, nystagmus, confusion, paradoxical agitation, disinhibition, amnesia	0–12 hours after last use: Shakiness, headache, anxiety, nausea, vomiting, tachycardia, tachypnea, diaphoresis 12–24 hours after last use: Confusion, hallucinations with intact reality-testing, tremor, agitation 24–48 hours after last use: Seizures, death 4–12 days after last use: Delirium tremens	Benzodiazepine taper Referral to substance use treatment

Contd.

Substance	Intoxication	Withdrawal	Treatment
Opiods	Sedation, euphoria, miosis, nausea, constipation, urinary retention, respiratory depression, hypotension, bradycardia, cardio-pulmonary collapse, respiratory arrest, coma, death	Flu-like symptoms, shaking, diaphoresis, gooseflesh, mydriasis, yawning, rhinorrhea, nausea, vomiting, diarrhea, anxiety, depression, akathisia, cramps	Supportive care Buprenorphine induction, Methadone, or clonidine Referral to substance use treatment
Stimulants	Tachycardia, hypertension, tachypnea, hyperthermia, diaphoresis, mydriasis, anorexia, euphoria, agitation, anxiety, decreased reality testing, hallucinations	Intense dysphoria, anxiety, fatigue, restlessness, increased appetite, cognitive slowing, vivid dreams, sexual dysfunction, suicidality	Supportive care Cardiac monitoring Benzodiazepines for acute agitation Referral to substance use treatment
Cannabis	Conjunctival injection, impaired short-term memory, impaired attention, impaired motivation, ataxia, perceptual disturbance, increased appetite, euphoria or relaxation	Decreased appetite, difficulty sleeping, irritability, anxiety, headaches, nausea, abdominal pain	Supportive care Benzodiazepines for acute agitation Referral to substance use treatment
Hallucinogens (PCP, MDMA, LSD, Psilocybin, Ketamine, GHB)	Altered level of consciousness, dissociation, perceptual disturbance, euphoria, agitation, aggression, tachycardia, hypertension, diaphoresis	Variable	Supportive care Referral to substance use treatment

treatment for various substances (Fader and Mroczkowski 2020). It is important to recognize and diagnose the problem and provide emergency care. Most of these require treatment in a specialized center for de-addiction services.

Abnormal Behaviour

Sudden appearance of abnormal behaviour in the form of psychomotor excitement, stupor, irrelevant speech, abnormal motor movements, inappropriate acts, amnesias (partial or total loss of memory), occurring in the background of a psychiatric disorder or emotional stress constitutes an emergency. The parents are generally overwhelmed by the gross abnormalities which they believe indicates child's helplessness in controlling his/her behaviour. Level of consciousness must be ascertained first and neurological assessment must be done. After the neurological causes are excluded, sudden abnormal behaviour can occur in acute onset functional psychosis like schizophrenia, affective disorder or acute and transient psychotic disorder. In these conditions psychotic symptoms are often present like delusions, hallucinations, gross psychomotor excitement, stupor, etc. Often schizophrenia and affective disorders take days or weeks to develop and parents may be able to give history of some disturbance retrospectively lasting over several weeks before on outbreak of acute psychosis. In certain situations, the onset of psychosis may be abrupt particularly when there is acute stress preceding the onset such as accident, trauma, bereavement; and in such cases patient's symptoms reflect the stress, and psychosis is brief and short lasting. Sometimes, drug intoxication or withdrawal might present as acute psychosis. Detailed history is sufficient to clarify the diagnosis.

Sometimes abnormal behaviour is not of psychotic proportions or there are no associated psychotic symptoms like delusions or hallucinations, etc. Such a condition can occur following acute emotional stress as in dissociative disorder or post-traumatic stress disorder. Patient does show some degree of control over his/her behaviour and it may be possible to engage the patient in normal conversation and exhibit normal behaviour by strong suggestion. The patient may reveal the cause of emotional distress which may or may not be known to parents. Such a child is handled with psychological support in the form of reassurance, ventilation and catharsis, encouragement and positive guidance. Change in the environmental circumstances like removal of the child from the stress situation would be necessary sometimes. Medication such as Fluoxetine or Sertraline may be given to counteract manifest anxiety or depression for a longer-term use. Psychotic behaviour is managed with anti-psychotic drugs like haloperidol, risperidone, or olanzapine. Need for hospitalization is assessed. Patients who show continuous or recurrent abnormal behaviour where environmental factors make significant contribution to abnormality need to be admitted.

Refusal to Eat and Severe Weight Loss

One of the rare, life-threatening emergencies, encountered in adolescent females is refusal to eat, anorexia or severe persistent vomiting, leading to weights dangerously lower than optimum for that age. This condition is called anorexia nervosa and is characterized by a body weight that is at least 15% lower than the expected, distorted body image, fear of becoming fat, and amenorrhoea. Many a times patients go into a medical emergency due to complications of starvation such a dehydration, electrolyte imbalance, hypoglycemia, cardiac arrhythmias vomiting and abdominal pain, etc. Mortality in severe anorexia nervosa is 15–20%. This condition is 10 times more common in females than in males. Behaviourally, these adolescent girls exhibit near normal level of activity which appears disproportionate to their physical condition, a tendency to minimize the dysfunction, denial of illness, abnormal attitude towards food like hiding or surreptitious eating, attempts at deception like attaching weights on body before weighing, and refusal of treatment, induced vomiting, purging, or excessive exercise.

There are secondary hormonal changes involving hypothalamic-pituitary-gonadal axis causing elevated levels of growth hormone, raised cortisol, delayed onset of puberty, primary or secondary amenorrhoea.

Sometimes, patients go into bouts of overeating followed by extreme steps to control body weight like vomiting (often induced), pruging, starvation, used of drugs, etc. This is called bulimia nervosa. It can be seen as sequelae to anorexia nervosa and is seen commonly in adolescent or young adult females. Repeated vomiting may lead to hypokalaemia, electrolyte disturbance, muscle weakness, seizures, etc.

Etiology of anorexia and bulimia is ill understood but appears to be caused by a complex interplay of biological and sociocultural factors.

Physical causes of weight loss, e.g. chronic debilitating illness, malabsorption syndrome, occult malignancy should be considered and distinguished. Other psychiatric disorders such as depression or psychotic disorder must be ruled out.

Such a patient requires hospitalization and immediate assessment of the functioning of the vital organs like ECG, complete blood count, serum electrolytes, kidney function tests, liver function tests, urinalysis. These patients are highly resistant to treatment and may have to be admitted against patient's wish. Any serious medical complication needs to be managed accordingly. Psychological management is lengthy, and multifaceted. Family members are explained the seriousness of the disease and that they need to pursue treatment rather than leave it to the judgement of the patient who obviously refuses it. Psychiatric evaluation is done in medical emergency and further treatment in the form of intensive psychotherapy, behaviour therapy, family therapy is carried out in the psychiatric ward or in outpatients service.

After stabilizing the medical condition, patient is engaged in therapeutic alliance, the patient is made to see the fallacy in her/his own judgement, discuss risk to life and patient's coveted goals, delineate objectives of treatment, and try to enter into a therapeutic contract for working towards those objectives. It is important to be non-judgemental, non-authoritarian, set small goals for each step in discussion with the patient, make the patient feel that the patient is in command of his life. Psychotherapy, behaviour therapy, or CBT are useful. Medication can be used in the form of SSRI's for depressive symptoms, very small dose antipsychotics for anxiety/agitation/anger, cyproheptadine as appetite stimulant, vitamins or hematinics as supplements.

Hyperventilation Syndrome

Hyperventilation syndrome is a form of dysfunctional breathing which is a changed breathing pattern leading to dyspnoea and other symptoms. Boulding et al (2016) proposed the classification of dysfunctional breathing disorders into hyperventilation syndrome, periodic deep sighing, thoracic dominant breathing, forced abdominal expiration and thoraco-abdominal asynchrony. The most widely recognized form of dysfunctional breathing is hyperventilation syndrome.

Sometimes, children are brought to emergency with rapid, deep or excessive breathing along with many psychological and physical symptoms. Hyperventilation is a state of breathing that exceeds metabolic requirement, may lead to respiratory alkalosis. Hyperventilation involves stimulation of the autonomic nervous system with consecutive arousal and stimulation of adrenaline secretion leading to an increase in heart rate, cardiac output and respiratory rate. Hyperventilation is a clinical syndrome and not a diagnosis. Medical causes of hyperventilation have to be ruled out. Common medical causes that one should consider are: Respiratory problems like infection, asthma; ketoacidosis; cardiac problems; drug overdose (stimulants, aspirin).

Most patients present with associated symptoms like anxiety, fear, paresthesia's, dizziness, chest pain, dyspnoea, light headedness, headache or even tetany. There may be dryness of mouth, muscle spasms in hands and feet, numbness and tingling around mouth or hands, and trouble sleeping. It is commonly seen in young age females. Majority of patients have a psychiatric co-morbidity such as anxiety disorder, panic disorder, depression, conversion/dissociation, somatization, hypochondriasis or obsessive traits. The episode may be triggered by some stress, bereavement, emotional upset.

Management

First and foremost is to make the patient calm and relaxed, reassure that all is ok, and that patient is not going to die. Keep the patient in a safe, quiet secluded place. Relatives and family members should be out. Ask the patient to breath slowly, breath from abdomen, breath with pursed lips or breath in a bag to allow accumulation of carbon dioxide in blood. Once this is settled, then take a detailed history, do mental state examination, look for stresses and proceed accordingly. Propranolol can be used for quick relief. Appropriate treatment of underlying psychiatric disorder needs to be done along with psychological management for psycho-social stresses.

Paralysis, Paresis, Loss of Bodily Sensations

Sometimes, patients are brought to emergency with sudden development of weakness of limbs or paralysis or loss of superficial sensations (pain, touch, temperature) or of special sensations like loss of vision, hearing, smell or taste. More dramatic presentations like aphonia, mutism, agraphia, paraesthesias, etc. are not uncommon. Although all these symptoms mimic neurological disorder but these can be easily distinguished from true neurological syndromes on the basis of a good history and clinical examination. Sudden development of these symptoms in the absence of any history of medical/ neurological illness preceding it, without any evidence of concomitant disease makes it unlikely to be a true neurological disorder. If the symptoms do not follow the known pattern of distribution, based on the anatomical and functional segments of the central nervous system; in a child who had been perfectly normal before the onset of present symptoms that generally occur following a stressful event, the symptoms are more likely to be pseudo-neurological and psychogenic. In such cases, the disability and distress are disproportionately lower than the severity of symptoms, and the function underlying the symptoms is preserved which can be demonstrated by encouraging the child, giving positive suggestion or by some sudden maneuver when the child is inattentive. These were earlier called as conversion disorders, now as a dissociative disorders. These are often construed as child's cry for help in a situation of emotional trauma or stress

which the child is trying to avoid or resolve. It generally occurs in children who have relatively low level of intelligence and who come from lower socioeconomic status families who have limited resources and are unable to handle their life problems in a more adaptive manner. Prevalence of such dramatic presentations has considerable reduced in recent times, and is commonly seen in patients from rural area.

Once the diagnosis is established, further approach towards management should be cautious and sensitive. Absence of organic pathology underlying the symptoms should not be understood as feigning or malingering. Such a child is troubled by emotional difficulties which should be understood by the physician and the family members. Using an empathic and supportive approach often brings out the underlying cause of emotional distress in the child. Such a child should be isolated and interviewed alone. Reassurance and positive suggestion, encouragement can be used to make the symptoms disappear. Rarely a noxious stimulus like deep pressure can bring about symptom removal. Once the symptom is removed the family feels reassured. The family members are then explained the nature of illness of the child. Parents should be congratulated for the absence of any physical illness in their child. Nevertheless, the genuineness of patient's symptoms should be emphasized because otherwise the parents are likely to develop a negative, hostile attitude towards the patient which will be further deleterious for mental health. Parents are explained the need for establishing a communication with the child where the child can express his desires and needs without fear. Parents should understand that the child's emotions and thoughts need to be respected and duly considered. It is not necessary that the parents must accept all the demands of the child but what is necessary is that there should be scope for free expression, discussion and negotiation. After the initial intervention, further treatment targeted at resolution of conflicts, improvement in interpersonal relationships, developing alternate and more adaptive ways of handling problems is to be carried out at outpatients' level by a psychiatrist. Drugs have no major role in this situation. Drugs are used as placebo sometime for quick removal of symptoms, and SSRIs can be used to tackle underlying anxiety or stress. Main mode of treatment is psychotherapy in various forms depending upon the age, education and maturity of the child. Comprehensive evaluation of the family functioning specially for evidence of hostile, abusive environment or family pathology should be done and adequate measures for correction should be applied.

Acute Anxiety and Panic

Acute anxiety can occur in many psychiatric disorders and may manifest as acute palpitation, sweating, trembling, choking, dizziness, numbness, tingling, hyperventilation, fainting or acute chest pain. All these symptoms may build up gradually or may start suddenly and remain for a variable period of time. A discrete period of intense fear or discomfort which builds-up to its peak intensity within less than 10 minutes and is accompanied by acute anxiety symptoms along with a sense of imminent danger or impending doom and a desire to escape is called as a "panic attack". Panic attacks occur in many anxiety disorders like generalized anxiety disorder, phobia, panic disorder, post-traumatic stress disorder, and acute stress reaction, etc. In children, it can occur as a manifestation of separation anxiety (separation from parent figure), school phobia, or sexual abuse.

Sometimes symptoms like derealization, i.e. a feeling of unreality, or depersonalization (as if there is some change in the person), fear of dying, light headedness, unsteadiness, nausea or abdominal distress may also be seen. All these symptoms pertaining to emotional, cognitive and somatic domains characterize underlying anxiety which when acute and intense may be brought to emergency service.

Children who have experienced severe catastrophic traumatic event may develop extreme fear of the specific trauma or of the situations or persons associated with the traumatic event. Such a child looks terrified, may even hallucinate, re-live traumatic situation, have illusions or dreams about it. This condition is easily recognized by the history of trauma and the characteristic symptoms reflecting the trauma.

Separation anxiety is commonly seen in young children who join the school first time or on when they are separated from the attachment figure usually the mothers. Children with separation anxiety have extreme fear or worry that something terrible or catastrophic will befall their mother or the attachment figure when they are separated. Such children may also present with somatic symptoms like headaches, stomachaches, nausea, vomiting.

When separation anxiety is first seen in adolescence it indicates presence of depressive and anxiety disorder or some other severe disorder like psychosis as the basic pathology.

Examination of physical and mental state of the child presenting with acute anxiety and panic, shows no evidence of an underlying medical disorder. There may be marked tachycardia or high blood pressure secondary to anxiety which settles down with lowering of general anxiety. Child should be placed in a calm, and comfortable non-threatening environment and reassured to reduce the distress. He/she should be asked to take regular, slow and deep breathes which immediately lowers the anxiety. Oral or parenteral use of a short acting anxiolytic may be required for quick relief.

The child and the family is reassured that the child has no physical ailment and that all the symptoms are due to emotional upset and anxiety, the cause of which needs to be understood and tackled. Many a times parental anxiety is so high that it is transmitted onto the child directly/indirectly making the condition worse. Therefore, the intervention must involve the family members. Various techniques of psychotherapies like supportive psychotherapy, behaviour therapy and play therapy are very useful in managing the acute as well as continuing problems of anxiety. Hospitalization may be necessary when the parents are unable to handle the problem at home due to their own anxiety, emotional upset or lack of ability to provide support to the child. In separation anxiety disorder and post-traumatic stress disorder, sertraline or escitalopram are effective and may be used as an adjunct to psychotherapy. Benzodiazepines alone are not recommended as it does not tackle the source of the problem and cause rebound anxiety and dependence. Propranolol is useful as adjunct. Buspirone can be used for long term management. Very small dose of antipsychotic may be required in patients with PTSD. Acute intervention should be followed by a multimodal long-term treatment plan oriented towards the child as well as the family.

Acute Non-Organic Pain

Pain is a subjective feeling of an unpleasant sensation that underlies a physical disease with an associated emotional upset. Presentation of acute pain in any part of the body, internal or external, in the emergency is not uncommon. However, the differentiation between somatic pain and the so called "psychogenic pain" or psychosomatic pain is not always easy and could be sometimes impossible. Term psychogenic pain is no more used because pain is caused by many factors and not any single cause. Physical symptom without underlying medical cause is called as somatization.

Factors attributed to pain can be multiple, can be present cross sectionally or in the past, can be conscious or unconscious. These factors can be individual's bodily threshold of pain sensitivity, or past experiences and memories, or person's mental state where negative affective states and thoughts intensify pain perception. Moreover, the experience of pain is unique for every individual. A thorough physical exam and clinical history should be taken in every case. Whereas the somatic pain is usually well-localized, conforms to a pattern and is consistent in nature and location, psychogenic pains is often variable and shifting in nature and is modified by situational stress and distraction. However, there are many exceptions where the knowledge about site, the character and associated aggravating and relieving factors does not help in differentiating the source or cause of pain.

A sudden, dramatic onset of pain in the absence of a known history of physical disorder, occurring in a stressful situation is likely to be pain arising in the brain due to mental health issues, particularly when it occurs in the background of conversion or dissociative disorder, anxiety, depression or histrionic behaviour. Pain may be a somatizing response to stress or an affective concomitant of stress. If there is evidence of underlying psychiatric disorder like anxiety, depression, hypochondriasis, etc. that should be treated as such by an expert psychiatrist. In case of pain manifesting only as a stress response, management of stress should be attempted. However, stress or motivation for symptom production is conscious and tangible in malingering, factitious disorder; and unconscious and intangible in conversion/dissociative disorders. Moreover, conversion/dissociative disorders are more often seen among patients with histrionic and borderline personality whereas malingering and factitious disorder is seen in antisocial personality. Although the clinician makes efforts at thwarting the fulfilment of patient's motives through symptoms, he/she is encouraged to talk about underlying desires, frustrations, and ambitions, etc. in order to provide a more adaptive framework for achievement of motives. Such patients need intensive and specialized treatment in a psychiatric set-up. Psychogenic pains are not relieved by anti-inflammatory analgesic drugs. However, these may respond to narcotic analgesics or to tricyclic antidepressants. SSRIs can also help in psychogenic pain. Use of narcotic analgesics is avoided in such patients as invariably leads to dependence. Anxiolytic drugs are also not effective. These days many such patients are put on pregabalin or gabapentin to the extent that there is almost an outbreak of epidemic.

After acute intervention, main treatment involves psychotherapy and medication such as SSRIs. Effort is made to understand the meaning of pain for the patient in the background of his/her emotional upsets and life circumstances. Patient is helped to acquire greater skills in handling emotions or life stresses.

Other treatments like biofeedback, yoga and meditation are also very useful for such patients.

Non-Accidental Injuries and Neglect

Non-accidental injuries like bruises, multiple fractures, burns due to physical abuse; rape, incest and other injuries to private parts in girls occurring as a result of sexual abuse are sometimes encountered in paediatric medical practice. There are reports of severe brain injuries, subdural hematomas, multiple fractures in children presenting in emergency. These children are brought with complaints of physical injury or damage that does not fit the pattern of history or the details of the accident given by relatives to account for the injury. Informants account of mode of injury is vague, unclear and inconsistent with the pattern of injury. Abuse is suspected by the clinician. There is often associated emotional abuse and neglect of long duration in the form of lack

of care of physical needs, hostility, rejection, threatening, ridiculing and harassment. Malnutrition and failure-to-thrive due to neglect, stunting and psychosocial dwarfism are more serious consequences of prolonged deprivation and lack of physical and emotional care taking of children.

Deliberate poisoning of children and deliberate suffocation of the child with pillow to cause smothering has been reported.

Munchausen syndrome by proxy is another phenomenon in which the mother induces or fabricates the illness in the child and brings him over to the doctors repeatedly. Fabricated illnesses are presented with many serious and sinister symptoms like poisoning, seizures, bleeding from various orifices, fever, injuries, etc. (Meadow 1989). Many instances (10%) of sudden infant death syndrome or cot death are due to deliberate suffocation (Meadow 1990).

For diagnosis of all these conditions it is necessary to have high index of suspicion. The judgement on whether the injuries presented are accidental or non-accidental is necessary. Some of the indications pointing towards injuries being non-accidental in nature are:

a. Delay in seeking medical help;
b. Details of accident provided do not sufficiently explain how the injuries could have been caused;
c. Parents do not show adequate concern or anxiety for the illness of the child;
d. The child may appear frightened of his parents, withdrawn;
e. Parents show hostility and anger towards the child and the doctors, and may even thwart the attempts of the doctors to directly talk to the child. They often reject or refuse treatment and may leave before investigations are complete.

Child may be repeatedly presented to different doctors and different hospitals without adequately pursuing diagnosis or treatment anywhere. All the above, is suggestive and not a pathognomonic evidence in favour of non-accidental injuries and neglect. Perpetrator of abuse could be biological parents, step parents or others in-charge of the care of the child. Emotional abuse and sexual abuse is more common than physical abuse. It may be an acute abuse or a chronic abuse. These are serious emergencies responsible for high mortality and morbidity in the form of brain damage, permanent physical deformities, emotional and behavioral disorders, suicide and even serious mental illness (Skuse and Bentovim 1994).

In cases of suspected abuse, the child and family members must be interviewed individually. Close observations of child's behaviour and emotional state, parent-child relationship are necessary to make a judgement about abuse. Many a times children are too frightened to open up or may even retract all information after disclosing abuse. This is a medicolegal problem requiring mandatory reporting. There is a strong risk of parents or family taking the child away without treatment which further risks the life of the child and also the child continues living in the abusive environment.

In all cases, child's safety and protection are the foremost concerns. Social and legal agencies need to be involved for taking the child into protection. The child generally requires strong reassurance and support before he/she can repose his faith or trust in the adults around. Further psychiatric intervention involves improving the parent-child relationship; improving the parenting skills and attitudes of parents; help to parents for poor impulse controls, inadequate social and problem solving skills.

Conclusion

Psychiatric and behavioral emergencies present in a variety of different ways and could pose an immediate threat to child's life or it could be non-life threatening. In all the situations, an emergency is an indication of the breakdown of an already compromised psychological, social, and family functioning and it serves as the contact point for initiation of steps for remedy and restoration of function. A comprehensive assessment of the biological, physical, psychosocial and family factors is necessary. An attitude of sensitivity, empathic understanding, unflustered composure and patient listening; an atmosphere of calmness, quietness, isolation and non-threatening environment and a holistic approach to the analysis and understanding of problems can bring down the emotional distress in the child as well as in the family members in most of the distressing or disruptive presentations. Simple supportive measures like ventilation, catharsis, reassurance and expression of regard for the patient is very helpful. Drugs have a for the treatment of medical complications or in cases of severe psychiatric illness like psychosis, depression or anxiety or in handling acutely distressing or disruptive symptoms. Psychiatric hospitalization may be necessary to tide over the crisis. Psychiatric consultation in emergency sets the tone for subsequent prolonged intervention for treatment of the basic pathology. Psycho-social interventions provide invaluable support.

BIBLIOGRAPHY

1. Fader RP, Mroczkowski MM. (2020) Child and adolescent psychiatric emergencies. In Rey JM & Martin A (eds), JM Rey's IACAPAP e-Textbook of Child and Adolescent Mental Health. Geneva: International Association for Child and Adolescent Psychiatry and Allied Professions.

2. Gerson R, Malas N, Feuer V et al (2019). Best practices for evaluation and treatment of agitated children and adolescents (BETA) in the emergency department: consensus statement of the American Association for Emergency Psychiatry. Western Journal of Emergency Medicine 20(2), 409.

3. Kaplan HI; Sadocks BJ, (1993). Psychiatric emergencies in children. In Pocket Handbook of Emergency Psychiatric Medicine. BI. Publications. pp 50–63.

4. Meadow R (1989). ABC of Child Abuse. British Medical Association, London.

5. Meadow R (1990). Suffocation, recurrent apnoea, and sudden infant death. Journal of Paediatrics 117, 351–357.

6. Richard Boulding, Rebecca Stacey, Rob Niven and Stephen J. Fowler (2016) Dysfunctional breathing: a review of the literature and proposal for classification. Eur Respir Rev; 25: 287–294.

7. Skuse D, Bentovim A (1994). Physical and Emotional Maltreatment. In Child and Adolescent Psychiatry. Modern Approaches. Eds. Michael Rutter, Eric Taylor and Lionel Hersov. III Edition. Blackwell Scientific Pub. pp 209–29.

8. Tomb DA. (1991). Child psychiatric emergencies. In Child and Adolescent Psychiatry: A Comprehensive Textbook. Ed. Melvin Lewin. Williams and Wilkins pp 930–40.

Sexual Abuse in Children and Adolescents

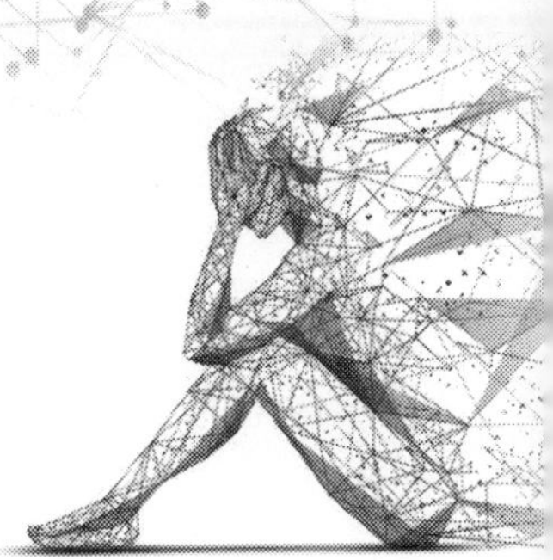

Sexual abuse in children and adolescents is an extremely serious, socially disruptive, psychologically devastating and medically damaging form of trauma which is commonly seen in families and society and generates strong emotional reactions. Child sexual abuse (CSA), also called child molestation, is a form of child abuse in which an adult or older adolescent uses a child for sexual gratification. The World Health Organization (WHO 1999) defines Child Sexual Abuse (CSA) as "the involvement of a child in sexual activity that he or she does not fully comprehend, is unable to give informed consent to, or for which the child is not developmentally prepared and cannot give consent, or that violates the laws or social taboos of society."

The phenomenon of child sexual abuse (CSA) has been well-recognized since ages but it is only recently that there is professional acceptance of its reality. Child sexual abuse can occur in a variety of settings, including home, school, or work. In recent years, CSA has been a subject of intensive research and clinical study by professionals in the fields of mental health as well as in medical and social sciences.

It has also been seen that sexual abuse in children occurs along with other forms of maltreatment, i.e. physical abuse, emotional abuse and neglect, making the actual experience of children very complicated, presenting challenges for the clinicians and researchers. Child sexual abuse contributes to child mortality and morbidity with long standing effects on mental health, alcohol and drug abuse, suicide, criminality, risky sexual behavior, eating disorders and so on that persists well into adulthood.

Most comprehensive definition of CSA is given by the Standing Committee on Sexually Abused Children (SCOSAC) which states "Any child below the age of consent may be deemed to have been sexually abused when a sexually mature person has, by design or by neglect of their usual societal or specific responsibilities in relation to the child, engaged or permitted the engagement of that child in any activity of a sexual nature which is intended to lead to the sexual gratification of the sexual mature person". By this definition, sexual activity between two sexually immature persons (e.g. children) cannot be termed CSA.

Broad concept of CSA substitute 'as defined' includes– sexual behavior between a child and an adult or between two children when one of whom is significantly older or uses coercion. The perpetrator and the victim may be of the same or opposite sex. Most sexual abuse offenders are acquainted with their victims; approximately 30% are relatives of the child, most often brothers, fathers, uncles, or cousins, around 60% are other acquaintances, such as "friends" of the family, babysitters, or neighbors; strangers are the offenders in approximately 10% of child sexual abuse cases. The sexual behaviors include touching breasts, buttocks, and genitals (whether the victim is dressed or undressed); exhibitionism, fellatio, cunnilingus, and penetration of the vagina or anus with sexual organs or with objects. Pornographic photography and sexual grooming are usually included. Sometimes, child is allured into a sexual relationship, i.e. provided "incentive" by the abuser (especially, if familiar/known to the child) to gain consent of the child. Children being cognitively and emotionally immature, may not be able to appreciate and/or recognize that allurement is a form of coercion. Child marriage is one of the main forms of child sexual abuse; UNICEF has stated that child marriage "represents perhaps the most prevalent form of sexual abuse and exploitation of girls".

Sexual abuse severity can be categorized into: severe forms of abuse which included sexual assault (including oral/vaginal/anal penetrative sexual activity); or less severe forms such as making child fondle private parts; making child exhibit private parts; photographing child nude; and other forms include forcible kissing; forcing child to view pornographic material/ private parts; or sexual advances in public places like travel/marriage situation.

Often children reporting CSA are not heard, not taken seriously, they are shunned and at times considered to be imagining things that were impossible. Under the circumstances, children are left with no one to confide in and they live their lives under persistent trauma of abuse.

PREVALENCE

The true prevalence of CSA is difficult to ascertain due to numerous factors like lack of reporting and lack of adequate data. It has been reported that the prevalence of CSA has assumed epidemic proportion affecting children and communities worldwide (Sapp and Vandeven 2005). A 2009 meta-analysis of 65 studies from 22 countries found a global prevalence of 19.7% for females and 7.9% for males. In that analysis, Africa had the highest prevalence rate of child sexual abuse (34.4%); Europe showed the lowest

prevalence rate (9.2%); and America and Asia had prevalence rates between 10.1% and 23.9% (Pereda, N et al 2009).

Epidemiological data that is now available suggests that the phenomenon of CSA is prevalent in India. The largest national level survey conducted by the Ministry of Women and Child Development, Government of India reported the prevalence of CSA in India (Kacker et al 2007). The sample consisted of 17220 children and adolescents in the age range of 5-18 years selected by a multistage purposive sampling design. This is the most authoritative report on child abuse in India. 53.22% children reported having faced one or more forms of sexual abuse, of which 21.9 % faced serious forms of sexual abuse like sexual assault, making the child fondle private parts, exposing or photographing the private parts of the child. Children on street, children at work and children in institutional care reported the highest incidence of sexual assault. In half of the cases abusers were persons known to the child or in a position of trust and responsibility and most children did not report the matter to anyone.

More recently, the problem of 'internet sex offenders' have gained ground, where the victim is targeted through the internet, which is a form of non-contact CSA. A comparison of internet sex offenders with actual sexual molesters showed that there were marked similarities in socio-affective traits and childhood physical abuse (Webb and Keen 2007).

Child sexual abuse can involve a variety of sexual offenses, such as:

- *Sexual assault:* Where an adult uses the minor sexual gratification, for example, rape (including sodomy), and sexual penetration with an object.
- *Sexual exploitation:* Where an adult victimizes a minor for advancement, sexual gratification, or profit; prostituting a child, live streaming, creating or trafficking in child pornography.

- *Sexual grooming:* Where the social conduct of a child sex offender seeks to make a minor more accepting of their advances, for example in an online chat.

Etiology

CSA is a complex social-psychological phenomenon where factors within the individual, the family, the community and the culture are embedded. There is a vulnerable child [young age, female, poor or broken family, lack of parent(s), presence of any disability, poor social support, child maltreatment]; presence of an offender or perpetrator (person usually known to the child's family, a relative, who can try to take advantage of the situation in child's life, who may enjoy the trust of the family and has access to the child); poorly supervised environment in the family or society (child lives in mostly in unsupervised environment); use of power, authority or threat, allurement, or promise by the offender to the child (the offender takes advantage of his closeness/ trust of the child's family/parents, antisocial traits); and societal attitudes towards sex and intimacy (permissiveness, treating children as adults); that creates a suitable scenario for CSA. Risk factors for CSA have been described as parental death, presence of stepfather, harsh punitive parenting, maternal sociopathy, unwanted pregnancy, female gender, parental history of childhood maltreatment, parental alcoholism. The adult sex offenders have a high prevalence of personality disorders, whereas, juveniles who commit sexual offenses are a heterogenous diverse population. Sex offenders against children were, by and large, not different from sex offenders against adults.

Consequences

Studies have found that 51% to 79% of sexually abused children exhibit psychological symptoms (Caffaro-Rouget A et al 1989; Conte JR; Schuerman JR 1987).

Trauma of CSA leads to serious, persistent and long-standing consequences that could persist through adulthood. During childhood, emotional disturbances, dissociation, sexually inappropriate behaviors, suicidal behavior, self-harm behavior, anxiety, panic, insomnia, somatoform complaints are some of the common and intensely disabling consequences. There can be physical complaints like headache, body aches, gastrointestinal problems, vomiting in some children. However, some children may not manifest with any psychiatric illnesses in the period immediately following sexual abuse, and these are not to be taken as well. Long-term outcome is more complex and disabling. Many psychiatric disorders emerging during adolescent or adult phase of life in these children have direct link with sexual abuse. Common outcomes are depression, PTSD, borderline personality disorders, drug abuse, dissociative disorders, somatization disorders, sexual disorders and even schizophrenia. There is a consistent association between CSA and sexual risk behavior such as sex trading, sexual promiscuity and early age of first sexual intercourse. There is little literature on CSA among boys, but psychological consequences such as anxiety, denial, dissociation, self-mutilation are common. Boys may cope with abuse by becoming the angry avenger, the passive victim, a daredevil, or a conformist. These children may exhibit self-blame, shame, guilt or avoidant behavior.

There may be physical complaints or ill health in the form of abdominal pain and gastrointestinal symptoms, pelvic pain and gynecological disturbances, headaches. There can be teenage pregnancy, sexually transmitted disease, genital warts or HPV (human papilloma virus) infection.

Age-inappropriate sexualized behavior is found significantly more commonly in, although not in most, sexually abused children and is an important unwanted outcome of child sexual abuse. It refers to repeated genital stimulation (touching, inserting finger or objects, or masturbation) and sexual behavior, often involving another child, a doll or sometimes an adult. There is propensity to further victimization in adulthood. Sexual abuse by a family member is a form of incest and can result in more serious and long-term psychological trauma, especially in the case of parental incest (Courtois, Christine A. 1988).

Diagnosis

Diagnosis of CSA is most frequently based on history. Assessment of the validity of CSA is a tedious task with legal and social implications. Considering that CSA occurs in private without much physical evidence, CSA can be very difficult to detect (Malhotra and Biswas 2006).

Children often do not disclose experiences of abuse for months and years. One has to be sensitive to pick up early indicators of abuse. Children do not disclose abuse due to several reasons like: Presence of feelings of shame, guilt or fear in the child; wish of the child to protect the abuser with whom the child may have developed a positive relationship; fear and threat by the abuser about negative consequences to disclosure like "if you tell anyone I will kill your parents"; fear of having to face negative responses from family, i.e. disbelief, denial or outright rejection. Many a times parents blame the child that "it must be your fault" or "this can't be true" or "you are lying". Sometimes, children report amnesia (memory loss) for such traumatic events; and sometimes the child tends not to label events of sexual abuse as "abusive", as the child has been "sexually groomed" and has started to enjoy sexual activity. The perpetrator and the victim may be of the same or opposite sex. The strongest indicator of sexual abuse is sexual "acting out" and inappropriate sexual knowledge and interest. There may be physical injuries such as bleeding, bruises, or swelling in

the genital area, bloody, torn, or stained underclothes, difficulty walking or sitting, frequent urinary infections, pain, itching, or burning in the genital area.

A causal relationship has been found between childhood sexual abuse and various adult psychopathologies, including crime and suicide, alcoholism and drug abuse, conflict in romantic or interpersonal relationships, fear of intimacy, and sexual dysfunction. So adult patients who present with these psychiatric conditions should be explored for CSA in retrospect. Males who were sexually abused as children more frequently appear in the criminal justice system than the clinical health care system.

Disclosure

Disclosure of abuse is both a diagnostic exercise as well as a part of management. Assessment and interview in CSA cases requires a considerable degree of experience, expertise, and tact on the part of clinicians. The interview should be conducted in a friendly, non-judgmental, and empathetic way and should not have an investigative overtone. Conduct the interview jointly with parents or care givers as children with CSA are very nervous to be alone with a stranger. Interview should occur in a neutral environment. Suspected offender should not be in the vicinity and there should be a reasonable degree of privacy, with facility for audio and video recording if possible. You have to elicit the details of the event, as to what happened, and what effect it had on the child. Child is to be reassured for safety and confidentiality. Use of drawings, play materials like dolls and psychological tests can be of additional help. Depending on the age and developmental level, the child may be able to verbally express and describe the events.

There has to be a high index of suspicion. Children who exhibit sudden change in behaviour such as avoidant behaviour, irritability, secretiveness, learning problems, cruelty to animals, oppositional defiant disorder, teenage pregnancy, inappropriate sexual knowledge and interest, or unusual behaviour, would raise suspicion about sexual abuse. Negative social reactions to disclosure have been found to be harmful to the child's mental health. In most cases when children disclose abuse, the person they talked to did not respond effectively, blamed or rejected the child, and took little or no action to stop the abuse. Disclosing abuse can be distressing and sometimes shameful, reassuring the child that he or she has done the right thing by telling and that the child is not bad and that the abuse was not the child's fault helps in disclosing more information. It has been reported that children who received a bad reaction from the first person they told, especially if the person was a close family member, had worse outcome as adults leading to general trauma symptoms, post-traumatic stress disorder symptoms, and dissociation. There can be a situation when a prepubescent child is sexually abused by one or more other children or adolescent youths, and no adult is directly involved, or there is sexual activity between children that occurs without coercion.

Treatment

Treatment is complex and has to be carried out in stages. Treatment is required for the affected child, as well as for the parents or other family members who are also affected by this event. Usually, a multi-disciplinary team involving experts from departments of obstetrics and gynecology, pediatrics/general medicine, pediatric surgery, psychiatry, and forensic medicine working together, can increase the probability of detection and is also required for management. Most of healthcare professionals are not sufficiently trained to evaluate or handle cases of CSA. If the abuse is reported within less than 72 hours of its occurrence, then the legal proceeding has to be started immediately before proceeding for treatment.

a. Adequate physical examination and management of any injuries or medical issues is the necessary first step. Forensic examination should simultaneously be carried out along with physical examination.

Thereafter, take steps to build rapport and establish therapeutic alliance.

b. *Protection of the child:* It is essential to immediately take measures to protect the child from further abuse, particularly when the perpetrator is a family member or a person known to the child, and the abuse has occurred at home or at school, hostel, sports club, neighborhood or any place that child regularly visits. Child must be immediately removed from being in contact with the perpetrator. Any relative or member of extended family can provide a safe and comfortable space. Alternative living arrangement has to be made which may not be always an ideal situation but is needed to remove the child away from the abusive environment. Seshadri and Ramaswamy (2019) have provided detailed guidelines for treatment of CSA.

c. *Management of psychological trauma:* Management of psychological trauma to the child requires to be done by experienced professional who has worked in this area, maintaining trust of the child, alleviating fear, and providing reassurance and needed confidentiality. The child has to be prepared to disclose the incident to police. A minimum requirement is to ascertain that the child is able to talk about their experiences to a parent or another identified person, who believes the child and is able to listen to the child supportively and uncritically. It has also been reported that children who are victims of sexual abuse might display secrecy, helplessness, entrapment, accommodation, delayed and conflicted disclosure or recantation, due to which the child may give inconsistent account of events. This makes the disclosure to happen slowly, in a piece-meal fashion. Treatment of young children generally requires strong parental involvement and can benefit from family therapy and play therapy. Adolescents tend to be more independent; they can benefit from individual therapy or group therapy. Psychotherapeutic approach has to be tailored to the individual child's level of development, cognitive maturity, verbal felicity, co-cooperativeness, emotional state and so on.

d. Supportive care in the form of reassurance, guidance, ventilation, catharsis is very helpful. CBT for older children works well. Art therapy, music therapy, activity therapy, relaxation therapy and yoga work for most children and adolescents.

e. *Pharmacotherapy:* By and large medication has no direct role in management of CSA. However, medication is invariably needed for acute symptoms of PTSD, depression, anxiety, agitation, fear, insomnia. SSRIs are helpful for treating depression, dissociation, anxiety, panic and self-harm behaviour. Small dose antipsychotic may be required for managing symptoms of intense anxiety or agitation in PTSD or psychosis.

f. *Allow time for healing and recovery:* Allow normal activities, play, normal sleep, some recreational activities. Encourage the child to express feelings and thoughts, even indirectly through stories, without directly touching the subject of child's experience. Use distraction methods using games, play materials, movies.

g. *Intervention for parents and family members:* Parents and families have to be helped to overcome the shock and disbelief, and accept the problem. Most important issue is validating the child's experience, and dealing with their own fears, shame, or threat of disruption or breakdown of family relationships, if the perpetrator is someone from within the family. Parents are more concerned about the social consequences for them rather than the consequences for the child and often want the status quo to be maintained. They are often hesitant to report the matter to police, and need help to prepare for reporting the matter to police or child Welfare committee or the judiciary.

Legal Issues

CSA is a legal issue and also an issue of human rights. In India, a new law has been enacted called "Protection of Children from Sexual Offences Act, 2012". Under this Act, CSA is a crime and stringent punishments are prescribed. Various child-friendly procedures are put in place at various stages of the judicial process for reporting of the crime, recording of evidence, investigation and trial of offences in this Act. The possibility of establishment of Special Courts for the trial of offences under the law has also been provided for. Also, the Special Court is to complete the trial within a period of one year, as far as possible. Disclosing the name of the child in the media is a punishable offence, punishable by up to one year. The law provides for relief and rehabilitation of the child, as soon as the complaint is made to the Special Juvenile Police Unit (SJPU) or to the local police. These agencies are required to make immediate arrangements to give the child adequate care and protection such as admitting the child into a shelter home or to the nearest hospital within twenty-four hours of the report. The Child Welfare Committee (CWC) is also required to be notified within 24 hours of recording the complaint.

There is a medico-legal obligation to report CSA to police, but the family and the child are invariably not prepared for it. On many occasions the family takes the child away to avoid reporting which is not in the interest of the child. The child and the family have to be assisted and gradually prepared psychologically to make a complaint and report the abuse to police, or child welfare officer or the magistrate.

The Ministry of Women and Child Development (MWCD), Govt. of India, has established Sakhi, a centrally funded scheme, as a One Stop Centers (OSC) preferably within a hospital/medical facility to provide support and assistance to victims of gender violence (Sakhi 2017, 2020), where holistic facilities, including medical, police, psychosocial counseling, legal assistance, shelter, referral, and video-conferencing are given under one roof.

Prevention

CSA is a major public health concern requiring a societal response in terms of breaking the silence, ensure respect for protection of the rights of children, fight stigma and socio-cultural taboos around CSA, making homes and public spaces safe for children, reporting the crime, and advocacy. Sex education to children is one of the preventive strategies being used. The child aged between 3 and 5 years can be told what is "good" touch or "okay touch," and "bad touch," and places over the body where nobody except the mother can touch or clean. Children above 10 years onwards need to be provided sex education in schools, should be informed about body parts, puberty, privacy, and private parts. Adolescents need more detailed knowledge of body physiology, sexual intercourse, pregnancy, healthy relationships. There is strong need to raise awareness and support advocacy against sex abuse of children and adolescents. Parents, families, teachers and civil society at large must overcome the inhibition and hesitation in acknowledging and accepting the presence of CSA in society and join hands to deal with it effectively. Children have to be protected from this crime and empowered to safeguard their mental and physical integrity. Sensitization workshops, life skills training workshops in schools can empower children to deal with the problems. Children, specially girls should learn and use self-defence skills for self-protection. CSA is a silent misery. There is need for more research into normal sexual behaviour among children and adolescents.

BIBLIOGRAPHY

1. Caffaro-Rouget, A.; Lang, R. A.; Van Santen, V. (1989). "The Impact of Child Sexual Abuse On Victims' Adjustment". Sexual Abuse: A Journal of Research and Treatment. 2: 29–47. doi:10.1177/107906328900200102. S2CID 145389337.

2. Courtois, Christine A. (1988). Healing the incest wound: adult survivors in therapy. New York: Norton. p. 208. ISBN 978-0-393-31356-7.

3. Conte, J.R.; Schuerman, J.R. (1987). "The Effects of Sexual Abuse on Children: A Multidimensional View". Journal of Interpersonal Violence. 2 (4): 380–390.

4. Julia Whealin (2007-05-22). "Child Sexual Abuse". National Centre for Post-Traumatic Stress Disorder, US Department of Veterans Affairs. Archived from the original on 2009-07-30.

5. Kacker L, Varadan S, Kumar P. Study on Child Abuse: INDIA 2007. Ministry of Women and Child Development, Government of India 2007.

6. Malhotra S, Biswas P (2006). Behavioural and psychological assessment of child sex abuse in clinical practice. International Journal of Behavioural and Consultation Therapy. Vol 2, no 1, 17-28.

7. Pereda N; Guilera G; Forns M and Gómez-Benito J. (2009). "The prevalence of child sexual abuse in community and student samples: A meta-analysis" Clinical Psychology Review. 29 (4): 328–338. doi:10.1016/j.cpr. 2009.02.007. hdl: 2445/27746. PMID 19371992.

8. Protection of Children from Sexual Offences Act, (Central) Complete Act–Bare Act. Government of India. 2012. Available from: http://www.wcd.nic.in/sites/default/files/childprotection31072012.pdf.

9. Sakhi: One Stop Centre Scheme. Implementation guidelines for states governments and union territories. Ministry of Women and Child Development. 2017. [cited 2021 Jan 26]. Available from: https://wcd.nic.in/sites/default/files/OSC_G.pdf.

10. Sakhi: One Stop Centre Directory. Ministry of Women and Child Development. 2020. [cited 2021 Jan 26]. Available from: https://wcd.nic.in/sites/default/files/OSC%20 Directory_0.pdf .

11. Sapp MV, Vandeven AM. Update on childhood sexual abuse. Curr Opin Pediatr 2005; 17: 258-64.

12. SCOSAC. Definition of Child Sexual Abuse. London, Standing Committee on Sexually Abused Children 1984.

13. Shekhar Seshadri and Sheila Ramaswamy (2019) Clinical Practice Guidelines for Child Sexual Abuse. Indian J Psychiatry. Jan; 61(Suppl 2): 317–332. doi: 10.4103/ psychiatry.IndianJPsychiatry_502_18

14. "UNICEF" (PDF). unicef.org. Archived from the original(PDF) on 2019-10-10. Retrieved 2014-01-03

15. Webb L, Craissati J, Keen S. Characteristics of internet child pornography offenders: a comparison with child molesters. Sex Abuse 2007; 19: 449–465.

16. World Health Organization. Report of the Consultation on Child Abuse and Neglect Prevention, 29-31 March. Geneva, Switzerland: World Health Organization; 1999.

Alcohol and Substance Abuse in Children and Adolescents

Use of alcohol and substances commonly starts in young age as an experimental or recreational use and may turn into regular or harmful use in many who are vulnerable. It is difficult to predict who will experiment and stop, who will become occasional user without harm and who will a become regular user with serious harm. Adolescent substance use has been a relatively neglected area in clinical practice and research studies. It has been shown that children from around age 4 years understand what alcohol is (they know it as a grown up drink) and that there are social norms related to its use. They see it as a norm for grownups. Thus, social acceptance and normalization of alcohol use among societies constitutes a huge risk per se.

Vulnerable persons become harmful users in early adolescence and this pattern can further develop into a chronic use disorder. Substance use disorders (SUD) are among the leading causes of health risks for adolescents and young adults worldwide (Mokdad et al 2013). Substance use is associated with several health and social problems, including drug use behaviour in later life, school failure, poor judgment, impulse dyscontrol, accidents, violence, unplanned and unsafe sex, mental disorders and suicide.

Pattern of Use

It varies across populations. In the West most common substances of abuse among children and adolescents are alcohol and cannabis. In most instances first drug of use is tobacco and alcohol between the ages of 13–15 years. All psychoactive substances are used more commonly by male than by female adolescents, with a sex ratio of 2:1. Heavy alcohol use is almost 3 times more frequent in men than women. Women who abused drugs had a higher incidence of internalizing problems, e.g, depression, anxiety, and withdrawn behaviors, during childhood and had more severe psychiatric symptoms as adults. Conduct disorders were found more frequently in men who were in treatment for drug abuse. The lifetime prevalence of e-cigarette use among adolescents is 14.5% and is especially high among male adolescents with a low level of education. Kessler et al (2012) reported life time prevalence in 11.4% and 12-month prevalence in 8.3%, of DSM IV SUD among 13 to 18-year-olds in USA. The younger a child is exposed to alcohol and other drug use, the higher the risk for serious health consequences and adult substance abuse.

National Drug Abuse Survey, an Indian study, conducted at AIIMS Delhi (Ambekar et al 2019), reported prevalence of current use among adolescents to be 1.8% for opioids, 1.3% for alcohol, 1.17% for volatile solvents, and 0.9% for cannabis. The Global Youth Tobacco Survey (GYTS-4 2019) conducted in 2019, among 80,772 students aged 13 to 15 years, reported the prevalence of tobacco use to be 8.5%. The commonest drugs of abuse among children below 18 years from 100 cities in 29 states and UTs, were tobacco (83.2%) and alcohol (67.7%), followed by cannabis (35.4%), inhalants (34.7%), pharmaceutical opioids (18.1%), sedatives (7.9%), and heroin/smack (7.9%) (Dhawan et al 2017).

In India, child helpline data (child line 1098) shows that the children typically use whitener, cough syrups, pain relief ointments, glue, paint, gasoline, cleaning fluids, and other hard drugs. There is also rampant use of alcohol and tobacco among children.

Initiation of Use

Common reasons for initiation of substance use among children include:
- Curiosity
- Experimentation
- Fun seeking
- Peer influence
- To show off
- Easy availability and access to drugs
- Poor Role Models: Parent(s) using alcohol or substances

In majority (60–80%) of adolescents, the use of substances is a temporary phenomenon and it stops after adolescence and early adulthood. Only a small minority who are at risk go on to develop a long-term addictive disorder.

Vulnerabilities and Risk

There are multiple factors determining vulnerabilities and risk, e.g. include genetic predisposition, prenatal exposure to psychotropic substances; high sensitivity to reward salience and environmental stimuli; low inhibitory control; high sensation seeking; temperament of low threshold for stress tolerance, low persistence, low emotional regulation and impulsiveness; early emotional trauma; an unfavorable family environment; abuse, trauma; family history of alcohol and substance use. Childhood abuse has been found as a significant risk factor for later substance abuse.

Early warning signs of alcohol and drug use are:
- **Physical:** Weight loss, fatigue, red or glazed eyes, droopy eyes, cough.
- **Emotional:** Sudden mood changes, irritability, irresponsible behavior, low self-esteem, poor judgment, disinterest, and personality change.
- **Behavioural:** Starting arguments, breaking rules, withdrawing from the family, finding faults in others, blaming others, change in looks like hair style or tattoos, poor grooming, irregular habits etc.
- **School:** Missing school/classes, decreased interest, negative attitude, drop in grades, truancy, discipline problems.
- **Social problems:** New friends who are school drop outs or have no work, problems with the law, staying away from home.

Consequences of Use

There are many health as well as socio-economic and legal consequences of SUDs depending upon the type, duration and quantity of substance used. About one-third of traffic accident deaths among 15– to 20-year-olds are related to substance use (Levy et al 2002). Substance use significantly increases the risk of being either a perpetrator or a victim of violence, victim of sex abuse among girls, school drop out and failure, suicide, criminality, traffic violations, early and un-natural death. Adolescents indulge in petty crimes for procuring the illicit drugs. There is higher rate of psychiatric morbidity among substance using adolescents like depression, anxiety, social phobia, bipolar disorder, personality disorders narcissistic and borderline types, ADHD, conduct disorder, impulse control disorders, and schizophrenia. High cannabis use can trigger psychosis (Hasan et al 2020) and high tetrahydrocannabinol (THC) content in cannabis products plays a major pathogenetic role in triggering psychosis (Hindley et al 2020). Psychiatric comorbidity is far more common in child and adolescent patients (76%) with SUDs than in older patients (>18 years: 23.4%) (Kandell et al 1999).

Illicit drug use is associated with an increased risk of contracting human immunodeficiency virus (HIV). Children can acquire HIV infection perinatally if any of the parents were intravenous drug abusers.

It has been seen that adolescent brain is more sensitive to the pleasurable effects of alcohol and substances, gets more easily hooked to substances, and develops neuropathological effects in cortical and subcortical brain areas by chronic or repetitive use of alcohol and substances. Approximately 9% of cannabis users develop dependence over a lifetime. Experimental studies suggest that the epigenetic effects of cannabinoids can impair myelination of the pubertal brain (Thomas-Roig et al 2016). High cannabis use in adolescence impairs memory, learning, recall, attention, problem solving, reasoning ability, and intelligence, coinciding with the age-related structural and functional changes in the cerebral grey and white matter (Ganzer et al 2016). Excessive alcohol use has been reported to be associated with neurocognitive deficits (Brown and Tappert, 2004). Liberalization of cannabis use in many countries has sent the message that perhaps cannabis is a safe substance, whereas, the research data provides the contrary evidence.

Aetiology

Aetiology of substance use disorders multifactorial. There are genetic factors, biological factors, temperamental factors, psychological factors, social factors, familial factors at work that lead to substance use.

Genetic Factors

It has been reported that biological children of alcohol-dependent parents who have been adopted continue to have a 2- to 9-fold increased risk of developing alcoholism. The transmission of type II alcoholism,

from father to son, demonstrated a high heritability despite environmental factors. Studies of siblings and twins born to parents who are drug dependent have confirmed the existence of a genetic predisposition not only for alcohol abuse but also for other drugs of abuse. In a study on event related potential P300 among children of alcoholic fathers from multiplex families, P3 amplitude was significantly reduced among high risk children indicating that it can be a potential biological marker of risk for alcoholism (Sharma et al 1997). However, there are very few number of genetic variants that have strong, and robust associations with substance use, which has led to increasing focus on the interplay between genetic predispositions and environmental exposures in the etiology of SUDs. It is the gene-environment interaction that significantly determines or mitigates the risk for alcohol or SUDs.

Biological Factors

Early exposure of brain to alcohol or addictive substances induces changes in prefrontal cortex activity (PFC) and PFC projections to subcortical regions, which may persist in adulthood and increase the risk of SUD. Adolescents have greater impulsivity and lower inhibitory control on behaviour due to an immature PFC leading to lesser control of the PFC control over subcortical and limbic urges. This is coupled with hyper-reactivity of reward system/salience and over stimulation of the limbic circuitry in adolescents which makes them use substances more often and repeatedly. Adolescents are more driven to pleasure seeking and pleasurable effect of substance use, which causes them to go for repeated use.

Temperamental Factors

There are temperamental factors which determine the behavioural individuality and uniqueness of neurophysiological and neuro behavioural reactivity and regulation in children and adolescents. Considerable research has been done on temperamental antecedents of alcohol and substance use disorders. Children who are over active, with low threshold of responsive ness, with intense reactions, low rhythmicity, and low attention span are more prone to develop alcohol and substance use problems. High activity level in infancy is consistently found to predict later substance abuse in both sexes. Children with high sensation seeking and novelty seeking are also more prone. Children with ADHD, Oppositional defiant disorders and conduct disorders are more prone. Children of substance dependent fathers have been found to have distinct temperamental characteristics (low rhythmicity, low adaptability, low threshold of responsiveness, withdrawal and negative emotionality) that makes them more prone to use substances themselves in later life (Malhotra et al 1993).

Social-psychological-familial Factors

Family influence is an extremely important determinant for early alcohol initiation, especially by younger children. In some families from the state of Panjab in north India, fathers who themselves use alcohol make their young sons 8–10 years olds taste alcohol as a matter of valour or pride. They do not realise that this is going to turn into a major alcohol use problem in later life. Other factors include parental drug use, dysfunctional family systems, physical abuse, neglect, sexual abuse, harsh punitive parenting, absent/negligent parenting, over indulgent or over protective parenting, family history of mental illness or psychopathy, parental criminality. Early maternal death or separation, institutionalisation and compromised care in early life are also risk factors. Substance abusing peers, poor neighbourhood, slum dwelling, exposure to criminality, and lack of bonding are other social factors associated with alcohol and SUDs.

Protective Factors

Children who have a stable, intact and optimally functioning family are generally protected. Children who have a close emotional bond with a parent or an adult member of the family, who have secure attachment with mother or primary care giver, who have consistent, high care and authoritative parenting, and close involvement with the child's life, have family cohesion, and adult supervision/monitoring, are protected against the risk. Positive self-esteem and self-concept, high self-control, presence of assertiveness and social competence, and academic achievement all promote resistance to drug use. Religious affiliation and moral compass also constitute protective factors. High intelligence, high resilience, absence of drug using peers protects the adolescents against drug use.

Assessment

Take a comprehensive psychiatric and drug use history from patient and family. Psychiatric history assessment must include information about child's prenatal, postnatal and early years of development, temperamental profile, family history, parenting practices, family functioning, social environment, educational history, peer group. Drug use history should include the age of first use, type of drug(s) used, current dose of each, route of administration, frequency of use and quit attempts if any. In some instances, patient is brought with some other mental health concern which may be some behavioural or emotional problem or legal problem. Patient may not disclose history of drug use. If a patient does not report substance use, the psychiatrist should have high index of suspicion and explore for presence of substance use.

Indicators of substance-use disorders are:

- Declining school performance, dropping out of school, missing school

- Social withdrawal, lying to adults, stealing, delinquency
- Substance use and delinquency among peers
- Early sexual contact, early pregnancy
- *Evidence of mental disorder, e.g.:* Conduct disorder, attention deficit disorder, affective disorder, anxiety disorder, suicidality
- *Family history:* Substance use by parents, antisocial behavior in the family, impaired parent–child relationships, mental illness of parents
- Socioeconomic disadvantage, deprived living environment, poverty and high crime rate

Drug testing is required to know the substance of abuse. Most patients would under report or mis report, so drug testing is useful. Testing can be done in urine, blood, saliva, hair, breath or sweat. Most common is urine testing because the mechanism and rate of excretion of the substances would vary with the sample used.

Treatment

Comprehensive treatment is most commonly done at outpatient level. Treatment planning requires detailed assessment that includes elaborate history of substance use, associated medical complications, psychological issues (e.g. attention deficit/hyperactivity disorders, conduct disorder, depression, other disorders, temperament, parenting issues, etc.), social, academic, and family issues, detailed mental state examination, assessment of motivation, locus of control, and social support (Gaur et al 2019).

The treatment of children and adolescents with SUD is highly structured and is intended to promote patient insight through a multimodal, interdisciplinary approach. Treatment is individualised depending upon the type of substance used, quantity, family situation, environmental issues, temperament qualities, presence of comorbid mental illness or physical problems. Biggest hurdle is the motivation for treatment. Those who have good motivation, they comply with treatment and do well, whereas those who are unsure or unmotivated have to be first prepared for treatment acceptance. Treatment generally starts with motivation enhancement therapy (MET).

The entire range of therapeutic spectrum from psychotherapy and environmental measures to somatic and pharmacological treatments is required to be used. A wide range of psychotherapeutic approaches are useful. Individual therapies, group therapies, family therapy, relapse prevention, social skills training, and other specialized therapies (movement therapy, music therapy, acupuncture, relaxation methods etc) can be used depending upon the suitability of the patient and therapist's skills. Psychotropic medications are often required simultaneously to treat psychiatric comorbidity, stabilise the patient in therapy, or for retention in the system.

Treatment goals include the following services depending upon the clinical staging, and most of these require specialized CAP centers for treatment of addictions.

1. Treatment of withdrawal
2. Treatment of comorbid mental illness
3. Restructuring of everyday life
4. Maintenance therapy and relapse prevention
5. Long term rehabilitation service
6. Educational and vocational training

Indications for hospitalization are:
- Heavy substance use
- Poly substance use
- Multiple failed treatment attempts
- Comorbid mental disorders
- Comorbid physical disorders requiring inpatient treatment
- Minimal family or social environmental support
- Acute danger to self or others
- Distance from treatment facility

Acute Treatment

Acute treatment involves treatment of intoxication, withdrawal from addictive substances or reduce the dose of substance used, and dependence. Treatment of withdrawal usually takes about 2–4 weeks. It can be done in outpatient if there is sufficient support in the family and social system. Otherwise, in most instances this is done in inpatient setting.

Table below gives symptoms of intoxication, withdrawal and recommended treatment for various substances (Fader and Mroczkowski 2020). It is important to recognize and diagnose the problem and provide emergency care. Most of these require treatment in a specialized center for de-addiction services.

Very few psychotropics have been studied and approved for use in children and adolescents with drug abuse. Buprenorphine-naloxone combination has been approved by FDA for opioid use disorder in adolescents above 16 years of

Substance	Intoxication	Withdrawal	Treatment
Alcohol Sedatives Hypnotics	Sedation, dizziness, ataxia, nystagmus, confusion, paradoxical agitation, disinhibition, amnesia	0–12 hours after last use: Shakiness, headache, anxiety, nausea, vomiting, tachycardia, tachypnea, diaphoresis 12–24 hours after last use: Confusion, hallucinations with intact reality-testing, tremor, agitation 24–48 hours after last use: Seizures, death 4–12 days after last use: Delirium tremens	Benzodiazepine taper Referral to substance use treatment
Opioids	Sedation, euphoria, miosis, nausea, constipation, urinary retention, respiratory depression, hypotension, bradycardia, cardiopulmonary collapse, respiratory arrest, coma, death	Flu-like symptoms, shaking, diaphoresis, gooseflesh, mydriasis, yawning, rhinorrhea, nausea, vomiting, diarrhea, anxiety, depression, akathisia, cramps	Supportive care Buprenorphine induction, Methadone, or clonidine Referral to substance use treatment
Stimulants	Tachycardia, hypertension, tachypnea, hyperthermia, diaphoresis, mydriasis, anorexia, euphoria, agitation, anxiety, decreased reality testing, hallucinations	Intense dysphoria, anxiety, fatigue, restlessness, increased appetite, cognitive slowing, vivid dreams, sexual dysfunction, suicidality	Supportive care Cardiac monitoring Benzodiazepines for acute agitation Referral to substance use treatment
Cannabis	Conjunctival injection, impaired short-term memory, impaired attention, impaired motivation, ataxia, perceptual disturbance, increased appetite, euphoria or relaxation	Decreased appetite, difficulty sleeping, irritability, anxiety, headaches, nausea, abdominal pain	Supportive care Benzodiazepines for acute agitation Referral to substance use treatment
Hallucinogens (PCP, MDMA, LSD, Psilocybin, Ketamine, GHB)	Altered level of consciousness, dissociation, perceptual disturbance, euphoria, agitation, aggression, tachycardia, hypertension, diaphoresis	Variable	Supportive care Referral to substance use treatment

age. There is some recommendation for use of methadone in those who have high risk of relapse. Benzodiazepines can be used in acute phase of alcohol withdrawal like that for adults. Long-acting BZDs such as chlordiazepoxide and clonazepam are preferred. Naltrexone and topiramate are also useful for alcohol use disorder. For nicotine withdrawal, varenicline and bupropion are recommended. For cannabis, N-acetyl cysteine has been used and found to show some benefit. Nutritional deficiencies are commonly seen with alcohol dependence and nutritional supplements in the form of thiamine, multivitamins, magnesium supplementation is recommended.

Along with withdrawal, treatment of comorbid psychiatric illness is started as part of acute treatment, and it takes longer, from few months to few years, depending upon the type of disorder. Comorbid psychiatric disorders such as ADHD, SLD, depression, Anxiety, which in most situations are likely to be primary conditions predating the alcohol or substance use, should be treated simultaneously using appropriate medications and psychosocial therapies. There has been some evidence that treating ADHD in childhood can mitigate the risk for developing alcohol or SUDs in later life. Treatment of associated psychiatric disorder should be done in full earnest in all cases. SSRIs, mood stabilizers are helpful for depression, anxiety, BPAD, impulse control disorders or emotional dysregulation; methylphenidate is helpful for ADHD; second generation antipsychotics in small doses are useful in treating aggression, violence, psychosis or delirium. The extent to which pharmacotherapy is effective in the treatment of adolescent SUDs remains uncertain due to insufficient research evidence. But in usual clinical practice all these drugs are found to be quite effective. More research is warranted for exploring pharmacotherapy options for adolescent SUDs, specifically as augmenting agents along with psychosocial treatments.

Maintenance Treatment

Once the acute crisis of intoxication and withdrawal is over, treatment shifts to maintenance phase and relapse prevention. Harm reduction is another strategy if complete abstinence is not possible. Naltrexone is used as anti-craving agent during maintenance phase.

Psychosocial interventions are essential. MET is needed in most cases. Further, there can be individual psychotherapy, CBT, or behaviour therapy, as suitable for the given patient. Group therapy or family therapy is also useful. Patient should be engaged in productive activity and daily activity scheduling. Life skills training is also effective.

Emphasis is placed on re-entry into school and addressing school issues. Many a times these children have specific learning disorders and are negatively treated in school by teachers and peers or even at times bullied. School liaison is important. Rehabilitation in education and vocational training with the aim to complete education, achieve autonomy and productive life remain the ultimate goals of therapy.

Relapse Prevention

The risk of relapse is highest in the first six months after treatment. Retaining the patient in treatment through maintenance phase is also a huge challenge. Many patients due to their typical personality or behavioural characteristics, get quickly bored, become impatient and want to return to their earlier patterns of behaviour and peer group activities. Adolescents may develop a false sense of self-confidence that they can control their behaviour and urges and want to stop treatment.

Based on previous work and examining the literature published between 2016–2019, (Fadus et al 2019) reported a synthesis of clinical interventions for adolescent SUDs and the general strength of recommendations for each. The results of this review are summarized in the table below (Fadus et al 2019).

Adolescent Substance-Use Disorder Treatment Recommendations

Well-established standalone interventions	Family based therapy, cognitive behavioral therapy, multicomponent psychosocial therapy
Probably efficacious standalone interventions	Motivational interviewing (MI)/motivational enhancement therapy (MET), third-wave cognitive behavioral therapies
Possibly efficacious standalone interventions	12-step programs
Possible adjunctive interventions	Pharmacotherapy, exercise, Yoga, mindfulness, recovery-specific educational settings, goal setting, progress monitoring
Modifications to improve existing approaches	Digital strategies, culturally-based programs

The clinician has to choose and adapt these intervention strategies to suit the given patient and circumstances. There is no standard formula.

Family-based interventions are well-established and first-line in the treatment of adolescent SUDs.

CBT is efficacious evidence based treatment for adolescent SUD used as stand-alone therapy.

Multicomponent psychosocial treatments is combinations of family-based therapy, cognitive behavioral therapy, motivational interviewing, and contingency management, and can be effective in treating adolescent SUDs.

Motivational interviewing and motivation enhancement therapy are effective interventions, as they may help change the adolescents attitudes toward treatment, but as a standalone treatment, motivational interviewing does not appear to be as strong as other more well-established interventions. However, given the convenience and brief nature (10–20 minutes) of MI and MET, these interventions are a key component in a comprehensive treatment of adolescent SUDs (Fadus et al 2019).

"Third-wave" CBTs, such as acceptance and commitment therapy (ACT) and mindfulness-based cognitive therapy, emphasize acceptance and mindfulness techniques.

There has been limited data regarding efficacy of 12-step programs for youth, and limited evidence to suggest that 12-step programs are effective as standalone treatments. However, much like MI/MET, it constitutes an effective component of a more comprehensive approach to treatment.

Exercise and yoga may be promising as potential adjunctive therapies, as some of the early studies have indicated that exercise among substance-using adolescents can help improve sleep, establish structure, strengthen relationships, and improve self-perception. These treatments could have benefits in a wide variety of other physical and mental health conditions and are therefore recommended despite the limited evidence.

Goal setting: According to social cognitive theory, individuals work harder and are more confident in their ability to achieve goals when they have actively formed them. Commitment to goal of abstinence in combination with other more established standalone or multicomponent therapies is highly useful and easily feasible.

Progress monitoring: Progress monitoring is a feasible way of knowing if the patient is responding to treatment and allows for adaptation of treatment strategies along the line.

Use of digital technologies: There are several innovative methods of intervention as computerized brief interventions. Web-based and mobile technologies are highly accessible and appealing to adolescents. Digital interventions are not only perceived as more private and less stigmatized than traditional clinical evaluations, but have also been found to facilitate participant motivation and self-efficacy. Digital technologies, may play a strong role in future in becoming adjunctive interventions for treating adolescent SUDs.

Cultural adaptations: Overall, treatment has to be culturally adapted to suit the patient, given that risk factors and response to treatment among adolescent substance users may vary based on ethnicity and race.

Prevention Strategies

Preventive strategies include programs for universal prevention, selective prevention, and indicated prevention. Universal interventions are designed to address the whole population, such as a community or school. Selective prevention targets 'at-risk' population, such as those children whose parents have drug or alcohol dependence. Indicated prevention programs targets individuals who already demonstrate the problem behavior or have other high-risk behaviors related to drug use. Information, education, life-skills training, assertiveness training, in schools, community centres, media constitute highly useful prevention methods. Prevention of access to alcohol and drugs to children as a state policy needs attention on a wider societal level. Implementing and enforcing minimum age limits and regulating access to alcohol and exposure of children to marketing should be regulated. Research suggests that the legalization of cannabis may be linked to an increase in use among adolescents as a result of increased accessibility and social acceptance. Policy and law must be in tandem with medical knowledge for dealing with a problem like alcohol and substance use disorders.

BIBLIOGRAPHY

1. Ambekar A, Agrawal A, Rao R, Mishra AK, Khandelwal SK, Chadda RK (2019) on Behalf of the Group of Investigators for the National Survey on Extent and Pattern of Substance Use in India. Magnitude of Substance Use in India. Ministry of Social Justice and Empowerment, Government of India.

2. Dhawan A, Pattanayak RD, Chopra A, Tikoo VK, Kumar R. (2017) Pattern and profile of children using substances in India: insights and recommendations. Natl Med J India.;30:224–229.

3. Fader RP, Mroczkowski MM. (2020) Child and adolescent psychiatric emergencies. In Rey JM and Martin A (eds), JM Rey's IACAPAP e-Textbook of Child and Adolescent Mental Health. Geneva: International Association for Child and Adolescent Psychiatry and Allied Professions.

4. Fadus MC, Squeglia LM, Valadez EA, Tomko RL, Bryant BE, Gray KM. (2019). Adolescent Substance Use Disorder Treatment: An Update on Evidence -Based Strategies. Curr Psychiatry Rep. Sept 14; 21(10):96.

5. Ganzer F, Bröning S, Kraft S, Sack PM, Thomasiusn R. (2016) Weighing the evidence: a systematic review on long-term neurocognitive effects of cannabis use in abstinent adolescents and adults. Neuropsychol Rev.;26:186–122.

6. Gaur N, Gautam M, Singh S, Raju VV, Sarkar S. (2019) Clinical practice guidelines on assessment and management of substance abuse disorder in children and adolescents. Indian J Psychiatry.;61:333–349.

7. Global Youth Tobacco Survey (GYTS-4), (2019) https://ntcp.nhp.gov.in/assets/document/National_Fact_Sheet_of_fourth_round_of_Global_Youth_Tobacco_Survey_GYTS-4.pdf.

8. Hasan A, von Keller R, Friemel CM, et al. (2020) Cannabis use and psychosis: a review of reviews. Eur Arch PsychiatryClin Neurosci.; 270:403–412.

9. Hindley G, Beck K, Borgan F, et al.(2020) Psychiatric symptoms caused by cannabis constituents: a systematic review and meta-analysis. Lancet Psychiatry. 7:344–353.

10. Kandel DB, Johnson JG, Bird HR, et al. (1999) Psychiatric comorbidity among adolescents with substance use disorders: findings from the MECA Study. J Acad Child Adolesc Psychiatry. 38:693–699.

11. Levy S, Vaughn BL, Knight JR. (2002) Office-based intervention for adolescent substance abuse. Pediatr Clin North Am. 49:329–343.

12. Malhotra S, Basu D, Bhagat A, Malhotra A. (1993). Temperament of children of Addicts: A preliminary report. Journal of Hong Kong College of Psychiatrists. 3, 5–8.

13. Mokdad AH, Forouzanfar MH, Daoud F, et al. (2016) Global burden of diseases, injuries, and risk factors for young people's health during 1990-2013: a systematic analysis for the Global Burden of Disease Study 2013. Lancet. 387:2383–2401

14. Kessler RC, Avenevoli S, Costello EJ, et al. (2012) Prevalence, persistence, and sociodemographic correlates of DSM-IV disorders in the National Comorbidity Survey Replication Adolescent Supplement. Arch Gen Psychiatry. 69:372–380.

15. Sharma A, Malhotra S, Raghunathan M, Malhotra A. (1997) A study of event related potential – P3 characteristics in children of alcoholics. Addiction Biology, 2, 43–438.

16. Tomas-Roig J, Benito E, Agis-Balboa RC, et al. (2016;) Chronic exposure to cannabinoids during adolescence causes long-lasting behavioral deficits in adult mice. Addict Biol. 22:1778–1789.

Glossary of Terms

A large number of psychiatric terms are used in the whole process of assessment and diagnosis. Some of these represent various symptoms and signs that the child presents with, some of these are the terms are used to denote types and levels of functioning, impairments, states, syndromes, deficits, interactions and so on. Brief definition and description of each of these as they appear in various chapters of the text, has been done. Readers may refer to this list according to their individual needs depending on their levels of familiarity and knowledge of these terms. It is neither a comprehensive nor an exhaustive list.

Many of the terms are common to adult as well as child psychiatric patients. Attempt is made to include those terms which are specific to working with children and adolescents or which may have a different connotation in the context of children. This glossary will also be useful to those psychiatrists who are predominantly dealing with adult psychiatric patients and occasionally have to deal with children or to paediatricians who come across several of these problems in their practice. Since many of the terms are also common words in English language, their specific meaning in psychiatric terminology needs to be defined and understood. Patient and relatives may use words in common usage which may not in fact mean what they denote in technical terms. Precision of definition and specificity of concepts involved in eliciting psychiatric signs and symptoms is the key to arriving at a reliable diagnosis.

Effort has been made to compile a list that includes most of the commonly used terms. Moreover, the consensus descriptions and definitions as currently accepted are presented. The terms are listed in an alphabetical order for the sake of convenience.

Abuse, substance: Use of a psychoactive substance which is harmful to the individual or the society.

Achievement age: Another term for educational age. It is established by standard achievement tests comprising a series of educational, rather than intelligence tests.

Acute psychotic agitation: Impaired state, characterised by severely increased psycho-motor activity, often associated with or produced by psychotic experiences such as delusions and hallucinations.

Addiction: Disease process characterized by continued use of a specific psychoactive substance despite physical, psychological or social harm (American Society of Addiction Medicine, 1990). Addiction is characterized by (a) inability to control amount and frequency of use; (b) irresistible cravings and urges; (c) continued use despite adverse effects; (d) denial of indisputable negative consequences; and (e) tendency to abuse other mood-altering drugs or alcohol, either concomitantly or in the absence of the abused substance.

Affect: Feeling tone, pleasurable or unplea-surable, that accompanies and/or determines the general attitude towards an idea. It includes inner feelings and their external manifestations. Affect and emotion are often used interchangeably. It is also described as experience of emotion expressed by the patient and observed by others.

Affective flattening: A disturbance of affective response, expressed as emotional blunting and indifference. It occurs as a symptom in schizophrenia or as part of certain neurological syndromes.

Aggresssion: Behaviour both physical and/or verbal that has potential for actual harm. Aggressive behaviour ranges from normal assertiveness and coping behaviour to acts of violence. It may be expressed overtly (abusing, cursing) or covertly (defiance, non-cooperation, gossiping), directly (physical assault) or indirectly (planned, systematic, hostile acts). Aggression includes diverse motivational, emotional and behavioural aspects.

Agitation, psychomotor: Generalised over activity occurring in the physical and emotional spheres. It is generally seen in response to either internal and/or external stimuli.

Agitation: Inability to sit still, pacing, fidgeting, movements of legs or fingers, wringing hands, and/or pulling at clothes, along with a feeling of uneasiness or restlessness.

Agoraphobia: Intense anxiety with a feeling of being trapped in a situation.

Amnesia, psychogenic: Loss of memory associated with or related to a traumatic situation or to important aspects of a traumatic event; probably mediated by dissociative process. Essential feature is sudden inability to recall important personal information (may be related to specific time duration). The patient may display perplexity, disorientation and wander aimlessly. In many cases, semantic (conceptual) memory and memory of skills remains intact.

Anger: Strong feeling elicited by real or supposed injury that is often accompanied by a desire to take revenge.

Anhedonia: Inability to derive pleasure from situations and stimuli that usually induce pleasure. It is a pathognomonic feature of major depressive disorder.

Anorexia nervosa (AN): Eating disorder that occurs commonly in prepubertal, adolescent, and young women. Distortion of body image is considered central to the diagnosis characterized by morbid fear of becoming fat, refusal to maintain normal body weight, and obsession with dieting, to the point of inducing profound weight loss, leading to body weight at least 15% below expected. Patients of AN suffer from widespread and serious medical complications, e.g. osteoporosis, hypothermia, arrhythmia, etc.

Anxiety-generalised: It is a feeling of tension or uneasiness arising from the anticipation of some external or internal danger.

Anxiety-free floating: Pervasive anxiety not attached to any particular ideational content or an object of fear. It is characteristic of generalised anxiety disorder.

Anxiety-psychic: Anxiety manifested predominantly by tension, apprehension, fear, irritability and excessive worry. It may or may not be accompanied by behavioural agitation.

Anxiety: Subjective unpleasant feeling or emotional state of apprehension, dread, or foreboding ranging from excessive concern about the present or future to feelings of panic, accompanied by a variety of autonomic signs and symptoms-palpitations, dry mouth, pupil dilatation, panting, shortness of breath, sweating with skin pallor, anorexia and abdominal discomfort, choking or tight feelings in throat, dizziness, trembling in the absence of external stimulus.

Apathy: Lack of feeling or absence of affect. This symptom is found in severe depression, schizophrenia and brain injury.

Aphonia-psychogenic: Loss of voice not caused by laryngeal or neurological abnormalities but as a symptom of conversion/dissociative disorder.

Assertiveness: Affirmative and confident behaviour that allows a child to meet his/her needs.

Astasia-abasia: Gait disorder characterised by bizarre staggering with abortive falls or collapse into the arms of medical staff personnel. Neurological examination confirms the absence of paralysis, ataxia, or sensory loss. It is generally a manifestation of hysteria or conversion disorder.

Ataxia: Inability to co-ordinate muscles for the execution of voluntary movement. It may be due to a disorder in the brain or spinal cord and is commonly found in cerebellar lesions. In the absence of neurological disorder, it can be a psychogenic symptom.

Attention: Ability to focus in a sustained manner on one activity. Disturbance in attention may be manifested by difficulty in finishing tasks that have been started, easy distracti-bility, or difficulty in concentrating on work.

Autism-infantile: Severe developmental disorder with probably a neurological basis characterized by disturbances in motility, perception, social interactions, speech, language and cognition that occurs before 30 months of age.

Autism: Behavioural syndrome characterised by poor social interaction, impaired communication and language, poor display of emotions, lack of empathy and atypical responses to people, objects and events. It is also associated with a hyper arousal state (e.g. hyperactivity, repetitive/stereotypic behaviour, self-stimulation, hyper vigilance). Autistic children often exhibit ritualised body movements, repeated touching and sniffing of objects, ritualistic ordering, checking and collecting, and insistence on precisely following routines:

Autistic fantasy: Mechanism in which the person substitutes excessive day dreaming for the pursuit of human relationships, more direct and effective action, or problem solving (DSM-IV).

Automatic behaviour: Stereotyped, repetitive actions that apparently occur without awareness.

Automatism: Repetitive stereotyped sensorimotor or verbal phenomena which occur episodically, associated with clouding of consciousness, over which the individual generally has no control and does not remember. It can be found in epilepsy and sleep disorders.

Behaviour disorder: Deviant or maladaptive behaviour inappropriate for the child's age or social expectations, causing nuisance or distress to people around but not to him/herself. These are differentiated from disorders of emotions where there is significant distress to the child. Behaviour disorder is a more generic and non-specific term that includes disorders such as attention deficit hyperkinetic disorders, conduct disorders, habit disorders.

Biological rhythms: The cyclical changes occurring in the physiological, psychological and emotional functioning, and the level of activity of an individual at regular intervals ranging from minutes to months. For example, circadian rhythm which is a cycle of about 24 hours.

Bulimia: Eating disorder manifested by insatiable hunger resulting in compulsive or binge eating of large quantities of calorie-rich food, followed by self-induced vomiting, excessively restricted dieting, or prolonged periods of fasting.

Catalepsy: It is a state of generalised unresponsiveness in which postures are held rigid for prolonged periods. In this condition, the person's limbs remain in the manner as they are placed, even uncomfortably. It is found in catatonic states which could be a part of schizophrenia, affective illnesses, organic brain syndromes or hysteria.

Cataplexy: It is a transient sudden loss of tone of the skeletal muscles which can result in fall and injury to the patient. It generally manifests as buckling of knees, sagging of head or complete collapse of the body. It is commonly found as a part of the syndrome of narcolepsy and can be precipitated by a variety of emotional states.

Catatonia: It is a syndrome characterised either by a state of stupor with marked muscular rigidity/flexibility or overactivity with verbal/motor stereotypies. It is found secondary to various medical, neurological and psychiatric disorders.

Catharsis: Relief due to release of pent-up emotions. It occurs when a child releases feelings (anger, affection, sorrow, grief) about past or present material that have previously been difficult or impossible to discharge.

Child-physical abuse: Acts that cause or could have caused physical injury to a child.

Child-psychological (emotional) abuse: Acts or omissions that caused or could have caused emotional strain or trauma that is inappro-priate for the developmental age of the child.

Child abuse: Physical abuse and neglect (often chronic) and harm of children, usually infants, toddlers or preschoolers, generally by those who are responsible for their care. They may present with minor or major injuries with explanations that often do not fit the injury.

Child neglect: Failure to provide care and nurturance to the child as is appropriate and necessary for his/her age.

Child sexual abuse (CSA): Acts in which dependent, developmentally immature children and adolescents are involved in sexual activities that they do not fully comprehend, are unable to give informed consent to, and that violate the social taboos of family roles. It includes acts from fondling to intercourse; intercourse between similarly aged adolescents just before the legal age of consent; sadistic, sexual assaults by adults on infants; single incidents perpetuated by strangers; and frequent contacts over many years by family members or well-known family friends. It also may involve exploitation for financial benefits.

Clanging: Speech in which associations are determined by sounds, rather than the meaning or the concept of the words. It may include rhyming and punning. The term is applied only when it is a manifestation of a pathological condition, e.g. schizophrenia and manic episodes. Children may exhibit this normally as in rhyming word play.

Clinging: It is the inability to end appropriately or unnecessary prolongation of an interaction or conversation. It is generally associated with circumstantiality and is found in temporal lobe epilepsy.

Clouding of consciousness: A state of impaired consciousness representing mild stages of disturbance on a continuum from full awareness to coma. It is found in the early stages of organic brain disease.

Cluttering: Disorder of speech fluency in which rate and rhythm of speech are affected and speech intelligibility is impaired. There are alternating pauses and bursts of speech that produce groups of words unrelated to the grammatical structure of the sentence (DSM-IV). Severity of cluttering ranges. Cluttering is distinct from stuffering.

Communication disorder: Form of speech or writing that impairs communication because of aberrant use of terms, content, or form. Examples include pressure of speech, tangentiality, echolalia, loose associations, flight of ideas and perseveration.

Compulsion: Repetitive, seemingly purposeful, behaviours performed according to a specific or stereotyped fashion (DSM-IV). Apparently, the purpose is to yield to or undo the obsessions. The compulsive activity is not a realistic way of achieving the purpose or is clearly excessive. The child may not recognize the senselessness of the behaviour.

Confabulation: Inventing stories and producing false and fluent answers to any question without regard to facts.

Confusion: It is a state of impaired conscious-ness associated with acute or chronic organic brain disease. Clinically it is characterised by disorientation, slowness of mental processes with scanty association of ideas, apathy, lack of initiative, fatigue and poor attention. In mild confusional states, rational responses and behaviour may be provoked by examination but more severe degree of disorder renders the subject unable to retain contact with the environment.

Consciousness: A complex mental state of vigilance with awareness of self and environment mediated by sensory and cognitive processes.

Conversion reaction: Somatic dysfunction without underlying organic cause, which represents an intrapsychic symbolic conflict or wish fulfilment.

Dangerousness: An estimate of the risk of inflicting serious violence on others, or causing serious psychological or physical harm or damaging property. It is subject to change according to the child's mental state and relationship with others.

Deja VU: "Already seen"; feeling of familiarity by a person who, when perceiving something never seen before, thinks he or she has had the experience in the past. It is not uncommon in normal persons and occurs more often in temporal lobe abnormalities.

Delinquency: A term applied to various forms of antisocial behaviour and conduct committed by children that constitutes legal offences.

Delirium: Transient organic mental syndrome characterised by global impairment of cognitive functions, including memory and perception; reduced and/or fluctuating levels of consciousness; disorientation and fear; impaired capacity to shift or maintain attention; increased or decreased psychomotor activity; disordered sleep–wake cycle; a variety of affective symptoms, including blunting or flattening of affect; and behavioural changes, including agitation, withdrawal and lack of interest. Delirium is a reversible disturbance of cerebral metabolism secondary to a cerebral insult (e.g. infection or a metabolic disturbance). The cardinal feature is fluctuation in brain dysfunction. Onset is acute, usually within 4–6 hours, although it may evolve over several days or weeks.

Delusion: Unfounded, unrealistic, idiosyncratic belief that is firmly held without supporting evidence and often in the presence of evidence to the contrary. It may be poorly formed, well-formed or highly systematized. Qualitatively and quantitatively, they are inconsistent with the patient's sociocultural or religious background. They often dominate the patient's life, resulting in inappropriate and irresponsible actions.

Denial: Mechanism in which a person fails to acknowledge some aspect of external reality that would be apparent to others.

Depersonalization: Perception or experience of the self is altered so that the subject feels as if personal identity is lost and that he or she, his or her body, and/or the environment is different or unreal. Other symptoms may include mood changes; difficulty in organising, collecting and arranging thoughts; and a feeling that the brain has been deadened. Also called 'feeling of unreality'. In this state, self awareness is heightened (but inanimate) in presence of a normal sensorium and an intact capacity for emotional expression. "As if" quality of experience is the key feature.

Depression: State of lowered or sad mood, often accompanied by feelings of unhappiness, social withdrawal, disturbances of sleep, energy, appetite, concentration and interest. There may be unexplained somatic symptoms, lowered levels of achievement or performance.

Derealization: A counterpart of depersonalization where a subjective experience of alienation occurs but involves the external world. The surroundings may seem to lack colour and life and appear as artificial, or as a stage on which people are acting contrived roles.

Developmental disability: Inability to perform certain roles and functions or acquire skills like normal individuals on account of mental handicap present early in childhood as in mental retardation, autism, cerebral palsy, specific learning disability, etc.

Developmental disorder, pervasive: A group of disorders with deviant and delayed development, abnormalities in reciprocal social interactions, patterns of communication and restricted, stereotyped, repetitive behaviour, involving child's functioning in all situations, and all areas. These are qualitative abnormalities, associated with varying degrees of general intellectual impairment manifesting within first 5 year of life. These are severe disorders with poor prognosis. Some of the common pervasive developmental disorders are childhood autism typical or atypical, Asperger's syndrome, disintegrative disorder, etc.

Developmental disorder, specific: Disorders associated with the biological dysmaturation of the central nervous system and characterised by impaired or delayed development of functions such as reading and writing language, visuospatial skills, motor coordination, associated with biological maturation of the central nervous system. Delay in the development of a specific function is apparent in early infancy or childhood (which is the appropriate age of normal development of that function) and the impairment decreases to some extent progressively with age. Some examples of specific developmental disorders are disorders of speech and language, of scholastic skills or of motor functions. These delays are not directly attributable to a neurological disorder, sensory impairment, mental retardation or environmental deprivations.

Deviance: Behaviour that is qualitatively different from the accepted norm or which is not relevant to a particular age or socio-cultural setting.

Disability: Restriction or lack (resulting from an impairment) of ability to perform an activity in the manner or within the range considered normal. It may hinder mobility, occupation, communication or ability to care for self. It can be continuous or intermittent and may be present from birth or acquired later.

Disintegrative psychosis: A condition, usually commencing at the age of three or four in a normally developing child. Over a few months, there is loss of speech and social skills, accompanied by hyperactivity, stereotyped motor behaviour and a severe impairment of emotional response and intellectual capacity. Clinical evidence of neurological disease may not always be present. The outcome is poor.

Disorientation: Lack of awareness of one's relationship to the milieu including persons, place and time. It can range in severity from mild to severe.

Dissociation: Mechanism in which the person sustains a temporary alteration in the integrative functions of consciousness or identity. Manifesting in states such as psychogenic amnesia, fugue trance, multiple personality.

Distractability: Frequently and/or easy shift of attention to unimportant or irrelevant external stimuli.

Disturbance of mood: A morbid change of affect extending beyond normal variation to subsume any of several reactions; including depression, elation, anxiety, irritability and anger.

Dyslexia: A form of difficulty in reading, writing or spellings despite having been taught to read and write in the absence of defective vision/hearing, mental handicap or brain damage. There is often a tendency to reverse letters and words in reading and writing. Dyslexia is more common in boys and tends to be associated with clumsiness and poor concentration.

Dysphoria: Unpleasant quality of mood in which acute transient changes in mood (e.g. feelings of sadness, sorrow, anguish, misery, mental malaise) accompanied by verbal complaints of feeling depressed, sad, blue, gloomy, down in the dumps and empty.

Dysthymia: It is a mild form of affective disorder where symptoms of depression persist for a longer time (>1 year in children) and may fluctuate from day-to-day or on an hour-to-hour basis.

Dystonia: Neurological condition characterized by slow, tonic, sustained muscle contractions often of the tongue, jaw, eyes and neck, frequently causing twisting and repetitive movements, or abnormal postures. There are five main types:

(a) focal, (b) segmental, (c) multifocal, (d) generalised, (e) hemidystonia. Most common manifestations are oculogyric crisis, cervical dystonia (torticollis), tongue contraction, trismus and opisthotonus.

Echolalia: Automatic repetition (echoing) of the words or phrases of others that is persistent. It is observed in some pervasive developmental disorders, organic mental disorders, schizophrenia, mental retardation, dysphasia or may be a feature of early normal speech development. It should not be confused with habitual repetition of questions, apparently to clarify the question and formulate its answer.

Elation: An affective state of joyous gaiety which is intensified and out of keeping with life circumstances. It is generally associated with increased motor activity and is classically seen in mania.

Elective mutism: A condition exhibited by children who, although being able to talk and comprehend language, remain silent (mute) in the presence of particular individuals and environments, usually related to school. It is associated with problems of temperament and emotion.

Emotion: Stirred up physiological state or a feeling state due to any stimulus, internal or external, tending to maintain or abolish the causative stimulus. It is often used interchangeably with affect.

Emotional incontinence: Involuntary sudden expression of feelings, such as weeping, grimacing and/or laughter, over which the person has no apparent control. It is frequently associated with neurological diseases, especially multiple sclerosis.

Emotional lability: Pattern of abrupt mood shifts from normal to one or more dysphoric states (depression, irritability, anger and anxiety).

Emotional neglect: Inadequate nurturance/affection and refusal or delay in psychological care.

Emotional withdrawal: Lack of interest in or involvement with events and happenings in life. It may range from mild-to-extreme.

Empathy: Capacity to understand what another person is experiencing in which one feels as the other person does, but recognises that other feelings are possible. Empathy is not sympathy, in which one person identifies with another while suspending critical intellect.

Encopresis: Involuntary functional fecal incontinence. Causes could be poor toilet training, emotional problems, constipation with overflow soiling, severe mental handicap and brain damage.

Enuresis: Involuntary passage of urine, usually at night during sleep, in the absence of a urological or neurological disorder. The term enuresis should not be used until a child is 4–5 years old. It generally occurs as an isolated symptom but it can be associated with poor toilet training, psychological problems, learning problems, emotional difficulties, problems with relationships and minor neurological dysfunction or may be a simple developmental lag in maturation.

Epileptic twilight state: A transient psychic or behavioural change occurring during or after an epileptic seizure and characterised by reduced alertness and blurred perception of surroundings. It is an organic condition with abrupt onset/off set, clouded consciousness, violent acts, emotional outbursts, variable duration, dream like state commonly seen in cases of temporal lobe epilepsy.

Euphoria: Morbid or abnormal sense of well-being.

Euthymia: Normal range of mood that is intermediate between an elevated and sad mood. The feelings of well-being are neither excessive nor pathological. Euthymia is more appropriately used as a description of the entire condition and not just mood (as opposed to dysthymia or hyperthymia).

Excitement: Hyperactivity as reflected in accelerated motor behaviour, heightened responsivity to stimuli, hypervigilance or excessive mood lability. It may range from mild-to-extreme.

Fatigue: It occurs during prolonged mental or physical activity that makes it difficult for the patient to sustain the same level of activity as normal and can be incapacitating.

Fear: An intense emotion in the face of a real external threat which is accompanied by sympathetic hyperarousal. It is accompanied by defensive patterns of behaviour associated with flight or escape.

Flashbacks: Vivid memories or recurring dreams of the stressful event occurring during sleep or when awake. These are associated with intense anxiety and are highly distressing. Common in Post Traumatic Stress Disorder and abuse of certain drugs, e.g. Cannabis, LSD, Mescaline.

Flight of ideas: A disordered form of thinking manifesting as rapid and incessant talk with speech associations that are facilitated or easily diverted by chance factors. Rhyming and punning often occur. It is manifested subjectively as pressure of thought and is seen in mania.

Fluctuation of mood: A morbidly unstable or labile pattern of affective response without external cause.

Functional disorder: Disorder without a physiological or anatomical cause which has purely psychological basis. The term has now been more or less abandoned because of difficulty of establishing the underlying causes or differentiating "organic" from "functional" disorders.

Ganser's syndrome: A form of pseudodementia with a core symptom of "approximate answers" or talking past the point (vorbeireden). Associated features include fluctuating disturbances of consciousness, hallucinosis and memory defects. It may be precipitated by emotional disturbance or accompanied by hysterical stigmata, resolving abruptly with subsequent amnesia for the episode. It can occur in organic brain disease, functional psychoses and dissociative disorders.

Guilt feelings: Sense of remorse or self-blame for real or imagined misdeeds in the past. Often seen in depression, it may be associated with suicidal thoughts and may go up to delusional level.

Habit: Behaviour pattern acquired by frequent repetition of the same.

Hallucination: A sensory perception occurring in the absence of an appropriate external stimulus to any of the sensory modalities and which occurs at the same time as the real perceptions. They can occur normally during awakening or dozing phases of sleep, fatigue and in various psychotic disorders.

Hallucinatory behaviour: Behavioural symptoms indicating the occurrence of perception in the absence of adequate external stimuli. It can manifest in the form of smiling to self, muttering to self and making gestures in the air.

Handicap: Disadvantage due to an impairment or disability that limits or prevents fulfilment of a role that is normal (depending on age, sex, social and cultural factors) for the individual.

Head banging: Rhythmic and monotonous striking of the head against a hard surface. It may be seen as a developmental problem in infants and young children up to age 4. However, it may be a behavioural symptom in the severely mentally retarded or psychotic children.

Hospitalism in children: A syndrome closely related to anaclitic depression developing in infants in hospital who are separated from their mothers or mother surrogates for a long period of time. It is characterised by listlessness, unresponsiveness, emaciation and pallor, poor appetite and disturbed sleep, febrile episodes, lack of sucking habits and an appearance of unhappiness. The disorder is reversible if the mother or mother surrogate and child are reunited within a few weeks.

Hostility: Verbal and nonverbal expression of anger and resentment towards others. It can be extreme, as manifested by extreme uncooperativeness or assault towards others.

Hyperactivity: Increased speed and frequency of motor responses, i.e. body movements and speech. It also denotes excessive physical activity in a child.

Hypergraphia: Excessive and/or compulsive writing in any form. The writings are often characterized by excessive and unnecessary details. It is seen in patients with temporal lobe epilepsy, mania or schizophrenia.

Hyperkinesia: Excessive muscular movements.

Hyperphagia: Excessive eating. It can be compulsive, forced or otherwise.

Hypersomnia: Excessive sleepiness, especially during the day. In this, the child does not usually feel refreshed on waking up. It is found in depression, sleep apnea syndrome, Klein-Levine syndrome, etc. It should be distinguished from narcolepsy.

Hypertonia: Presence of greater degree of tension (tone) in the muscles than usual. It is found in upper motor neuron lesions and presents as spasticity.

Hyperventilation: A condition of longer, deeper or more rapid respiratory movements eventually leading to dizziness and cramps. It may be associated with paraesthesias, light-headedness, numbness, palpitations and apprehension. Hyperventilation is a physiological response to hypoxia but can occur in states of anxiety. However, it is probably the most common but least recognised anxiety reaction.

Hypervigilance: Excessive attention and focus on all internal and external stimuli.

Hypokinesis: Slow or diminished body movements. It may be drug-induced or a symptom of depression or Parkinson's disease.

Hypomania: Milder form of mania. The patient may appear very confident, talkative, fast and unusually productive and may indulge in prankish behaviour.

Hyposomnia: Significant decrease in sleep, ranging from sleep lasting only a few hours per night to total insomnia up to 1–2 days.

Hysteria: Apparent presence of bodily dysfunction which reduces the psychological distress and for which the typical organic causes are not applicable. Hysteria should be differentiated form malingering.

Hysterical tremor: The presence of tremors of irregular frequency or variable intensity associated with movement. They tend to diminish or disappear when the child's attention is diverted. If the child is asked to perform a manual task with one hand, there is associated suppression of the tremor in the other hand.

Idea of reference: Idea, held less firmly than a delusion, that events, objects or other people in the person's immediate environment have a particular and unusual meaning specifically for him or her (DSM-IV).

Illogical thinking: Thinking that contains obvious internal contradictions or in which clearly erroneous conclusions are reached, given the initial premises (DSM-IV). It may be seen in normal people who are distracted or fatigued. It has psychopathological significance only when it is marked.

Illusion: An erroneous or distorted perception that may relate to an object or a sensory stimulus. Illusions are experienced by most people and do not necessarily indicate mental disorder. They may occur in any sensory modality.

Impairment: Any loss or abnormality of psychological, physiological or anatomical.

Impulse control-poor: Poor control over one's inner urges, resulting in sudden or mis-directed acts or emotional outbursts without forethought or concern about consequences.

Impulsivity: Behaviour characterised by lack of deliberation and failure to consider risks and consequences before acting. It is a temperamental factor related to extra-version.

Inappropriate mood: A discrepancy between affect and thought-content or experience; seen in schizophrenia and organic brain syndromes.

Incoherence: Speech that, for the most part, is not understandable because of distorted syntax (grammar) and idiosyncratic word usage.

Incontinence: Inability to control excretory function.

Inner restlessness: Subjective feeling of psychic unrest or uneasiness. It may be associated with agitation or tension in patients who are depressed, fearful and can be part of drug-induced akathisia.

Insight, lack of: Impaired awareness or understanding of one's own psychiatric condition and life situation in which the patient refuses treatment or help.

Insight: Recognition by the patient that there is presence of an illness or maladaptive behaviours and requires treatment.

Insomnia: Subjective dissatisfaction with or poor quality and decreased quantity of, or non-refreshing nature of sleep arising from a variety of intrinsic (stress, emotional disturbance, physical disease) and/or extrinsic (noise) factors. It is likely to cause impaired concentration, short-term memory problems, inability to handle minor irritations and decreased ability to accomplish tasks.

Intelligence: Intelligence refers to the ability of the individual and is variously defined as ability to learn, ability to adjust to novel situation, ability for abstract thinking, etc. A comprehensive and most accepted definition, however, is that it is a global capacity to think rationally, act purposefully and deal effectively with the environment.

Irritability: A feeling state of reduced control over temper or undue state of excitability to annoyance, impatience or anger which may appear as brief episodes in certain situations such as fatigue. It can be more prolonged or generalised as a clinical feature of temperamental anomalies.

Kleptomania: Compulsive stealing due to a conscious, irresistable urge to steal. The child may not plan to steal, may steal articles that are not of much use to him/her and may consider this as a problem behaviour.

It is a type of impulse control disorder and different from ordinary stealing.

La belle indifference: Inappropriate lack of emotion or concern for the implications of one's disability. Commonly seen in hysteria.

Mannerism: Repetitive involuntary or semivoluntary movements that once served a useful purpose in the past. They are less insistently repeated and are more in keeping with the subject's personality. They should be differentiated from stereotypies.

Melancholia: Major depressive episode with agitation or retardation, severe mood lowering unresponsive to environmental changes, and depressive delusions. Term is retained in DSM-IV but replaced by 'somatic symptoms' in ICD-10.

Mental age: Age corresponding to the actual ablilities of the child which may be higher or lower than the chronological age. During the course of develompment, children are able to achieve certain abilities at different age levels. Some are brighter than others and achieve them earlier, others slower and achieve them later. Mental age is the chronological age of the child, at which majority of the children are able to perform the designated tasks. For example, if a child of say 8 years is able to perform tasks which can be done by majority (75%) of children at 9 years, then his mental age would be 9 years. But, if he can do only the tasks which can be done by majority of children at 6 years, then his mental age would 6 years.

Microcephaly: Abnormal smallness of the head.

Mood congruent: Symptoms and behaviour consistent with the patient's expressed or prevailing mood.

Mood: Degree of well-being experienced more or less habitually over long periods of time. It is influenced by affects. Mood has also been used to indicate the entire gamut of affects and emotions.

Motor retardation: Slowing/lessening of movements and speech, diminished responsiveness to stimuli and reduced body tone. Extreme motor retardation can lead to stupor.

Mutism-akinetic: State of disturbed consciousness and severe apathy in which the patient is alert, conscious of surroundings and able to see and hear, but is completely paralysed and unable to communicate except through eye blinks. It may be due to lesions of the third ventricle and pons, certain acute brain syndromes, Guillain-Barre syndrome and potent neuroleptics.

Mutism: Condition in which a patient is unable to produce sound despite being capable of phonation. There is no evidence for aphasia or laryngeal or labial dysfunction. Mutism accompanied by akinesia suggests the possibility of organic brain damage.

Negativism: Contrary or opposite behaviour or attitude. It can be active (where the child actively resists or does the opposite of what is asked) or passive (where the child refuses compliance or cooperation).

Neologism: New word invented by the subject, distorted word, or standard word to which the subject has given a new, highly idiosyncratic meaning. The judgement that the subject uses neologism should be made cautiously, taking into account his or her educational and cultural background (DSM-IV).

Night terrors: A sleep disorder in which there is awakening with a frightening dream in which there is no recall or only vague perception of a frightening dream-like experience. The child appears confused and may show signs of autonomic arousal.

Nightmare: A sleep disorder characterised by awakening with a frightening or bad dream that must be differentiated from night terror. In nightmares there is vivid and detailed dream recall.

Obsession: Recurrent, persistent, intrusive idea, thought, image or impulse that is recognized as one's own, felt to be senseless/absurd/repugnant, hence resisted, more often than not unsuccessfully, resulting in considerable anxiety and distress.

Oculogyric crisis: Form of abnormal movement that begins with a fixed stare for a few moments, followed by the eyes rotating upwards and to the side and remaining fixed in that position. This is associated with backward head movements, opening of mouth and protrusion of tongue. It may last from minutes to hours and is induced by neuroleptic.

Oppositional disorder: Pervasive opposition to all in authority regardless of self-interest, continuous argumentativeness, and un-willingness to respond to reasonable persuasion (DSM-IV).

Orientation: Awareness of where one is in relation to time, place and person (DSM-IV).

Palilalia: A type of verbal perseveration in which there is repetition of one's own last words or phrases.

Panic attack: A sudden attack, lasting usually for 15–20 minutes, of fear and alarm in which the signs and symptoms of morbid anxiety become dominant and are often accompanied by irrational behaviour and the fear of one going crazy or about to die. They are generally of two types, i.e. cardiac and respiratory. These commonly occur in panic disorder, depression and phobic disorders.

Paramnesia: Falsification of memory by distortion of recall.

Paresis: Partial loss of motor function due to a neurological disease.

Perplexity: A state of puzzled bewilderment in which verbal responses are desultory and disjointed and reminiscent of confusion.

Perseveration: Continuation of a response or inability to change 'set' after it is no longer appropriate. It should be suspected if a patient repeats certain words, phrases or gestures. It is usually elicited by a stimulus where initial response is appropriate followed by senseless repetition after it serves its purpose. It can be both verbal and motor. It is a common feature of frontal lobe dysfunction that may be tested by asking the patient to copy alternating letters or repetitive sequential patterns of hand movements. It is classically elicited when the patient gives the same answers to a number of different questions.

Phobia, simple: Unreasonable fear of a specific object or situation, such as animals, snakes, heights or thunderstorms. These are often triggered by an actual frightening experience and generally disappear as the child gets older.

Phobia, social: Disorder characterised by fear of being judged by others and embarrassing oneself in public where the person will be subject to scrutiny while performing a specific task or interacting with other people (e.g. public speaking, eating in restaurants, using public restrooms).

Phobia: An irrational involuntary fear which may be diffuse or focused on one or more objects or situations and is out of proportion of external danger or threat. It is usually accompanied by feelings of apprehension or intense dread, which may lead to avoidance of such objects or situations. In other words, it is severe anxiety evoked by a circumscribed object/event/set of circumstances.

Physical disability: Difficulty performing one or more activities that are generally accepted as essential components of daily living (e.g. self-care, social relations, economic activity) (WHO).

Pica: Compulsive eating of non-nutritive unusual substances. It can be due to anaemia in a child.

Poor attention is failure in focused alertness manifested by poor concentration, distractability from internal and external stimuli and difficulty in harnessing, sustaining or shifting focus to new stimuli.

Pressure of speech: Speech that is increased in amount, accelerated, difficult or impossible to interrupt, and usually loud and emphatic (DSM-IV). The child may talk spontaneously. It is most often seen in manic episodes.

Pretend play: Play in which objects are used as if they have other properties or identities. It is normally present by age 12–15 months, but is absent or abnormal in autism.

Pseudohallucination: Hallucination like experience different from true hallucinations in that the person is fully aware of the unreality of the experience. In this, the perception appears in subjective space rather than objective space.

Pseudoseizure: Seizure like episode of non-epileptic nature during which the EEG remains normal. Also called "hysterical seizure".

Psychological autopsy: Retrospective examination of a suicide death, reconstructed by examining medical, psychiatric and social records and by interviewing family and friends.

Psychomotor activity: It is a term used for both verbal and non-verbal behaviour including reaction time, speed of movement, flow of speech, involuntary movements and hand writing.

Psychomotor agitation: Generalised physical and emotional overactivity in response to internal and/or external stimuli.

Psychomotor retardation: Generalised slowing of physical, mental and emotional reactions, especially movements such as walking and eye-blinking.

Psychosis: Heterogeneous group of conditions showing a severe impairment of mental functioning (excluding retardation) associated with disordered psychological contact with reality and, usually, aberrant social behaviour. Disorders of consciousness, memory, mood, perception, thinking or psychomotor behaviour are prominent clinical phenomena depending on the nature of psychosis, and insight is often grossly deficient. It can be either organic or functional.

Rapport: Intrapersonal relationship characterised by emotional affinity and the ability to communicate freely, meaningfully and emotionally.

Reactive psychosis: A term employed to designate a group of psychoses causally related to a preceding external event, e.g. personal loss, bereavement, insult, natural disaster. The psychoses are mostly of brief duration, often but not always remitting with the recession of the provoking factor. Their form and content tend to reflect the nature of the precipitant.

Reactive: Secondary to, resulting from, or precipitated by an identifiable event; generally reactivity is an ambiguous concept, often equated with psychogenicity, applied to those neurotic and psychotic disorders that are supposedly caused or precipitated by psychosocial factors.

Reading disability: Specific difficulty or inability to read properly that is disproportionate to the general intelligence level.

Rigidity: Increased muscle tone with increased resistance to passive movement. It is seen as an extrapyramidal side effect of neuroleptics.

Ritualistic behaviour: Interactive, often complex, and usually symbolic actions carried out in a certain manner, that may acquire ceremonial significance for collective religious observances, and constitute a feature of play and normal development in childhood. It can be a morbid phenomenon.

Selective amnesia: A form of psychogenic memory loss which is restricted to the specific psychologically traumatic event.

Self-injurious behaviour: Self-destructive behaviour causing obvious tissue damage, without lethal intent or severity, resulting in a temporary relief of dysphoric feelings.

Self-mutilation: Deliberate damage to one's own body, without conscious intent to die. It may or may not be lethal.

Sensorium: Consciousness, actual awareness of the nature of one's self and surroundings.

Separation anxiety: Inability of the child to remain alone without the presence of the prominent figure in his/her life, most commonly parents. The fear of being alone leads to generation of intense apprehension and anxiety due to which the child tries to stop the prominent figure from going away.

Sexual exploitation: Sexual act by a person on an individual who is unable to consent to, or make an informed choice because of lack of knowledge.

Shallowness of affect: A state of morbid insufficiency of emotional response, presenting as an indifference to external events and situations.

Sleep talking: Phenomenon in which the person talks incomprehensibly while sleeping. Full consciousness is not achieved, and no memory of the event remains.

Sleep walking: Disorder in which walking and other motor acts are performed during sleep. The patient does not respond to verbal commands and has no recollection of them.

Social withdrawal: The retreat from social and personal contact leading to aloof detachment and an impaired capacity to communicate with others. It is commonly encountered in schizophrenia.

Somatization: Tendency to experience and communicate physical distress and symptoms unaccounted for by pathological findings. The patient attributes them to physical illness and seeks medical help for them.

Somnolence: Excessive daytime sleepiness. This is found frequently in several sleep disorders.

Startle reflex: Any jerky movement due to loud sound or other stimuli. It is an orienting response to stimuli associated with autonomic changes aimed at readiness for movement. It can be seen in a newborn infant where it is not considered pathological. Exaggerated startle response may be pathological or otherwise normal even in adults. It is generally found in association with fear and anxiety. It increases in frequency with the severity of the anxiety.

Stereopathy: Behaviours in which there are repetitive actions or words associated with self-injurious behaviours occurring parti-cularly in severely/profoundly mentally handicapped people. These include rocking, swaying, head banging, eye-poking, hand waving and finger movements.

Stereotypy: Persistent, spontaneous, abnormal repetition of gestures or movements that are not goal directed. They include repetitive acts, repetitive speech, locomotion, etc. They are found in severe mental retardation, brain damage and autism. Structure or function (WHO).

Stupor: A state characterized by mutism, an absence or profound diminution or blocking of voluntary movement, and psychomotor unresponsiveness.

Stuttering: Frequent repetitions or prolongation of sounds or syllables that markedly impair speech fluency (DSM-IV). Secondary symptoms include interruption in the flow of speech sounds, tremors of the lips, rapid blinking, etc.

Subdelirium: Prodromal form of a fully established delirium, manifested by restlessness, headache, hypersensitivity to auditory and visual stimuli, irritability and emotional lability.

Suicidal ideation: Thoughts, ideas or ruminations about suicide or overt verbal threats to kill oneself. They fall intermediate between extreme ideas of hopelessness and suicidal acts.

Suicide attempt: Life-threatening act requiring medical attention that is committed with a conscious intent to end one's life. Suicide attempts may develop at different times during the illness and fluctuate in severity independent of the severity of the depression.

Suicide pact: Agreement or pledge between two or more persons to take their own lives simultaneously.

Suicide: It is a conscious act of self-induced annihilation or an act of killing oneself deliberately.

Suspiciousness: Unrealistic or exaggerated ideas of feeling persecuted by others, reflected in guardedness, a distrustful attitude, suspicious hypervigilance, or frank delusions that others mean harm.

Temperament: Innate, and constitutional behavioural tendencies of an individual that characterise his/her unique style of behaviour arising from individual differences in the emotional, attentional and motoric reactivity and response patterns. It is underlying property of the individual that organizes interactions with the environment over a wide range of situations rather than the behaviour itself. Temperament is a biological concept, which manifest itself in interaction with the environment and is measured as phenomenological characteristics of the individual, that are relatively stable. Specific temperament variables have been empirically described by various authors varying from simple, micro level dimensions such as attention span, threhsold of responsiveness, amount and speed of motor activity, regularity of biological functions (rhythmicity) or reaction.

Tension: Unpleasant increased motor (rapid pacing) and psychological activity, with overt physical manifestations of fear, anxiety and agitation.

Tic: Brief muscle contractions that are repetitive and stereotyped. Tics appear suddenly in intermittently. They can be motor or vocal; simple or complex to new stimulus, or as more complex and macro level variable such as difficultness, soothability, sociability and emotionality.

Trance: Temporary alteration of the state of consciousness manifested by loss of usual sense of personal identity, narrowing of awareness of immediate surroundings and limited movements and speech to a specific and small repertoire. Commonly seen in dissociative disorders.

Trichophagia: Hair eating; an activity often engaged in by trichotillomania patients.

Trichotillomania: Disorder characterised by impulses to pull out one's hair. Is basically an impulse control disorder.

Trismus: Firm closing of the jaw secondary to tonic spasm of masticatory muscles. A common symptom of tetanus and acute drug-induced extrapyramidal reaction.

Twilight state: Faint or indistinct mental perception, or a transitory disturbance of consciousness, during which complicated and noncomplicated acts may be performed without the patient's conscious volition or memory of them. It can be a postepileptic phenomenon.

Twitch: Very small body movement involving small groups of peripheral muscles.

Uncooperativeness: Active refusal to comply with the will of significant others. The patient may refuse to join in any social activities, tend to personal hygiene, converse with family or staff, or participate briefly in an interview.

Violence: Any act of aggression involving physical contact; irrespective of outcome.

Child and Adolescent Psychiatry Case History

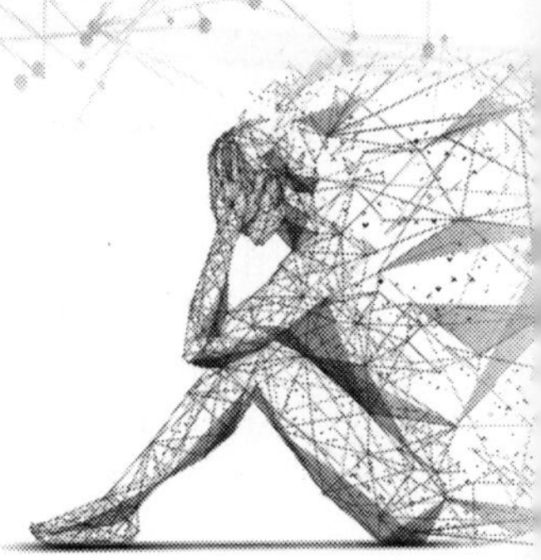

Dr Savita Malhotra MD, PhD, FAMS, FACPsych

No.____Date________________________

Child's Name______________________________Age__________________Date of Birth________________

Sex______________________________________Education____

Informant Mother/Father/Any other (specify)____

Informant's Name______________________________Age__________________Sex__________________

Education______________________________Occupation__________________________________

Family Income____

Residence (Address)____

Rural/Urban____

CHIEF COMPLAINTS (IN CHRONOLOGICAL ORDER)

History of Present Illness

(If the symptoms are present since birth, start history from conception through early and later development. Give chronological account of symptoms. Mention details of treatment). Functioning/Impairment: A global assessment of the child's functioning in the areas of interpersonal relations with parents, other adults, peers, household work: leisure activities. If impaired—mention moderately or severely.

Past History

a. Physical illness
b. Psychiatric problems

Personal and Developmental History

History of Early Development

1. Parental attitude towards pregnancy: Wanted/Unwanted
2. Mother's health during pregnancy
    i. Generally good
    ii. Exanthematous fever in first trimester
    iii. Serious illness
    iv. X-ray exposure
    v. Prolonged drug administration
    vi. Attempted abortion
    vii. Any other
3. Nature of birth:
    i. FTND
    ii. Premature birth
    iii. Instrumental or operation
    iv. Complicated delivery
    v. Head injury
    vi. Jaundice, cyanosis, delayed cry after birth
4. Feeding habits (till age):
    i. Breast
    ii. Bottle
    iii. Breast and bottle mixed
    iv. Weaning age
5. Age of:
    i. Neck holding
    ii. Tooth eruption
    iii. Sitting
    iv. Standing (unsupported)
    v. Walking
    vi. First word
    vii. Three-word sentence
    viii. Bowel control
    ix. Bladder control
6. Developmental problems (if any) of speech, language, motor function.

Social and Personal History

1. Habits
    a. Sleep: (i) Normal ___________, (ii) Fearful _________, (iii) Bruxism ____________
       (iv) Any other ___________
    b. Feeding: (i) Normal _________, (ii) Fussy __________, (iii) Overeating __________
       (vi) Others ___________
    c. Personal care: (i) Adequate ___________ (ii) Unkempt ___________
2. Neurotic traits
    a. Nail biting
    b. Thumb sucking
    c. Morbid fears of persons, animals, darkness
    d. Nightmares
    e. Night terrors
    f. Obstinacy
    g. Temper tantrums
    h. Enuresis, encopresis beyond 3 years

3. Behaviour problems
   Stealing, lying, truancy, disobedience, others
4. Play; individual/group, companies: A few/many, older/younger/same age, good/bad/both/others
5. Sexual history
   Normal/Malpractices

Educational History

1. Qualified up to ____________
2. Educated at (i) Home, (ii) School, (iii) Hostel ____________
3. Started reading at ____________ years
4. Educational problems (if any)
     i. Poor progress
    ii. Financial difficulties
   iii. Repeated absences
    iv. Poor peer relationships
     v. Problem with teachers
    vi. Scholastic skills development
   vii. Any others (also make a global assessment of functioning at school here)

5. Failures if any
   Class ____ No. of failures

TEMPERAMENT CHARACTERISTICS

Activity, rhythmicity, approach—withdrawal, adaptability, mood, intensity of reaction, threshold of responsiveness, attention-span, persistence, distractibility in infancy and later stages.

Family History

1. Family tree (with age, sex, personality, descriptions and any history of mental illness in the family).
2. Family functioning (any discord between family members, lack of communication, any problems with the family as a whole, e.g. isolated family).
3. Parent–child interaction (lack of warmth, hostility towards/scapegoating of child, abuse).

Patterns of Parental Functioning (follow the guidelines given below to elicit information)
- Permissiveness/rigidity
- Consistency/inconsistency
- Strictness of discipline/liberal (any appropriate supervision)
- Approval of interests/disapproval
- Protectiveness/non-protectiveness (any overprotection)
- Toleration of deviance/non-toleration
- Expectations from the child (any pressures, deprivation)
- Reactions towards the illness

Social and Environmental Conditions (mention any aspect of living conditions which you might consider stressful for the child)
- Type of dwelling
- Degree of crowding

- Type and amount of help in the care of child
- Affluence of the family/degree of financial stress

SPECIAL ENVIRONMENTAL CIRCUMSTANCES

Like birth, death, illness, accident, divorce, hospitalization, etc. in the family. If present, mention the effect of the life event on the child, e.g. on self-esteem

Physical Examination

____

____

____

Mental Examination

General appearance and behavior: Describe

____

____

Relationship capacity (response to separation from parents, reaction to interview situation)

____

____

Spontaneous motility and speech (flow form, level of development of speech)

____

____

Affective behaviour (any evidence of anxiety, fear, depression, shyness, including the child's attitude towards the examiner):

____

____

Attitude towards family, school, playmates:

____

____

Stated interests and content of thought: _______________________

Attention span and distractibility: _______________________

Intellectual capacity: _______________________

Motivation insight (child's knowledge of the reasons for his attendance, his desire for help, his sense of own capacity to change):

____

____

____

PROVISIONAL DIAGNOSIS

Try, as far as possible, to make multiaxial diagnosis according to
ICD-10, see under final diagnosis.

Discussion with the Consultant

Final Diagnosis (ICD-10)
Axis I: Clinical syndrome including pervasive development disorders
Axis II: Disorders of psychological development
Axis III: Intellectual level
Axis IV: Medical/physical conditions
Axis V: Rate 0/1/2 associated abnormal psychosocial situations
Axis VI: Global assessment of psychosocial disability

Management Planned

Strategy   *Objective*
 1. Drugs
 2. Further exploration
 3. Psychotherapy
 4. Behaviour therapy
 5. Play therapy
 6. Speech therapy
 7. Occupational therapy
 8. Special education/remediation
 9. Parental counselling
10. Family therapy
11. Environmental manipulation
12. Hospitalization
13. Investigations—Psychological (Psychometry)/ Physical
14. Consultation with other disciplines of medicine
15. Referred to other departments for further management
16. Other (specify)

Advice

____

____

Consultant's signature   Resident signature
(Name in Block letters)   (Name in Block letters)

Follow-up Notes (Date and Sign each note)

____

____

____

Temperament Measurement Schedule

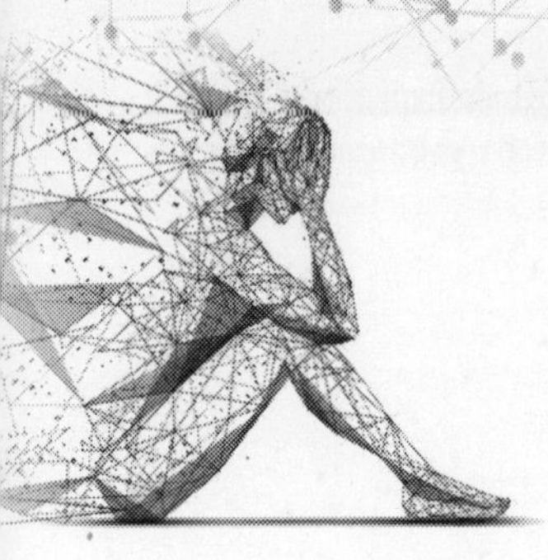

Dr Savita Malhotra MD, PhD, FAMS, FACPsych

No.____Date__________________________

Child's Name________________________________Age______________Date of Birth____________

Sex____Education__________________________________

Informant Mother/Father/Any other (specify)____

Informant's Name________________________________Age______________Sex__________________

Education____Occupation__________________________

Family Income____

Residence (Address)____

Rural/Urban____

TEMPERAMENT MEASUREMENT SCHEDULE

Instructions

Information is to be obtained regarding the child's temperament before the onset of symptoms if he has an illness or about when the child has been his most usual self if he has no illness. Informant should be one of the parents, preferably the mother. Each item explores into some area of routine activities of the child which may be repetitious at places but measures different aspects of temperament. Items are general probes and minor elaborations are permitted wherever necessary. Score all items on a five-point scale, where 3 denotes the average; 1 and 2 indicate lower and 4 and 5 are higher than the average frequency and intensity of the concerned behaviour.

निर्देश

हमारा उद्देश्य बच्चे के स्वभाव की जानकारी प्राप्त करना है। बच्चे का आमतौर पर स्वभाव अथवा बीमारी (यदि बच्चे को बीमारी के लक्षण है) होने से पहले उसका स्वभाव कैसा रहता है के बारे मे जानकारी दे। यह जानकारी माता या पिता कोई भी दे सकता है परन्तु यदि माता जानकारी दे तो बेहतर होगा। हर प्रश्न बच्चे के रोज के अलग-अलग व्यवहार से सम्बन्धित हैं जो कि दोहराया भी जा सकता है परन्तु यह स्वभाव के अलग-अलग पहलू की जानकारी देता है। स्वभाव से सम्वन्धित विषय अधिकतर प्रश्नों के रूप मे है। सरलता के लिए यदि आवश्यक है तो थोड़ा विस्तार किया जा सकता है। हर प्रश्न का उत्तर पांच अंकों पर दिया जा सकता है। आम बच्चो के व्यवहार को सामान्य मान कर इस बच्चे का व्यवहार अक्सर कैसा रहता है? यदि वह भी आम बच्चो जैसा है तो अंक तीन पर गोला लगाए। अंक तीन उस व्यवहार की बारम्वारता और तीव्रता के आधार पर सामान्यता को प्रकट करता है। अंक एक और दो सामान्य से कम और अंक चार और पांच सामान्य से अधिक बारम्बारता और तीव्रता को प्रकट करते है। जो अंक बच्चे के स्वभाव को सही प्रकट करता है उस पर गोला लगाएं।

FACTOR I: SOCIABILITY

a. Approach—Withdrawal

Score:

1. Feels frightened, cries, withdraws physically
5. Goes and talks spontaneously, rushes into new places, spontaneously holds or touches new things.

1. अत्यन्त डरता, शर्माता व संकोच करता है।
5. निसंकोच एकदम अपने आप पास जाता है खुलकर बातचीत करता है।

1. What is your child's first reaction when he meets a stranger (relative,   1 2 3 4 5
   neighbour, doctor, shopkeeper, bus-conductor, etc.)? Does he approach
   the stranger, talk to him or does he feel shy, frightened?

   जब इसको नये लोग मिलें (रिश्तेदार, पड़ोसी, डॉक्टर, दुकानदार, बस कंडक्टर, इत्यादि) तो यह एकदम क्या करता है? कैसे व्यवहार करता है? उनके पास जाता है उनसे बातचीत करता है या डरता, शर्माता है।

2. What is your child's first reaction when he meets children of his age   1 2 3 4 5
   for the first time? Does he approach them, get friendly or does
   he feel hesitant, shy, frightened?

   अगर पहली बार अपनी उमर के बच्चों से मिले तो शुरू-शुरू में क्या करता है उनके पास जाता है उनसे घुल-मिल जाता है या डरता, शर्माता है?

3. If he is given a new food (or placed in a new situation) what is his   1 2 3 4 5
   first reaction, will he try it or does he refuse to do so?

   जब इसे कोई नई तरह का खाना दिया जाए या कोई नई स्थिति में हो तो क्या करता है? एकदम खा लेता है या पहले मना करता है?

4. When your child is introduced to a new game or activity does he join   1 2 3 4 5
   in at once or initially prefers to sit on the side and watch?

   जब इसे कोई नया खेल/activity बताई जाए तो क्या फटाफट से उसमे भाग लेने के लिए तैयार हो जाता है या पहले दूसरो को खेलते देखना पसंद करता है?

Average score:

b. Adaptability

Score:

1. No adaptability—does not accept change at all
5. Initial reaction of withdrawal is only momentary

1. नई चीज या बदलाव को अपनाता ही नहीं।
5. संकोच केवल क्षण भर रहता है। बहुत जल्दी अपना लेता है।

1. Food that he refused earlier or disliked earlier does he still refuse it   1 2 3 4 5
   or has he now accepted it? After how long did he accept?

   जो खाना इसे पहले पसन्द नही था क्या यह अब वो खाना खा लेता है? कितनी देर बाद आराम (खुशी) से
   खाने लग जाता है?

2. If your child has been shy with some stranger earlier, how long   1 2 3 4 5
   does it take him to get friendly—just a few minutes or a long time?

   अगर यह किसी से शुरू-शुरू मे शर्माता हो तो कितनी देर के बाद उनसे दोस्ती कर लेता है या घुल-मिल जाता है?
   जल्दी से या काफी देर बाद?

3. If your child has been shy with some children earlier how long does   1 2 3 4 5
   it take him to mix up and get friendly, just a couple of minutes or a
   long time?

   यह शुरू-शुरू में जिन बच्चो से शर्माता था क्या अब उनसे बातचीत करता है घुल-मिल गया है? कितनी देर के बाद
   उनसे दोस्ती कर लेता है?

4. If he initially hesitates to join a game how long does it take him to   1 2 3 4 5
   start participating in it? Immediately, after sometime or never?

   अगर यह कोई नये खेल मे भाग लेने से आनाकानी करता है तो कितनी देर के बाद यह खेल मे अपने आप भाग लेना
   शुरू कर देता है? बहुत जल्दी ही या कुछ देर के बाद या बिल्कुल ही भाग नही लेता है?

5. Does he settle back into school routine quickly after a long holiday   1 2 3 4 5
   or does it take him a long time to do so?

   लम्बी छुट्टियो के बाद क्या यह स्कूल के कार्यक्रम मे जल्दी घुल-मिल जाता है या कुछ समय लेता है?

Average score:

c. Threshold of Responsiveness

Score:

1. Low threshold—easily bothered by noise, comments on temperature of food, etc.
5. High threshold—not bothered by noise, ignores temperature of food, etc.

1. आवाज, तापमान, दर्द, इत्यादि बहुत अधिक महसूस करता है।
5. बिल्कुल महसूस नहीं करता।

1. Does he seem to bother about the minor noises or sounds around or
   does he ignore these?

   अगर आस पास छोटी मोटी आवाजें या शोर हो तो क्या ये उनकी परवाह करता है या इसे कोई फर्क नही पड़ता–
   जैसे कि ध्यान नही देता?   1 2 3 4 5

2. Does he ignore the temperature of food—hot or cold?

   अगर खाना बहुत गर्म हो या ठंडा हो तो क्या यह उसके बारे मे कहता है या बिना कुछ कहे चुपचाप खा लेता है?

3. Does the child have to be seriously injured before he comments, cries   1 2 3 4 5
   about cuts, bruises?

   जब इसे कोई छोटी मोटी चोट लग जाए तो क्या यह आकर बताता है या तभी जिक्र करता है जब कि
   चोट/ज़ख्म ज़्यादा हो?

4. Does the child not react if accidentally touched pushed or lightly   1 2 3 4 5
   brushed by another child?

   खेलते समय अगर इसको कोई धक्का दे दे या छू दे तो क्या यह उसकी शिकायत करता है रोता है या परवाह नही करता?

5. If there is something new or different about things or people at   1 2 3 4 5
   home, does he notice it immediately or not?

   यदि घर मे कोई नई चीजे या घर के लोगो के पास कोई नई तरह का सामान हो तो क्या इसका ध्यान एक दम
   उस तरफ जाता है या नहीं?

Average score:

Sociability score (add average scores of approach—withdrawl, adaptability and
threshold of responsiveness or a+b+c):

FACTOR II: EMOTIONALITY

d. Mood

Score

1. Always crying, angry, annoyed, irritable, discontented.
5. Always laughing, giggling, contented, happy.
1. हर समय गुस्से मे अप्रसन्न, असन्तुष्ट व चिड़चिड़ा रहता है।
5. हर समय प्रसन्न सन्तुष्ट रहता है।

1. Is your child generally happy, satisfied or generally unhappy discontented?   1 2 3 4 5
   आमतौर पर यह बच्चा खुश, हंसता, मुस्कुराता रहता है या चिड़चिड़ा व असन्तुष्ट रहता है?
2. When with other children does he seem to be happy and having a good time? Is he generally dissatisfied, angry, irritable?   1 2 3 4 5
   जब यह दूसरे बच्चो के साथ होता है तो क्या यह खुश होता है लगता है कि मजे मे है या आमतौर पर चिड़चिड़ा और गुस्से मे लगने लगता है?
3. When playing with other children does he argue/fight with them or does he not?   1 2 3 4 5
   जब यह दूसरे बच्चो के साथ खेलता है तो उनसे बहस झगड़ा करता है या बड़े प्यार व आराम से खेलता है?
4. If your child cannot have or do something that he wants, then for how long does he remain annoyed-only momentarily or for a long time?   1 2 3 4 5
   जब इसे कोई चीज़ जो यह चाहता हो न दी जाए या कोई चीज़ जो यह करना चाहता हो और उससे मना किया जाए तो यह कितनी देर तक गुस्से मे या नाराज रहता है? कुछ ही पल या काफ़ी देर तक?

Average score:

e. Persistence

Score:

1. No persistence—no effort at all.
5. Continues till he achieves what he sets out to.
1. बिल्कुल कोशिश नहीं करता।
5. अंत तक कोशिश करता है।

1. When your child starts on some project like painting, etc. does he work at it completing it no matter how long it takes or does he give it up without completing it?   1 2 3 4 5
   जब कभी यह कोई मनपसन्द काम शुरू करता है जैसे कोई तस्वीर बनाना इत्यादि तो क्या यह उसको पूरा करता है चाहे कितना भी समय लग जाए या उसके जल्दी ही बिना पूरा किए छोड़ देता है?
2. If your child finds a game or a piece of work difficult, what does he do? Does he quickly turn to another activity or does he keep on trying until he learns that particular game or activity?   1 2 3 4 5
   अगर बच्चे को कोई काम या खेल मे मुश्किल लगे तो क्या करता है? छोड़कर कुछ और करने लग जाता है या उसको किसी तरह सीखने की कोशिश करता है?
3. For how long can he continue on the same activity? For about an hour or less than that?   1 2 3 4 5
   अगर यह किसी काम मे लगा हो तो कितनी देर तक उसे ध्यान लगाकर करता रहेगा? आमतौर पर अन्दाज़न एक घंटा या उससे कम?

4. If he gets angry or annoyed how long does it take him to come out   1 2 3 4 5
   of it—just a few moments or long time?

   अगर बच्चा कभी नाराज़ हो या गुस्सा हो जाए तो कितनी देर मे मूड ठीक हो जाता है? जल्दी ही या

   कुछ पल मे या बहुत देर मे ठीक होता है?

5. If you interrupt your child's activity does he try to go back to it or   1 2 3 4 5
   does he forget it?

   अगर बच्चा कोई काम कर रहा हो या खेल मे लगा हो और उस को कुछ समय के लिए हटा लिया जाये तो क्या करता है?

   उस काम या खेल पर दोबारा लग जाता है या उसे भूल जाता है?

Average score:

Emotionality Score (add average scores of mood and persistence or d+e):

FACTOR III: ENERGEY

f. Activity Level

Score:

1. Completely still or very little movement
5. Always on the move, jumps rather than walks always fidgeting

1. बहुत कम हिलता जुलता है।
5. हर समय उछल कूद करता रहता है।

1. How active is your child? Do you find him so active that he runs   1 2 3 4 5
   rather than walks or is he so inactive that he hardly moves?

   आपका बच्चा कितना चुस्त है? क्या आपको ऐसा लगता है कि यह इतना चुस्त है कि चलने की बजाए भागता है

   या इतना सुस्त है कि हिलता ही नहीं?

2. Can he keep still or does he have difficulty in doing so and   1 2 3 4 5
   keeps moving and fidgeting?

   क्या यह टिककर बैठ सकता है या हर समय हिलता-जुलता ही रहता है?

3. Can he sit still while listening to story, joke or some interesting   1 2 3 4 5
   happening?

   जब यह कोई कहानी चुटकुला या मज़ेदार बात सुन रहा हो तो क्या यह टिककर सुनता है या घूमता-फिरता ही सुनता है?

4. While playing does he run and jump about being actively   1 2 3 4 5
   involved or does he quietly move about?

   खेलते समय यह काफी उछल कूद भाग दौड करता है या चुपचाप एक तरफ रहता है?

5. While eating does he eat staying still or does he keep moving about?   1 2 3 4 5

   खाना खाते समय यह कितना हिलता-जुलता है? आराम से बैठकर खाता है या पूरा समय हिलता-जुलता छेड़ाखानी

   करता रहता है?

Average score:

g. Intensity

Score:

1. Hardly any reaction
5. Roaring with laughter screaming with anger, crying loudly

1. बिल्कुल कोई प्रतिक्रिया नहीं करता।
5. अधिकतर प्रतिक्रिया दिखाता है जैसे कि चिल्लाना उछलना।

1. What is his reaction if he is given some food which he likes very   1 2 3 4 5
   much? Is he very happy and eats it with relish or does it not make
   much of a difference to him?

   अगर इसे कोई खाना बहुत अच्छा लगे तो यह क्या करता है—बहुत खुशी से मजे से खाता है या कोई खास फर्क नहीं पड़ता?

2. If your child is taken away or stopped from an activity that he   1 2 3 4 5
   enjoys very much, how does he react? Does he protest mildy,
   gets annoyed, angry or starts crying?
   यदि आप इसे कोई खेल या किसी कार्य से जो इसे बहुत पसन्द हो हटा दे तो यह क्या करता है? सिर्फ मना करता है,
   नाराज होता है, बहुत गुस्सा होता है, या फिर रोने लग जाता है?

3. When he is not given something that he wants then how does he   1 2 3 4 5
   behave? Does not matter very much, gets a little annoyed, gets angry,
   cries and yells?
   अगर इसे कोई चीज जो यह चाहता हो न दी जाए तो यह क्या करता है? सिर्फ मुंह बनाता है, बहुत गुस्सा करता है,
   रोता चिल्लाता है या इसे कोई फर्क नहीं पड़ता?

4. What is his reaction if he or his team loses a game? Does not mind   1 2 3 4 5
   very much, takes it lightly or gets upset, cries?
   अगर यह बच्चा या इसकी टीम किसी खेल मे हार जाए तो यह कैसा महसूस करता है, एकदम झगड़ा करने या रोने लग
   जाता है या बहुत महसूस नहीं करता?

5. What is his reaction if another child takes away his toy or book or   1 2 3 4 5
   any other possession? Does not matter much, gets upset, cries,
   fights with the other child?
   अगर कोई दूसरा बच्चा इसकी कोई चीज़ या खिलौना किताब ले ले तो यह क्या करता है, नाराज होता है, रोता है
   मारपीट करता है या इसे कोई फर्क नहीं पड़ता?

Average score:
Energy score (add average scores of activity and intensity or f+g):

FACTOR IV: DISTRACTIBILITY

h. Distractibility

Score:

1. Low distractibility, even on frustration and active effort can't be distracted
5. Highly distractible on his own
1. बहुत कोशिश के बावजूद भी ध्यान बटाया नही जा सकता।
5. अपने आप ही एकदम ध्यान बंट जाता है।

1. If he is annoyed or is in a bad mood can he be easily joked out of it   1 2 3 4 5
   or is it very difficult to do so?
   अगर यह कभी नाराज़ हो जाये या कुछ चिड़चिड़े मिजाज में हो तो क्या इसका मज़ाक इत्यादि करने से मन बहल
   जाता है या बहुत मुश्किल होती है?

2. What does he generally do, if he is playing or is absorbed in some   1 2 3 4 5
   work and there is a noise outside his window or on the road, will
   he keep on with his activity or will he be easily drawn away from it?
   अगर यह खेल रहा हो या और कोई काम मे लगा हो और खिड़की के बाहर या सड़क पर कोई शोर या ऊंची आवाजे
   सुनाई दे तो क्या करता है, अपने काम मे ध्यान लगाकर बैठा रहता है, ध्यान नहीं देता या एकदम उठकर देखने जाता है?

3. Is it easy or difficult to console him with a toy or story when he is crying? 1 2 3 4 5
   जब कभी यह रोने लग जाये तब इसको खिलौना देकर कहानी सुनाकर आसानी से बहलाया जा सकता है या
   बहुत मुश्किल होती है?

4. Do you find that when he is engrossed in an interesting task, you   1 2 3 4 5
   have to call out several time before he hears or responds?
   अगर यह किसी दिलचस्प काम मे लगा हो तो क्या ऐसा भी होता है कि जब तक आप इसे दो चार आवाजे
   न लगाए इसे सुनाई ही नही देता?

5. While the child is eating or reading if someone knocks at the door   1 2 3 4 5
   or comes does he immediately stop eating or reading or does he
   continue to do it?

   मान लो यह पढ़ रहा हो या खाना खा रहा हो और घर मे मेहमान आ जाए तो क्या यह खाना या पढ़ाई छोड़ देता है
   या उनसे पल दो पल बात करने के बाद अपनी पढ़ाई खाने पर वापिस आ जाता है?

Average score

Distractibility score (average score for h)

FACTOR V: RHYTHMICITY

i. Rhythmicity

Score:

1. Very and always irregular
5. Very fussy about time even when away from home

1. हमेशा अनियमित रहता है।
5. किसी भी स्थिति मे इसका नियमित समय नही बदलता।

1. Does your child feel hungry at approximately the same time every   1 2 3 4 5
   day? Are you able to tell roughly at what time he is bound
   to feel hungry?

   इसके भूख लगने का कोई नियमित (खास) समय होता है या किसी भी समय भूख लग जाती है? क्या आपको
   पता होता है कि इसे किस समय भूख लगेगी?

2. Does your child eat roughly the same amount of food every day or   1 2 3 4 5
   does it vary from one day to the next? Do you have an idea of how
   big or small an appetite he generally has?

   आमतौर पर यह खाना रोज जितना ही खाता है या किसी दिन बहुत ज्यादा और किसी दिन बहुत कम खाता है?
   क्या आपको इसकी भूख का अन्दाजा रहता है कि यह कितना खाना खाएगा?

3. Does your child go to sleep at approximately the same time   1 2 3 4 5
   every night? What time does he generally go to sleep?

   क्या इसके सोने का कोई नियमित (ख़ास) समय होता है? हर रोज कितने बजे सोता है? रोज इसी समय सोता है
   या इसके सोने का समय बदल जाता है?

4. At what time does your child wake up every morning? On   1 2 3 4 5
   weekends or holidays does your child wake up at the same time as
   on other (school) days or does the time change?

   आपका बच्चा सुबह कितने बजे उठता है? इतवार को या छुटिटयो मे यह किस समय उठ जाता है—हर रोज की तरह
   या समय बदल जाता है?

5. Does your child have the bowel movement at about the same   1 2 3 4 5
   time every day?

   यह हर रोज टट्टी किस समय जाता है? इसका समय रोज वही रहता है या बदल जाता है?

Average score

Rhythmicity score (average score for g)

Childhood Psychopathology Measurement Schedule

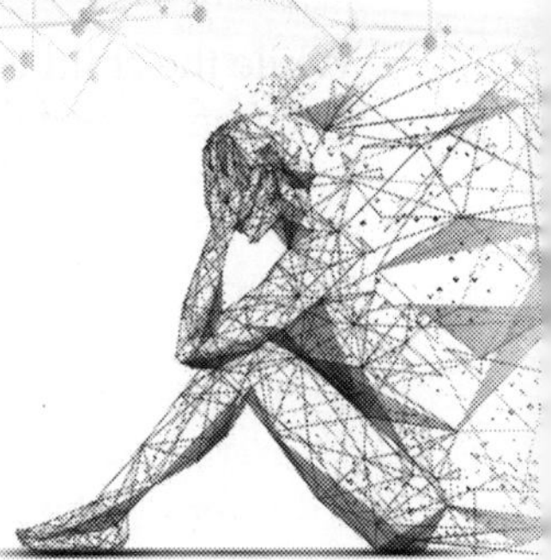

Dr Savita Malhotra MD, PhD, FAMS, FACPsych

No.____Date_________________

Child's Name_____________________________Age_____________Date of Birth_____________

Sex____Education___________________________

Informant Mother/Father/Any other (specify)____

Informant's Name_____________________________Age_______________Sex__________________

Education____________________________________Occupation_______________________

Family Income____

Residence (Address)____

Rural/Urban____

CHILDHOOD PSYCHOPATHOLOGY MEASUREMENT SCHEDULE

Instruction

I will ask you certain questions regarding the child's illness and behaviour during the last 12 months. All the questions may not be applicable to your child but these are to be asked for the sake of completion. Please answer whether it is often true or very much true (score 1) or often not true (score 0). (Items given below are in the form of questions. Please use additional probes wherever necessary.)

निर्देश

आपसे बच्चे के पिछले एक साल के व्यवहार और बीमारी के बारे में कुछ प्रश्न पूछे जाएंगे। ज़रूरी नही है कि हर सवाल आपके बच्चे पर लागू होता हो। आप हां या ना मे जवाब दे। अगर यह व्यवहार आपके बच्चे मे अक्सर पाया जाता है तो अंक एक (1) पर गोला लगाइए और अगर यह नहीं पाया जाता तो अंक शून्य (0) पर गोला लगाइए। सभी विषय प्रश्नों के रूप मे पूछे गए है जहां ज़रूरी हो थोड़ा विस्तार किया जा सकता है।

FACTOR I: LOW INTELLIGENCE WITH BEHAVIOUR PROBLEMS

1. Acts too young for his age.   0   1
   इसकी हरकते अपनी उमर के या अपने से छोटों जैसी है।

2. Does he go to school, if yes, is he poor at school work?   0   1
   यह पढ़ाई मे कैसा है? क्या कमज़ोर है?

3. Has your child ever repeated a grade?   0   1
   क्या आपका बच्चा कभी फेल हुआ है?

4. Prefers playing with younger children.   0   1
   क्या यह अपनी उमर से छोटे बच्चो के साथ खेलना पसन्द करता है?

5. Steals at home.   0   1
   क्या यह घर मे चोरी करता है?

6. Steals outside home.   0   1
   क्या यह कभी घर से बाहर चोरी करता है?

7. Impulsive or acts without thinking.   0   1
   क्या यह बिना सोचे समझे अचानक कुछ कर बैठता है?

8. Runs away from home.   0   1
   क्या यह कभी घर से भाग जाता है?

9. Can't concentrate or pay attention for long.   0   1
   क्या इसको ध्यान लगाकर काम करने में मुश्किल होती है?

10. Confused or seems to be in a fog.   0   1
    क्या कभी ऐसा लगता है कि यह कुछ खोया-खोया सा है कुछ समझ नही पा रहा है?

11. Day dreams or gets lost in his/her thoughts.   0   1
    क्या यह आमतौर पर अपने विचारों मे खोया व मग्न रहता है?

12. Secretive, keeps things to self.   0   1
    क्या यह अपने मन की बात बता देता है या उसे मन मे ही रखता है?

13. Irrelevant talking.   0   1
    क्या कभी कोई बेमतलब (न समझ आनेवाली) बाते करता है?

14. Talks too much.   0   1
    क्या यह ज़्यादा बोलता है?

15. Poor memory.   0   1
    क्या इसकी याद्दाश्त कमज़ोर है?

16. Uses alcohol, tobacco or drugs.   0   1
    क्या शराब व सिगरेट पीने या और नशीली चीज़े प्रयोग करने की आदत है?

Factor I score

FACTOR II: CONDUCT DISORDER

1. Argues a lot.   0   1
   क्या उसको ज़्यादा बहस करने की आदत है?

2. Destroys his or her own things.   0   1
   क्या यह कभी अपनी चीज़ों की तोड-फोड करता है?

3. Destroys things belonging to other family members or children.   0   1
   क्या यह दूसरे बच्चों या घरवालों की चीज़े तोड-फोड़ करता है?

4. Disobedience at school.   0   1
   क्या यह स्कूल में कहना मानता है या नहीं?

5. Disobedience at home.   0   1
   क्या यह घर वालों का कहना मानता है या नहीं?

6. Cruel to animals.   0   1
क्या इसको जानवरों/कीड़े-मकौड़ो को मारने व परेशान करने की आदत है?

7. Cruelty, bullying, meanness to others.   0   1
क्या इसको और बच्चों को तंग करने व चिढ़ाने की आदत है?

8. Physically attacks people.   0   1
क्या यह मारपीट करता है?

9. Stubborn, obstinate, irritable.   0   1
क्या यह ज़िद्दी व चिड़चिड़े स्वभाव का है?

10. Threatens people.   0   1
क्या यह कभी औरो को धमकिया देता है?

11. Gets in many fights.   0   1
क्या यह आमतौर पर लड़ाई-झगडे कर बैठता है?

12. Cries a lot.   0   1
क्या यह बहुत रोता है?

13. Screams a lot.   0   1
क्या यह बहुत चिल्लाता है?

14. Temper tantrum or hot temper.   0   1
क्या यह बहुत गुस्सा करता है?

15. Teases a lot.   0   1
क्या यह औरो को बहुत चिढ़ाता है?

16. Sets fire.   0   1
क्या यह कभी आग लगाता है?

17. Swearing or obscene language.   0   1
क्या यह गंदी गालिया निकालता है?

Factor II score

FACTOR III: ANXIETY

1. Nervous, high-strung, tense.   0   1
क्या यह जल्दी घबरा जाता है व परेशान रहता है?

2. Too fearful or anxious.   0   1
क्या यह बहुत डरा या घबराया रहता है?

3. Bites finger nails.   0   1
क्या इसको नाखून चबाने की आदत है?

4. Nightmares.   0   1
क्या यह रात मे डरकर चिल्लाता है?

Factor III score

FACTOR IV: DEPRESSION

1. Withdrawn, does not get involved with others.   0   1
क्या यह आमतौर पर बिना किसी से मिले-जुले अकेला रहता है?

2. Likes to be alone.   0   1
क्या यह आमतौर पर अकेला रहना पसन्द करता है?

3. Deliberately harms self or attempts suicide.   0   1
क्या इसने कभी अपने आपको जानबूझ कर नुकसान पहुंचाने की या खुदकुशी करने की कोशिश की है?

4. Shy or timid.   0   1
क्या यह बहुत शर्माता है?

5. Unhappy, sad or depressed.   0   1
क्या यह अकसर उदास रहता है?

6. Worrying.   0   1
क्या यह ज़्यादा फ़िक्र करता है?

7. Feels and complains no one loves him.   0   1
क्या यह महसूस करता है कि कोई इसे प्यार नहीं करता?

8. Feels others are out to get him.   0   1
क्या यह महसूस करता है कि लोग इसके पीछे पड़े है?

9. Feels worthless and inferior.   0   1
क्या यह महसूस करता है कि यह बेकार (हीन) है?

10. Talks about killing self.   0   1
क्या कभी यह खुदकुशी करने की बात करता है?

11. Over eating.   0   1
इसकी भूख कैसी है? क्या ठीक खाना खाता है या ज़्यादा खाता है?

12. Gets teased a lot.   0   1
क्या यह खुद जल्दी चिढ़ जाता है?

13. Sleeps more than most children.   0   1
क्या यह और बच्च्यो से ज़्यादा सोता है?

Factor IV score

FACTOR V: PSYCHOTIC SYMPTOMS

1. Fears going to school.   0   1
क्या यह स्कूल जाने से डरता है?

2. Can't get his mind off certain thoughts (obsession).   0   1
क्या इसके मन में विचार बार-बार आते है जिन्हे कि यह मन से नही निकाल सकता?

3. Strange behaviour, specify.   0   1
क्या इसने कभी अजीब हरकते की यदि हां तो किस तरह की हरकते करता है?

4. Strange ideas, specify.   0   1
क्या इसने कभी अजीब विचार जाहिर किये—किस तरह के विचार?

5. Stares blankly.   0   1
क्या यह कभी टकटकी लगाकर खाली काफ़ी देर तक देखता रहता है?

6. Too concerned with neatness or cleanliness.   0   1
क्या यह सफाई का बहुत अधिक ध्यान रखता है?

7. Hangs around with children who get in trouble.   0   1
क्या यह बुरे बच्च्यो जो कि लड़ाई-झगडे मे पड़ जाते है की संगति मे रहता है?

8. Trouble sleeping.   0   1
क्या इसको सोने मे कोई मुश्किल होती है?

9. Sleep less than most children.   0   1
दूसरे बच्च्यो से कम सोता है?

Factor V score

FACTOR VI: SPECIAL SYMPTOMS

1. Repeats certain acts over and over (compulsions).   0   1
क्या यह कुछ काम अपनी मर्ज़ी के खिलाफ बार-बार करता है जिससे इसको परेशानी होती है?

2. Eats or drinks things that are't food.   0   1
क्या यह कोई ऐसी चीजे खाता है जो कि खाने की नही है जैसे कि मिट्टी कागज़ लकड़ी?

3. Thumb sucking.   0   1
क्या इसे अंगूठा चूसने की आदत है?

4. Wets the bed.   0   1
   क्या रात को बिस्तर पर पेशाब करता है?
5. Wets self during the day.   0   1
   क्या कभी दिन में कपड़ों में पेशाब कर लेता है?

Factor VI score

FACTOR VII: PHYSICAL ILLNESS WITH EMOTIONAL PROBLEMS

1. Fears certain animals, situations, places other than school.   0   1
   क्या यह कई जानवरों या जगहों से बहुत डरता है इतना कि उनके पास जाने से बहुत घबराता व कतराता है?
2. Complaining of loneliness.   0   1
   क्या यह अकेलापन महसूस करता है?
3. Does not eat well.   0   1
   क्या यह खाना ठीक से नहीं खाता है?
4. Any other physical complaints (specify), e.g. allergy, asthma, diarrhea, epileptic fits.   0   1
   क्या इसको और शारीरिक बिमारी है (जैसे कि दमा, दस्त, मिर्गी के दौरे इत्यादि), क्या है?

Factor VII score

FACTOR VIII: SOMATIZATION

1. Poorly co-ordinated or clumsy.   0   1
   क्या यह सलीके से काम करता है या बेसलीके से करता है जैसे कि चीज़ों को ठीक ढंग से नहीं पकड़ सकना या चीज़ें अक्सर हाथ से छूट जाती है, बिखर जाती है या यह काम करते समय अक्सर इधर-उधर टकरा जाता है?
2. Clings to adults or too dependent.   0   1
   क्या यह आम-तौर पर माँ-बाप या बड़ों से चिपका रहता है और उनका सहारा ढूंढता है ?
3. Demand a lot of attention.   0   1
   क्या यह चाहता है कि इसकी बहुत देखभाल की जाए या हर समय घर के लोग इसी का ध्यान रखे?
4. Abnormal movements.   0   1
   क्या यह कभी गलत हरकते करता है?
5. Gets hurt a lot, accident prone.   0   1
   कुछ बच्चे रोज के खेल व कामो मे बहुत चोटे खाते है क्या यह कभी ज़्यादा चोटे खाता है?
6. Physical problem without known medical cause   0   1
   क्या इसको (बिना किसी शारीरिक बीमारी के) कुछ शारीरिक तकलीफे रहती है जैसे कि
   • Aches and pains—दर्द
   • Nausea—मतली मचली
   • Headache—सरदर्द
   • Stomach aches—पेट दर्द
   • Fits—दौरा
   • Vomiting—उल्टी
   • Overtired—ज़्यादा थकावट
   • Constipated—कब्ज़
   • Feels dizzy—चक्कर
   • Over weight—मोटापा

Nervous movements and twitching, tics, others

Factor VIII score
Total score (sum total of all the factors scores)

Life Events Scale for Indian Children

Dr Savita Malhotra MD, PhD, FAMS, FACPsych

No.____Date_______________________

Child's Name_______________________________Age_______________Date of Birth_______________

Sex____Education_______________________________

Informant Mother/Father/Any other (specify)_______________________________________

Informant's Name_______________________________Age_______________Sex_______________________

Education_______________________________Occupation_______________________________

Family Income____

Residence (Address)____

Rural/Urban____

Instructions

Can you recall any significant events in child's life which may have affected the child? Specify with year and month.

निर्देश

क्या आप बच्चे के जीवन मे घटित हुई किसी महत्वपूर्ण घटना के बारे मे बताएंगे जिसका बच्चे पर प्रभाव पड़ा होगा कृपया संक्षेप मे बताएं महीना एव वर्ष सूचित करे?

How stressful do you think these events were for your child (subjective stressfulness score)?

आपके अनुसार इस घटना का बच्चे पर कितना प्रभाव पड़ा है?

0	1	2	3
Not at all	to some extent	to a greater extent	to considerable extent
बिल्कुल नहीं	कुछ-कुछ	अधिक	बहुत अधिक

Given below is a set of events that take place normally during the course of life. Some of these may also apply to you. Kindly indicate by yes or no, whether the event has occurred ever or in the last one year and approximate date/month/year if it has occurred. Mark separately for occurrence of events in the last one year or ever in life. Corresponding stress scores are given in the column B of the scale.

Also indicate how stressful it was for your child. Score 0,1,2,3 (in column A of the scale) as explained above to obtain subjective stressfulness score.

नीचे जीवन मे घटित होने वाली कुछ घटनाओ का वर्णन है। इनमे से वो घटनाए जो आपके बच्चे के साथ घटी है उनको तिथि-महीना-वर्ष के साथ सूचित करे। कृपया यह भी बताए कि इस घटना का बच्चे पर कितना प्रभाव पड़ा है।

Life events	Yes/ No	Date/ Month/Year	**A** Subjective stress-fulness score (0,1,2,3)	**B** Stress score
1. Decrease in number of arguments with brothers and sisters भाई/बहन का साथ बहस/विवाद मे कमी				18
2. Beginning another school year स्कूल मे नये साल की शुरूवात				21
3. Visit of relatives रिश्तेदारो का घर मे आना				30
4. Decrease in number of arguments between parents. माता पिता की आपसी बहस मे कमी				28
5. Move to a new house नये घर मे जाना				31
6. Change in parent's financial status माता पिता की आर्थिक स्थिति मे परिवर्तन				34
7. Outstanding achievement of brother or sister भाई/बहन की विशेष उपलब्धि				35
8. Acquisition of TV by family/going for a picnic or excursion परिवार का टेलिविज़न खरीदना/पिकनिक अथवा घूमने जाना				43
9. Increase in number of arguments with brothers and sisters भाई/बहन के साथ बहस में वृद्धि				39
10. Outstanding personal achievement बच्चे की विशेष उपलब्धि या व्यक्तिगत सफलता				40
11. Not being sent to school (against child's wish) बच्चे की इच्छा के विरूद्ध स्कूल न भेजे जाना				42
12. Serious illness of brother/sister requiring hospital treatment भाई/बहन की गम्भीर बीमारी एवं अस्पताल में इलाज				42
13. Loss of job by parent माता-पिता की नौकरी छूट जाना				43
14. Mother beginning full time work माता का पूरे दिन की नौकरी शुरू करना				45
15. Witnessing a serious mishap (traffic accident, fire) or death procession गम्भीर दुर्घटना देखना जैसे शव यात्रा, सड़क दुर्घटना, आग लगना, आदि				55

Life events No	A Yes/ Month/Year (0,1,2,3)	B Date/	Subjective stress-fulness score	Stress score
16. Examinations परीक्षा				45
17. Close brother or sister leaving home निकटतम भाई-बहन का घर छोड़ना				49
18. Change of schools स्कूल का बदलना				49
19. Change in father's job requiring increased absence from home पिता का व्यवसाय में परिवर्तन के कारण अधिक समय घर से बाहर रहना				48
20. Physical punishment by parents माता-पिता द्वारा शारीरिक दण्ड				48
21. Problems with teacher or school work स्कूल मे अध्यापकों अथवा काम सम्बन्धी कठिनाई				49
22. Quarrel between parents/parent and neighbour/relative माता-पिता का पड़ोसी अथवा रिश्तेदारो के साथ झगड़ा				47
23. Prison sentence of parent माता-पिता को जेल की सज़ा				50
24. Death of a grand parent दादा/दादी अथवा नाना-नानी की मृत्यु				51
25. Birth of a brother or sister भाई/बहन का जन्म				50
26. Increase in number of arguments with parents माता-पिता के साथ बहस में वृद्धि				51
27. Suspension from school स्कूल से कुछ समय के लिए निकाले जाना				53
28. Increase in number of arguments between parents माता-पिता के बीच बहस मे वृद्धि				54
29. Expulsion from school स्कूल से निकाले जाना				58
30. Beginning school स्कूल जाना शुरू करना				58
31. Excessive use of alcohol by parent leading to undesirable behaviour माता-पिता का ज़रूरत से ज़्यादा शराब पीकर बुरा व्यवहार करना				60
32. Death of child's close friend or relative बच्चे के नज़दीकी मित्र अथवा रिश्तेदार की मृत्यु				60
33. Change in child's popularity with friends बच्चे की अपने मित्रों के बीच लोकप्रियता में परिवर्तन				57
34. Being kept down a year at school कक्षा मे एक साल पिछड़ जाना				60
35. Attaining menarche/puberty माहवारी शुरू होना/यौवन अवस्था को प्राप्त करना				63

Life events No	A Yes/ Month/Year (0,1,2,3)	B Date/	Subjective stress-fulness score	Stress score
36. Being responsible for another child's death (accidental or homicidal) किसी दूसरे बच्चे की मृत्यु के लिए ज़िम्मेवार होना				68
37. Being sent to hostel हॉस्टल में भेजे जाना				67
38. Seeing the sexual activity of parents माता-पिता की सैक्स/यौन सम्बन्धी गतिविधियों को देखना				67
39. Serious illness of parent requiring hospital treatment माता-पिता की गम्भीर बीमारी एव अस्पताल में इलाज				67
40. Psychiatric disturbance of parent माता-पिता की मानसिक बीमारी				69
41. Being a battered child अक्सर बेरहमी से पीटे जाना/सताए जाना				74
42. Marriage of parent to step parent माता-पिता की दूसरी शादी होना				72
43. Discovery of being an adopted child बच्चे को जानकारी मिलना कि वह गोद लिया हुआ है				72
44. Serious illness of child requiring hospital treatment बच्चे की गम्भीर बीमारी एवं अस्पताल मे इलाज				73
45. Death of a brother or sister भाई/बहन की मृत्यु				77
46. Acquiring a visible deformity अपंग होना				76
47. Sexual assault on child बच्चे के साथ सैक्स सम्बन्धी दुराचरण				78
48. Divorce of parents माता-पिता का तलाक होना				83
49. Separation of parents माता-पिता का अलग हो जाना				86
50. Death of a parent माता-पिता की मृत्यु				94

Where will you place the event(s) you told me in the beginning (if it is not already covered by the list of questions above) in the above list in term of its seriousness and impact on the child/family?

जो घटना प्रारम्भ मे आपने बताई थी अगर वह इस सूची मे नही है तो आप इसे बच्चे एव परिवार पर पडे प्रभाव के अनुसार इस सूची मे किस स्थान पर रखेंगे?

____

____

____

____

Total stress score (add the scores of marked items in column B) _______________ _______

Total subjective Stressfulness Score (add scores of marked items in column A) _________

Parental Handling Questionnaire

Dr Savita Malhotra MD, PhD, FAMS, FACPsych

No.____Date__________________________

Child's Name____________________________Age______________Date of Birth______________

Sex_________________________________Education____________________________________

Informant Mother/Father/Any other (specify)_______________________________________

Informant's Name____________________________Age________________Sex________________

Education____________________________Occupation________________________________

Family Income____

Residence (Address)____

Rural/Urban____

TEMPERAMENT MEASUREMENT SCHEDULE

Instructions

Below is a set of questions inquiring about the way you deal with your child. Every parent has his/her own ways of handling the child. So, please circle '0' if you answer is 'No', '1' if your answer is Sometimes and '2' if your answer is 'Yes'.

निर्देश

हर माता-पिता का अपने बच्चे की देखभाल का एक तरीका होता है। नीचे कुछ प्रश्न दिये गए हैं। जिसमे बच्चे की सम्भाल के तरीको के बारे मे पूछा गया है। यदि आपका उत्तर नही है तो 0 पर गोला लगाएं। यदि आपका उत्तर अक्सर कभी कभी है तो 1 पर गोला लगाए और यदि आपका उत्तर हा है तो 2 पर गोला लगाए।

1. Do you frequently smile at your child?   0 1 2
   क्या आप अक्सर बच्चे को देखकर मुस्कुराते है?

2. Do you praise your child often?   0 1 2
   क्या आप अक्सर बच्चे की प्रशंसा करते है?

3. Do you help your child as much as he needs?   0 1 2
   क्या आप बच्चे की आवश्यकता अनुसार मदद करते है?

4. Do you often talk to (spend time with) your child?   0 1 2
   क्या आप अक्सर बच्चे से बात करते है। अथवा उसके साथ समय व्यतीत करते है?

5. Are you able to make the child feel better when he is upset?   0 1 2
   जब बच्चा परेशान हो तो क्या आप उसका मन बहला सकते है?

6. Does your child come to you whenever in distress?   0 1 2
   जब बच्चे को कोई परेशानी हो तो क्या वह आपके पास आता है?

7. Do you feel that your spouse is unduly strict/lenient towards the child?   0 1 2
   क्या आप महसूस करते है कि आपके पति/पत्नी बच्चे से साथ अधिक नरम/सख्त हैं?

8. Do you often reprimand your child?   0 1 2
   क्या आप अक्सर अपने बच्चे को डांटते है?

9. Do you (or some other family member) often console or protect   0 1 2
   the child when he is reprimanded by the other parent?
   क्या आप (अथवा परिवार का कोई और सदस्य) जब बच्चे को डांट पड़ रही हो तो उस वक्त
   उसे बचाते है या पुचकारते है?

10. Do you get very angry when the child does not behave well?   0 1 2
    जब बच्चा उचित व्यवहार न कर रहा हो तब क्या आपको बहुत ज़्यादा गुस्सा आता है?
                                                   Parental care (add scores)

11. Do you let your child do things he likes doing?   0 1 2
    क्या आप बच्चे को उसकी पसन्द के काम करने देते है?

12. Do you let him make his own decisions?   0 1 2
    क्या आप बच्चे को स्वंय निर्णय लेने देते है?

13. Do you think that the child cannot look after himself unless   0 1 2
    you are around?
    क्या आप सोचते हैं कि आपके बिना बच्चा अपनी देखभाल स्वंय नहीं कर सकता है?

14. Do you try to control everything the child does?   0 1 2
    क्या आप बच्चे की हर कार्य/बात पर नियन्त्रण रखने की कोशिश करते है?
                                                 Parental control (add scores)

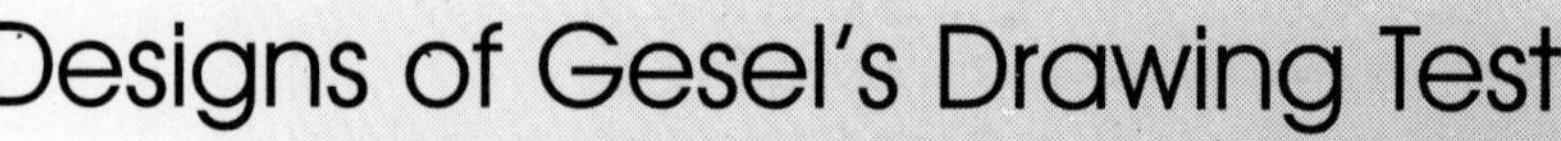

Designs of Gesel's Drawing Test

Design	Age level
◯	3 years
+	4 years
▭	5 years
△	6 years

Design   **Age level**

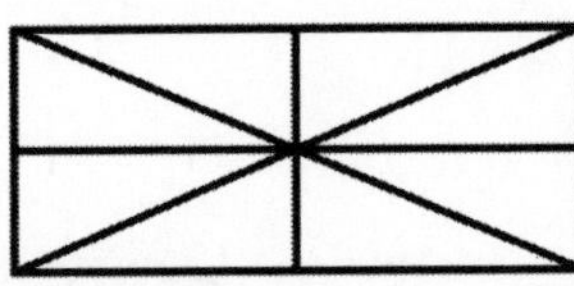

7 years

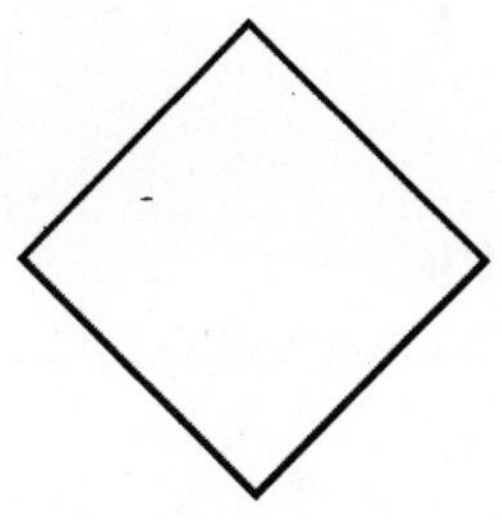

8 years

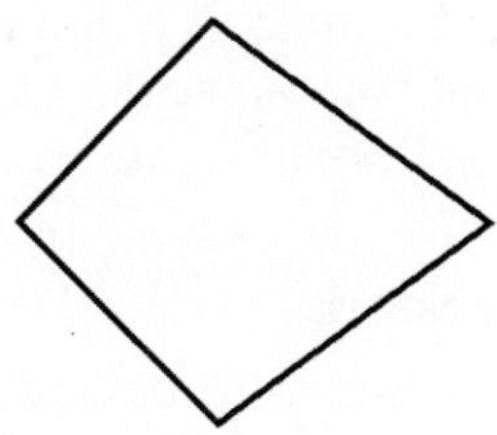

9 years

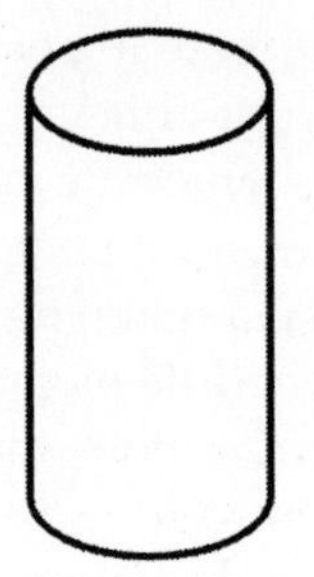

10 years

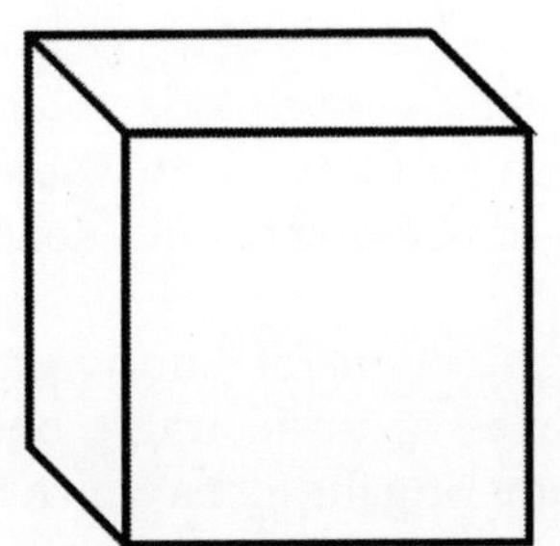

12 years

Guidelines for Healthy Parenting

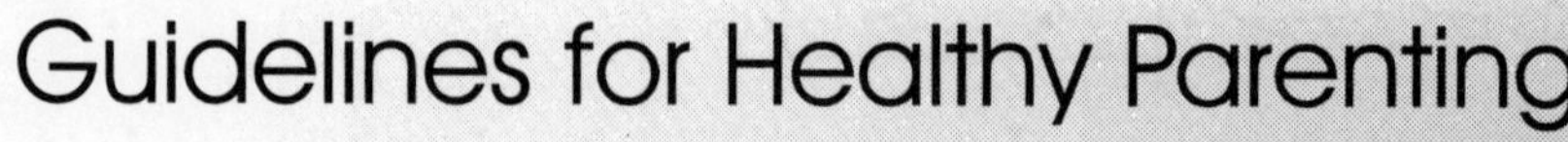

Always Remember

- To be a good role model.
- Not to indulge in behaviour that you do not want the child to learn—try to be as you would like your child to be.
- To develop a positive relationship with your child and nurture it.

> Child is a gift of God and
> not an object of possession
> So, Handle with care

What does your child need? Do you really know about it?

Here are certain tips for you. Child needs:
- To express lineself/herself
- To communicate
- Your time, your availability
- To interact with you

> - Give ample time to the child when the child needs it
> - Listen to your child
> - Do not overcompensate for non-availability of time

Child Needs

Your timely praise, smile and reassurance. Some degree of assistance

> - Do not think that it would spoil your child
> - Remember child is not an adult

Child Needs

To play. To enjoy with children of his/her age

> - Allow time and opportunity to the child to play and interact with peers
> - Remember that some degree of freedom is a basic human right.

Child Also Needs

To be disciplined. To be checked for undesirable/socially incorrect behaviour

> - Be gentle rather than being too harsh or strict with your child.
> - Try methods which are not too punitive.
> - Use behavioural principles, i.e. encourage the child when he/she follows a desirable schedule of activities.
> - Encourage the child by praise or a small token or reward for good behavior
> - For undesirable behaviour convey it to the child clearly that the particular behaviour is not desirable of him/her.
> - Use behavioural strategies, viz. time-out (wherein the child is not given the attention by making him/her face the wall or not talking to him/her for some time.
> - Over-correction for undoing the consequences of undesirable behaviour (e.g. gathering the items which the child had thrown in anger and putting them back in place).

Child Needs: A Role Model

Be one !

Growing, developing and reliving with your child is a wonderful experience

Enjoy your parenthood !

In order to deal effectively with your child, it is important that you.

Know Your Child

You must know your child in terms of his/her?

i. *Intelligence:* Each child is different in terms of his/her intelligence, i.e. the sum total of the intellectual and cognitive abilities that include the child's pick up, grasp, comprehension, ability to think rationally and solve problems, judgement, abstraction, skills and scholastic adequacy with respect to his/her age. Each child has a certain level of intelligence and there is a limit to what the child can achieve.

ii. *Temperament:* Temperament refers to the inborn characteristics of behavioral style such as activity level, intensity of emotional reactions, approach or withdrawal reaction in face of new situation or person, adaptability, distractibility, attention span and persistence in tasks, etc. making him unique and different from others. For example some children may be more outspoken and the others may be shy and slow to warm up. Each child has a behavioral style of his/her own that distinguishes him/her from other children.

iii. *Interests:* Child's interests vary and also depend on his/her intelligence and temperament.

iv. *Assets:* Children do have talents or strengths which need to be recognized or encouraged.

In Order to Care for Your Child Better

Be observant about the needs and temperament of your child. Each child has his/her own individuality in terms of intelligence, temperament, interests and assets. Avoid making comparisons with sibs and friends in front of your child as it may lead onto:

a. Negative feelings in the child's mind towards those with whom the child is compared; and

b. An unhealthy competition.

Be considerate of your child's interests. Listen to your child and let the child express his/her viewpoint. Do not nag and check the child all the time as it can decrease the importance/impact of checking the child for a more objectionable behaviour as, e.g. the child may associate the parents with nagging behaviour and may stop caring about it. Avoid your child getting such a feeling.

Be patient in dealing with your child. Listen to your child's views and problems. Give adequate explanations to satisfy the child's queries (of course keeping in mind the child's age and understanding ability). Wrong explanations can mislead the child leading to formation of wrong concepts in the child's mind. Postponements cannot satisfy the child, rather leave the child more inquisitive to explore into other undesirable/inappropriate ways.

Be fulfilling of the child's demands that are genuine and appropriate for age or development level.

Do not make false promises to your child. False promises can lead to resentment and also provide a wrong model to the child.

Do not postpone the child's rational demands indefinitely, as the child is cannot wait too long.

Reward the child appropriately and consistently for the child's achievements in order to boost his/her morale and to maintain the desired behavior.

Be a playful teacher: Teach your child in a playful manner.

Consider your child's age before sending the child to school. For example—by the age of four years child has sufficient motoric and linguistic development to manage sitting in class, handling objects, understanding instructions; withstand separation from mother; and have interest in peer group.

Be rational: Make rational expectations from your child. Keep in mind the child's level of development, age, intelligence, temperament and interests.

In Disciplining the Child

1. Be clear
2. Be consistent in your approach in handling your child.
   Never scold or punish the child when it's not the child's fault.
   Do not punish the child just because your mood is upset.
   If you are angry with your boss or if you have a quarrel with your partner never make the mistake of displacing your anger onto your child. Remember this can confuse the child about the behaviour desired/expected of him/her.
3. Be judicious in use of punishment.
4. Do not be too punitive/harsh in dealing with your child. Do not instill fear in the child's mind in order to make your child obedient. Avoid statements like "We will take you to a doctor—get you an injection" to check the child's behaviour. Such a statement may lead the child to develop fear towards the doctor and the child may refuse to visit the doctor when required. If your child indulges in a wrong behaviour, express to the child that he/she is behaving in a wrong manner and is thereby making you feel angry.
5. Be firm and clear in your stance: You can also say that "this behaviour will not be tolerated". These statements need to be used judiciously and firmly in order to maintain their impact. Repeated non-judicious use of such statements may reduce their impact over time. Then the child may think "Oh! my parents are always after me, no matter what I do or indulge in"; or "my parents check me just for the sake of checking and are not so serious about it".

If the child does not listen to you despite your having checked him/her, you can follow behavioural management strategies like:

a. Time-out, i.e. withdrawing attention from the child. For example—by making the child stand in a corner or not talking to your child for a few minutes. This is a principle often employed by primary school teachers to curb undesirable behaviour in the child wherein the teacher makes the student face the wall at one corner of the room. It helps in checking the inappropriate behaviour in the child as well as serves as a warning for the rest of the students in the class so as not to indulge in inappropriate behaviour.

b. *Over-correction:* Let the child correct what he/she has spoiled. For example if your child deliberately throws away an article, let him/her gather the same and put it back in place.

c. *Punishment:* Even when you punish the child, do no forget to praise or reward the child later when the child shows desirable behaviour. Remember that intense punishment carries the risk of development of strong conditioned emotional responses towards the punisher. If the punisher is a parent, it becomes an unfortunate situation.

- Mild punishment to guide behaviour, if used judiciously, may be more effective in the long run.
- Thus while using punishment, remember to administer it more consistently, closer in time to the behaviour being punished.

- Mild punishment contingent to an incorrect or socially undesirable response can serve as a cue signaling incorrectness of the response.
- Similarly, positive reinforcement (i.e. the use of praise/reward on occurrence of desirable behaviour) can be used to signal the correctness of a response.

Disciplining is not synonymous with punishment.

If you need to keep a check on undesirable behaviour, you also need to reward the child timely and appropriately for his/her desirable behaviour.

This encourages the child to inculcate good habits in his/her life.

Index